Your Child with Arthritis

A Johns Hopkins Press Health Book

Your Child with Arthritis

A Family Guide for Caregiving

•

Lori B. Tucker, M.D.

Bethany A. DeNardo, M.P.H., P.T.

Judith A. Stebulis, M.A.

Jane G. Schaller, M.D.

Foreword by Barbara M. Ansell, M.D.

THE JOHNS HOPKINS UNIVERSITY PRESS

BALTIMORE AND LONDON

Note to the reader:
We wrote this book to help parents and others to provide better care for
their children who have arthritis. We also hope that this book will promote
and facilitate the conversation between parents and health care
professionals. This book is not intended to substitute for medical care, however,
and treatment should not be based solely on its contents.

© 1996 The Johns Hopkins University Press
All rights reserved. Published 1996
Printed in the United States of America on acid-free paper
05 04 03 02 01 00 99 98 97 96   5 4 3 2 1

The Johns Hopkins University Press
2715 North Charles Street
Baltimore, Maryland 21218-4319
The Johns Hopkins Press Ltd., London

Illustrations by Domenic S. DeNardo

Library of Congress Cataloging-in-Publication Data
will be found at the end of this book.
A catalog record for this book is available from the British Library.

ISBN 0-8018-5293-5

This book is dedicated to the many parents and children who have taught us so much throughout the years

Contents

Foreword

Rheumatic diseases in childhood are relatively rare, and therefore many people have never heard of the illness from which their child suffers until the diagnosis is made. Indeed their family physician or pediatrician may also not have a good working knowledge of the particular disease. Informed responsibility in the management of chronic disease is essential if a satisfactory outcome is to be attained, not just in control of the disease, but also in the integration of the young person into society.

This book will be of enormous help to family doctors, pediatricians, parents, and older patients, giving as it does the background of what is known about rheumatic diseases in childhood today. It also covers drugs in general use, as well as the principles of management of the various chronic inflammatory states that are subsumed under the term "rheumatic diseases of childhood." Of these diseases, juvenile rheumatoid arthritis in one of its forms is the most common.

This book, co-authored by two leading pediatric rheumatologists, their physical therapist, and a parent of one of their patients, provides the knowledge and understanding which are necessary for effective management.

It begins by describing the various diseases that may be encountered, including such varieties as dermatomyositis, and then goes on to discuss the problems faced by children with these diseases, as well as such health care solutions as medication and physiotherapy.

Barbara M. Ansell, C.B.E., M.D., F.R.C.S., F.R.C.

Preface

Raising a child is a joyous but daunting adventure. Just when you think you have everything figured out, new challenges arise. Toilet training, the first day of school, driving, dating, and similar milestones keep parents busy coming up with new approaches to dealing with daily challenges. Fortunately, most of us have personal experiences and family and community role models on whom we can draw in designing our own strategies for handling each stage in our children's and our family's development. Chronic childhood illness, however, is not something with which most parents have any experience. Specific information and new skills are needed to meet its unique challenges.

In *Your Child with Arthritis: A Family Guide for Caregiving*, health care professionals and parents of children with rheumatic disease provide the information you need to help make decisions regarding your child's health care and to develop your own techniques for dealing with the broader impact of rheumatic illness on other aspects of family life. This is a comprehensive resource, with information on juvenile rheumatoid arthritis, systemic lupus erythematosus, dermatomyositis, scleroderma, and other childhood rheumatic diseases. Each of the childhood rheumatic diseases is discussed in detail, including how it is diagnosed and treated, the possible course of the disease, and possible outcomes.

With rheumatic illnesses, even children with the same diagnosis can have very different disease courses and very different responses to treatment, and you may find that your own child's illness differs in some respects from the descriptions provided here. Because of this tremendous variation in the way the rheumatic diseases affect children, your role in health care decision making is especially important. For one thing, you will have choices to make about treatment options. Your observations about your child will help health care providers to evaluate the effectiveness of treatment decisions and determine new treatment plans to help your child achieve his or her goals in home, school, and community activities.

We believe that children do best when they and their parents are involved in all of the decisions regarding their health care. The information provided here about medications, exercise programs, nutrition, and surgical procedures can help you understand the various treatment options available. The section on laboratory tests and other diagnostic procedures explains what test results mean and how they are used to aid in diagnosing and monitoring your child's response to treatments. Understanding more about your child's illness and medical care can help you work with your child's health care providers to make the best decisions about your child.

Routine frequent doctor visits and continuing medical treatments are only a part of the adjustment families make when a child is diagnosed with a rheumatic disease. Chronic illness can affect all aspects of family life. Most important, children with rheumatic diseases may need special accommodations to help them attend and benefit from school. We have included a chapter on school issues that provides suggestions for dealing with the kinds of problems children with rheumatic diseases are likely to encounter. We also provide information about federal laws that guarantee a free, appropriate public education for all children who have disabilities. The chapter on health care financing can help you understand your current health insurance policy, identify gaps in your coverage, and negotiate for medically necessary services. Private health insurance and public medical assistance programs are described.

Finally, there is a chapter that deals with the emotional impact of childhood rheumatic diseases on individual family members and on relationships within the family. No one can say precisely how your family will be affected. But we *can* provide insights gathered from our personal experiences and from those of the hundreds of families we have known. We hope that these insights can help you anticipate and understand your own family's response to your child's illness.

Your Child with Arthritis: A Family Guide for Caregiving can be read in its entirety for an overview of the diseases and their treatments, or you can use it as a reference throughout the course of your child's illness, when new therapies are tried or as new situations (such as a change in schools or health insurance) arise. The checklists and blank forms that appear throughout the book are included to help you keep track of changes in your child's illness, to organize tasks, and to schedule appointments—and record their outcome.

Just as there is no single treatment that is effective for every child with a rheumatic disease, there is no single "best way" for families to deal with their child's illness. *Your Child with Arthritis: A Family Guide for Caregiving* provides information and tools that we hope you will find useful in fashioning your own family's response. We hope that it will make your job as the parent of a child with a chronic rheumatic illness a little easier, so that you can concentrate on the joyous adventure of parenting.

Acknowledgments

We thank the many parents, children, and colleagues who helped us to create this book. We could not have done it alone.

Many of the questions and answers, and some other parts of this book, first appeared in slightly different form in *The Joint Report,* a newsletter that we published for parents and professionals from 1988 to 1993. We particularly thank the following individuals for their contributions: Erica Almeida, Eva Aquino, Bradley J. Bloom, M.D., Maria V. Bruno, Domenic S. DeNardo, Judith DiNardo, R.N., M.S., Andrea Dubois, Beth Gibbons, P.T., Dena Goldberg, Ph.D., R.D., Audie Hittle, Molly Holland, M.P.H., R.D., Susan S. Hollis, L.C.S.W., Darryl T. Hubbard, Larry Jung, M.D., Lynne K. Karlson, M.D., Marybeth Kiernan, O.T.R./L., Marisa Klein-Gitelman, M.D., Judith S. Meaney, Laurie C. Miller, M.D., Erika Lessard Mundor, Robyn M. Nichols, James J. Nocton, M.D., Carol Ferguson Page, P.N.P., Ann Pardee, Agnes Pont, O.T.R./L., Elizabeth Ramsey, David Reese, M.D., Virgina Rice, L.I.C.S.W., Deborah Rothman, M.D., Sheila Rubino, Christopher Sadler, Michael T. Scalli, Paul A. Scanlon, Melissa S. Schaffer, Amy C. Sharples, R.N., M.S., Kendra Staudinger, Ilona S. Szer, M.D., Madelon Visser, O.T.R./L., Carol Watson, L.I.C.S.W., Lindsley Wilkerson, Martin H. Young, Ph.D., and Lawrence S. Zemel, M.D.

In addition, we thank the Federation for Children with Special Needs, in Boston, Massachusetts, and the Children's Hospital of Los Angeles, in Los Angeles, California, which gave us permission to reprint their materials in this book.

Your Child with Arthritis

Chapter 1

•

The Rheumatic Diseases of Childhood

This chapter introduces the rheumatic diseases of childhood, describing how they are similar to each other, how they differ, and, most importantly, how they affect children. The more common diseases will be discussed in detail. They are:

- Juvenile rheumatoid arthritis (JRA) and its three onset subtypes, pauciarticular JRA, polyarticular JRA, and systemic JRA
- Juvenile spondyloarthropathy syndromes, including juvenile ankylosing spondylitis, seronegative enthesopathy and arthropathy syndrome, arthritis associated with inflammatory bowel disease, reactive arthritis, Reiter's syndrome, and psoriatic arthritis
- Systemic lupus erythematosus (SLE)
- Dermatomyositis
- Scleroderma, including both localized and systemic disease
- Vasculitis, including cutaneous polyarteritis, Kawasaki disease, and Henoch-Schönlein purpura

In addition to describing each of these diseases, this chapter explains how each disease is diagnosed, its course and outcome, and how it is treated. The many different laboratory tests and procedures used to diagnose and monitor the rheumatic diseases are described in a section at the end of this chapter.

About the Rheumatic Diseases

The rheumatic diseases are a group of illnesses characterized by the presence of *inflammation* in the body's tissues. Some of the rheumatic diseases, such as JRA, cause inflammation within the joints (the knees, the wrists, or the ankles, for example). Others, such as SLE or dermatomyositis, cause inflammation in other parts of the body (such as the internal organs or muscles).

Although *controlled and limited inflammation* is a normal bodily response to infection or injury that occurs in healthy people, the inflammation that occurs in the rheumatic diseases is not normal. The common thread that links the rheumatic diseases is inflammation that can cause damage to healthy body tissues.

What Is Inflammation?

Normal inflammation. Inflammation is a normal and essential response of the immune system in healthy people. Inflammation is one outcome of the way the body responds to heal injury or to fight foreign invaders such as bacteria or viruses. When the healthy immune system detects injury or infection, it sends white blood cells to the injured site, where a variety of chemical substances are made. These chemical substances promote healing of the injury. When the injury has healed or the foreign invader has been eliminated, the immune system "turns off" the inflammatory response, and the inflammation goes away.

Inflammation in the rheumatic diseases. The immune system does not function properly in children with rheumatic diseases. In these children, the immune system directs the inflammatory response against the body's own healthy tissues rather than against infections. Rheumatic diseases are often referred to as *autoimmune;* that is, the immune system is directed against the self. Once started, the inflammation in a person with rheumatic disease is not turned off as a normal inflammatory response would be once a foreign invader was destroyed. We do not know what triggers the unusual inflammation that leads to a rheumatic disease, or why the inflammation cannot be halted by normal mechanisms.

Signs of inflammation. Everyone has noticed that an infected area near the surface of the skin is red, swollen, warm, and painful. These are the signs and symptoms of inflammation and are also associated with inflamed joints in children with arthritis.

What Causes the Rheumatic Diseases?

No one knows why some children develop rheumatic disease, or what triggers the immune system to malfunction. We do know that these diseases are not contagious. Your child did not "catch" this disease, he will not pass it on to someone else, and he did not get it because of anything that you or he did.

It is unusual for more than one child in a family to develop a childhood rheumatic disease, although there seems to be a family tendency toward some kinds of rheumatic diseases. In particular, SLE may occur in more than one family member. In contrast, JRA is rarely seen in siblings or close relatives. We believe that the combination of having some type of inherited gene and then being exposed to another (as yet unidentified) factor may dispose a person to get a rheumatic disease.

Researchers are studying whether the presence of certain genes can cause a child to have a predisposition to develop a rheumatic disease. People with SLE, for example, are more likely to have certain immune genes. Children and adults with spondyloarthropathy commonly have a gene called HLA-B27—although the gene does not cause the disease all by itself. This type of research is complicated, because humans have a huge number of genes, and the kinds of genes we have vary between different ethnic and racial groups.

What Is the Usual Course of Childhood Rheumatic Diseases?

The rheumatic diseases of childhood are extremely variable. The different diseases have different symptoms, and even within a single disease symptoms and severity may vary. Some children have very mild symptoms while others are severely affected. Some children experience severe pain while others have very little discomfort; some take many medications while others need little or none; some have disease that lasts for only a few months while others have disease activity for years. Most children fall somewhere in the middle.

When your child is diagnosed with a rheumatic illness, your physician may not be able to predict the course of his illness. Instead, it will take time to determine how things will progress. There is often no correlation between how severely ill a child is at the time of disease diagnosis and the eventual outcome. Many children with severe illness recover completely.

About Flares and Remissions

All of the rheumatic diseases are characterized by unpredictable periods of flares and remissions. There will be times when the rheumatic disease is quite active—a period called a *flare*—and there will be times when the rheumatic disease is quiet, a period that is often referred to as a *remission*. There is no way to predict when your child's disease will flare up, nor is there anything that you or he can do to prevent this from happening. Once a flare occurs, it's usually impossible to say why it occurred when it did.

Some children have only one flare, some have none, and others have multiple episodes. Some flares are mild, with an increase in only a few symptoms, and some flares are severe. Some children may have a flare after several years of remission.

A true remission occurs when your child is no longer taking any medicine and has had no signs of active disease for a period of time. Some diseases, like JRA and dermatomyosis, are known to have permanent remissions, but not all children with these diseases will have a permanent remission. There is no way to predict whether your child will have a permanent remission of his disease, but it is something that all parents hope for.

Flares are difficult for both children and families. Sheila Rubino wrote the following description of how she felt when her daughter had a flare of JRA after a long remission:

A Flare after All This Time

In the last 3 years, I was finally able to make long-range plans. My daughter Michelle was in remission. I did not have to worry if she would be able to walk or if she would be feeling okay. I took two part-time jobs so I could still have some flexibility (even though I didn't need as much now), and everything looked good. Michelle's sister, 15-year-old Karen, didn't have to adjust her "just blooming" social life anymore because of hospital commitments for Michelle or my need to have Karen help take care of her sister. Everything was going great, and life was beginning to become smooth and normal.

Then *it* happened. *The flare.* The physical pain Michelle experienced was terrible; it was both knees this time, instead of just one, and they were so swollen she could not walk. She was frightened because she didn't know if something was seriously wrong with her. "Why would my knees swell after all this time?" she asked.

The most difficult aspect for me was the emotional impact. I was frightened and angry. Frightened because I didn't want my daughter to suffer any more and I didn't know what course this flare was going to take. I was angry because I didn't want to give up the newfound freedom we had all discovered. Life was good, and I didn't want to go back to the way it had been before. I had instant fears of Michelle being on crutches and using a wheelchair.

Our doctors were great; they immediately took steps to get the flare under control. Michelle is doing much better now but she will need further treatment to keep the arthritis under control. I thought the fight was over, but I guess we're just in for another round. This experience has been an eye-opener for me because it reinforced the fact that each flare is a traumatic experience not only for the child but for the entire family. The family, as a unit, has to make adjustments and compromises. It isn't fair, but that's the way it is when you have a child with a rheumatic disease.

What Is Arthritis?

Arthritis is a general term that refers to inflammation within a joint. When a joint develops arthritis, it becomes hot, swollen, and painful. Arthritis can develop as a response to many different circumstances; it is not unusual for arthritis to develop briefly when a child is recovering from a viral illness, for example, or as a

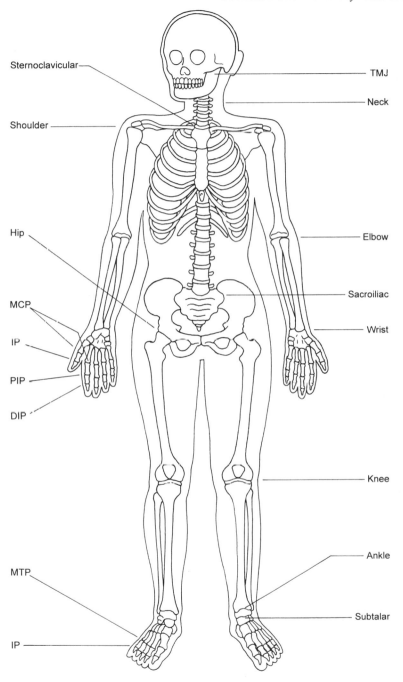

FIGURE 1. The joints of the body.

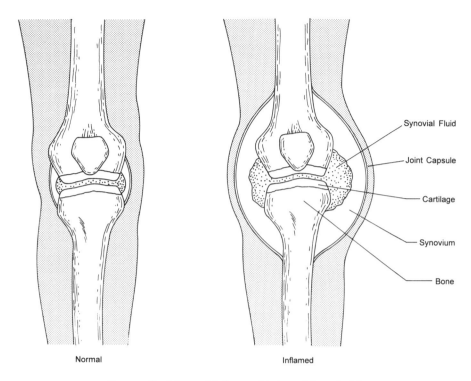

Normal

Inflamed

Synovial Fluid

Joint Capsule

Cartilage

Synovium

Bone

FIGURE 2. Normal joint and joint with arthritis.

result of an injury, such as a fall. These types of arthritis are temporary, and they heal quickly; they are not rheumatic disease.

Unlike the temporary arthritis described above, *chronic arthritis* is a common feature of nearly every kind of childhood rheumatic disease. In some diseases, like JRA, chronic arthritis is the main feature of the disease. Children with other rheumatic illnesses (SLE, dermatomyositis, scleroderma, and so on) may develop arthritis at some point in their illness. Because arthritis can cause significant problems for children with any type of rheumatic disease, the effects and treatment of arthritis will be discussed throughout this book.

Arthritis is a term which means inflammation in the joints. The joints allow smooth motion between adjacent bones. Figure 1 shows the joints of the body and their names.

All joints have a lining of tissue called *synovium* (Figure 2). This synovium secretes a special fluid, called *synovial fluid.* In healthy joints, the synovial fluid lubricates the joint, allowing it to move easily. Synovial fluid works the same way as motor oil does in a car engine; it allows all of the internal parts to move freely and easily without sticking against one another.

When a joint develops arthritis, the synovium becomes swollen and overgrown, in a process called *synovitis*. The inflamed synovium produces too much synovial fluid, resulting in swelling. The synovial fluid produced by a joint with arthritis is not normal. Inflammatory cells build up in the joint fluid, releasing substances that may destroy joint tissues. Instead of being a lubricating fluid, like oil, this joint fluid is more like water. You can imagine what would happen if you put water in your car engine instead of oil. Similarly, the abnormal synovial fluid causes the joint to become stiff and hard to move, and that hurts!

Arthritis affects the involved extremity (arm, leg, fingers) in several ways. For one thing, arthritis makes the joint difficult to move, and it is particularly hard to move the joint into its end ranges, or full range, of movement. As a result, the joints often become fixed in a bent position, called a *contracture*. It is also hard to use a joint that hurts. If the arthritis is in a leg joint, the child may limp. If the arthritis is in an arm joint, the child may have trouble writing, dressing, or performing other activities. Finally, all of this abnormal movement will cause the muscles that normally support the joint to become weak. Severe arthritis that lasts for a long time can damage the joint surface, causing it to be rough instead of smooth; this is called *joint erosion*. Arthritis is treated with a combination of medications and exercise. Medicines reduce the inflammation, and exercises preserve joint motion and muscle strength.

Juvenile Rheumatoid Arthritis

JRA is the most common rheumatic disease affecting children. About half of all children with rheumatic diseases have some type of JRA. To be diagnosed with JRA, a child must meet three criteria:

- Arthritis must be present in the same joint (or joints) for 6 consecutive weeks. As noted above, many illnesses can cause a child to have arthritis for a short time. But JRA is strictly a chronic disease.
- The onset of the child's disease must have been before his sixteenth birthday. JRA is a condition of childhood. Young adults who develop symptoms after the age of 16 are considered to have adult-onset arthritis. It is important to remember that JRA is an entirely different set of diseases from rheumatoid arthritis that occurs in adults.
- All other known causes of arthritis must be ruled out. There is no blood test that makes the diagnosis of JRA. Because there are many different illnesses that can cause arthritis in a child (infections, Lyme disease, and even cancer, to name a

few), the diagnosis of JRA can only be made when the doctor can prove that none of these other conditions are present.

Once a child is diagnosed with JRA, the next step for the doctor is to try to determine what *type* of JRA it is. There are three different onset subtypes of JRA: pauciarticular JRA, polyarticular JRA, and systemic JRA. These different types of JRA are called *onset subtypes.* Each onset subtype has a different set of symptoms, a different course, and a different outcome. Your child's onset subtype will be determined during the first 6 months of his disease. After that, your child's disease may change as time goes on, but his diagnostic category will not change. Here are some quick facts about the three subtypes of JRA:

PAUCIARTICULAR JRA
- Arthritis in four or fewer joints
- Usually younger children (average age 3 years)
- Often only one joint is involved; the knee is the most common
- No fever, rash, or generalized signs of illness
- Watch for eye inflammation!

POLYARTICULAR JRA
- Five or more joints involved
- Positive rheumatoid factor, called *seropositive disease,* means more severe disease
- Negative rheumatoid factor, called *seronegative disease,* means a milder course
- Arthritis is usually symmetric, often involving hands and feet

SYSTEMIC JRA
- Prominent symptoms outside joints, including high spiking fever, pink fleeting rash, enlarged lymph nodes, and anemia
- May not develop arthritis until later
- Arthritis may be mild and remitting or progressive and severe

JRA is treated with a combination of medications and physical therapy. The goal of medical therapy is to decrease pain and stiffness and improve functioning, not necessarily to eliminate joint swelling entirely.

Most pediatric rheumatologists begin therapy with *nonsteroidal anti-inflammatory drugs (NSAIDs).* If the inflammation is difficult to control, or if X rays show erosions, more aggressive medications, such as methotrexate or gold, may be suggested. Injection of steroids directly into an inflamed joint is often an effective treatment if a particular joint is causing significant problems.

This approach to treatment is a conservative one that makes sense based on some data showing that 80 percent of children with JRA will be free of the inflammation and will have no disability when they reach adulthood. With such an optimistic long-term outlook, it seems prudent to avoid treatments that may have serious long-term effects of their own. More recent research, however, suggests that the long-term outlook for children with JRA may not be quite so positive. The few long-term studies that have been done suggest that 10 to 45 percent of children with JRA may have a less positive functional outcome 10 to 15 years after the onset of disease.

Interpretation of the available data on long-term outcomes is difficult for the following reasons: there are too few studies; outcomes for children with different JRA subtypes are not compared; the definition of "functional outcome assessment" is vague; and there is no accepted definition of remission. Despite these interpretive difficulties, if it is true that a significant number of children go on to develop disability or continue to have joint inflammation in adulthood, then a more aggressive approach in medical treatment may be warranted. Further research is needed to determine accurate long-term outcomes of large numbers of children with JRA and to identify possible predictive factors for poor outcome.

If we accept the idea that many children with JRA are at risk for disability in adulthood, we may then consider initiating a more aggressive approach to treatment, with a combination of medications begun at the earliest stages of disease. After the disease is brought under control, a maintenance course of treatment would then be prescribed. These ideas, while new to pediatric rheumatology, have been voiced by many adult rheumatologists with regard to treatment for rheumatoid arthritis. (Pharmaceutical treatment of the rheumatic diseases is discussed in detail in chapter 3.)

Physical and occupational therapy are important elements of the treatment plan for JRA. Physical therapy will help to improve joint mobility so that the joints do not develop contractures and muscles stay strong. A daily exercise program is critical to prevent flexion contractures and to maintain muscle strength.

In most cases, parents can perform the exercises at home with their child, although if a simple exercise program is not proving effective, it may be necessary to follow more aggressive therapy techniques with the help of a therapist. Splints worn at night, or even traction, may be helpful. On rare occasions, children with JRA must have corrective surgery or other more invasive treatments, but the majority of children do well with medications and physical therapy.

Pauciarticular JRA

Pauciarticular JRA is the most common form of JRA, accounting for about half of all children with JRA. Most children with pauciarticular JRA are quite young at the start of their disease: the average age at onset is 3 years, but it is not unusual for a child with pauciarticular JRA to be as young as 1 year. Girls are affected more often than boys.

The word *pauciarticular* means "few joints." By definition, children with pauciarticular JRA have arthritis in four or fewer joints during the first 6 months of their disease. In fact, the majority of children with pauciarticular JRA have only one joint involved.

The arthritis of pauciarticular JRA is often *asymmetrical*; it affects one joint on one side of the body, but it usually does not affect the same joint on the opposite side of the body (for example, a child may have arthritis in the right knee but not in the left). The most frequently affected joint is the knee, although an ankle, elbow, wrist, or a small joint in the hand can also be affected.

Children with pauciarticular JRA often develop arthritis rather acutely and are otherwise healthy. They do not have fever, a skin rash, or other systemic symptoms (symptoms affecting all parts of the body). Some children with pauciarticular JRA have surprisingly little pain despite the presence of a large joint swelling or inability to move the joint properly. Some children may have stiffness or a limp, and some may refuse to walk.

Children with pauciarticular JRA usually have mild inflammation that does not lead to joint damage, even if the arthritis is present for several years. NSAIDs are generally sufficient to treat this disorder, although some children do better with joint injections. More aggressive medications, such as methotrexate, are usually not required.

It is impossible to predict at the outset what the course of an individual child's disease will be. Statistically, pauciarticular JRA is likely to be a relatively mild form of arthritis that may resolve completely at some point during childhood. Most children (about 80 to 90 percent) are completely well after a few years. Many children will have only one episode of arthritis lasting anywhere from 6 months to a few years. Other children will have several flares of arthritis, with involvement of the same or different joints. A small number of children with pauciarticular JRA will develop a severe flare involving more than four joints at some time during their disease, and a few of these children may go on to have more severe arthritis.

Children with pauciarticular JRA are susceptible to developing a form of eye inflammation called *iritis* (see chapter 5). Iritis is most common in children with pauciarticular JRA who also have a positive antinuclear antibody (ANA) blood test (see below). This eye inflammation can be silent for a long time and will not cause obvious symptoms such as eye pain, redness, or changes in vision early in its course. Iritis is easily treated with eye drops if it is detected early. If iritis is not detected early, permanent vision loss and even blindness may result.

Iritis can only be detected by an ophthalmologist (a physician who specializes in eye disease) who examines the child's eyes with an instrument called a slit lamp. Pediatric rheumatologists recommend that all children with pauciarticular JRA have their eyes examined by an ophthalmologist every 3 months. Eye screening should continue for several years after the arthritis has resolved, because a small risk of the child developing iritis continues even after the arthritis is gone. Some children have problems with eye inflammation for a long time after their arthritis has completely resolved; even in those children, though, loss of vision is rare if careful ophthalmology care continues.

Because pauciarticular JRA often affects one leg and not the other, it is common for the two legs to grow at different rates, resulting in a *leg length discrepancy*. Typically, the leg with arthritis will grow *faster* than the uninvolved leg because it has an increased blood supply. The shorter leg usually catches up after the inflammation has subsided. If the difference in leg length is large enough to cause changes in posture or gait, a shoe lift may be prescribed to be worn on the shoe on the shorter leg. It is important that the length of the child's legs be measured and monitored by his doctor or therapist to detect early signs of a leg length difference.

Polyarticular JRA

About one-third of children with JRA have polyarticular disease. The word *polyarticular* means "many joints." By definition, these children have arthritis in five or more joints during the first 6 months of their illness. Except for the joint inflammation, these children usually do not appear particularly ill. High fevers and skin rashes are not seen in this form of JRA, although the child may have mild anemia, loss of appetite, and decreased overall growth (children with polyarticular JRA tend to be small and thin for their age).

Polyarticular JRA usually results in *symmetrical* arthritis. That is, the same joints are usually affected on both sides of the body (both knees, both wrists, both index fingers, etc.). Small finger joints, wrists, ankles, neck, and toes are often involved, although any joints can be affected.

A wide variety of treatments are used in children with polyarticular JRA, depending on the extent and severity of disease. Many children respond well to NSAIDs. If the inflammation is difficult to control or if there is early evidence of joint erosions (damage to cartilage and bone in the joint), second-line medications such as methotrexate or gold may be suggested. Oral corticosteroid medications such as prednisone are rarely indicated because of the serious potential long-term side effects of these drugs.

There are two types of polyarticular JRA. They are defined by whether or not the child has a positive *rheumatoid factor* (RF) blood test. Children who have a negative rheumatoid factor test are called *seronegative.* Those with a positive test are called *seropositive.* The expected course and outcome of the disease are different depending on whether the rheumatoid factor is positive or negative.

Seronegative polyarticular JRA is more common. About 95 percent of children with polyarticular JRA are seronegative. Girls are affected about four times as often as boys, and children are generally young when the disease starts (the average age is 5). The course of seronegative polyarticular JRA is generally one of flares and remissions. The arthritis tends to be more active in the first 3 to 5 years and may quiet down after that.

Some children have surprisingly little joint damage over time despite long periods of active arthritis; there is a risk that joint damage will develop, however. More aggressive treatment may be needed if bony damage begins to become evident on X rays. Many children with polyarticular JRA have a remission after several years, although they may be left with some residual limitation of joint motion even after the active arthritis is gone. The residual joint stiffness is like a "scar" in the joint, and full joint motion may never return. Children who participate in a vigorous physical and occupational therapy program to maintain joint mobility during the active stages of disease are most likely to have a minimum of long-lasting effects of their JRA into adulthood.

Seropositive polyarticular JRA is less common. Only about 5 percent of children with polyarticular JRA have a positive Rf test. In adults with rheumatoid arthritis, the Rf test is usually positive, and seropositive polyarticular JRA often follows a course more like this adult-onset disease. Children with seropositive polyarticular JRA are generally teenagers at the time their disease begins. Girls are affected more often than boys.

This kind of arthritis tends to be persistent and aggressive, and for this reason pediatric rheumatologists recommend aggressive therapy early in the course of disease to try to minimize its damage. There is a risk of permanent joint damage in children with seropositive JRA, and many of these children will have arthritis that lasts into adulthood.

Systemic JRA

About 10 percent of children with JRA have systemic disease. Systemic JRA is equally common among girls and boys. This form of JRA is very different from the other types of childhood arthritis, in that it causes dramatic symptoms in body systems other than the joints. Children with systemic JRA have a characteristic high spiking fever and a rash that may come and go rather quickly. The body temperature becomes elevated once or twice a day and is normal in between; it is not unusual for the fever to be as high as 103 degrees or more. Chills and shaking may occur when the child has the fever, and he may feel very sick. A characteristic pink rash may come and go throughout the day; it is likely to be present when the fever occurs. The lymph nodes, liver, and spleen may become enlarged, and inflammation may develop around the heart (*pericarditis*) or lungs (*pleuritis*).

When laboratory tests are performed on children with systemic JRA, the results are usually abnormal. Most children with systemic JRA develop a severely low red blood cell count (*anemia*) and have a high white blood cell count and a high platelet count. A highly elevated erythrocyte sedimentation rate (ESR) is nearly always present. None of these tests, however, is diagnostic for systemic JRA. They are merely consistent with a high level of inflammation in the body.

The diagnosis of systemic JRA requires a careful and difficult workup. All other causes of inflammation, including infection, other inflammatory diseases, and cancer must be ruled out. Among the procedures that may be performed in order to exclude other illnesses are a bone scan, sonograms, gastrointestinal studies, studies of blood and urine, and a bone marrow examination.

Arthritis may not be present early in the course of systemic JRA, which makes the diagnosis of this illness quite difficult. Children with systemic JRA may have joint and muscle aching without actual joint swelling or decreased range of motion. A definite diagnosis of systemic JRA cannot be made until the arthritis appears.

Many children with systemic JRA do well when treated with NSAIDs alone, though some children need to take steroids to control fever or anemia. The steroids may be given daily by mouth or periodically by intravenous infusion (there is no strong evidence that one method is more effective than the other). It is important that the smallest effective dose be used to control the disease. Children should be weaned from steroids *as soon as* the inflammation is controlled.

The course of systemic JRA is variable. The systemic symptoms of fever and rash eventually disappear, sometimes within months and sometimes after a year. Some children have only one episode of disease, followed by complete remission. Some children have flares and remissions repeatedly over time, and a small percentage of children have severe, persistent arthritis.

Many children with systemic JRA recover completely after several months, although about half of these children will have a recurrence of disease. About 25 to 40 percent of children with systemic JRA develop arthritis in many joints that is progressively destructive and has severe effects on their functioning. The arthritis may continue even after other symptoms are gone, and it can involve many joints.

Juvenile Spondyloarthropathy Syndromes

The juvenile spondyloarthropathy syndromes are a group of related conditions that include:

- Juvenile spondyloarthritis
- Juvenile ankylosing spondylitis
- Seronegative enthesopathy and arthropathy syndrome
- Arthritis of inflammatory bowel disease
- Reactive arthritis
- Reiter's syndrome
- Psoriatic arthritis

This group of conditions is diverse and it is difficult to characterize them. Many individuals affected with one of these disorders have a particular genetic marker called HLA-B27. Having this genetic marker does not mean that a person will develop a spondyloarthropathy syndrome, but someone who has the HLA-B27 marker is more likely to develop it than someone who doesn't. Many children with a spondyloarthropathy syndrome have other family members who are affected with one of these conditions, even if the HLA-B27 marker is not present.

Most of the spondyloarthropathy syndromes are characterized by asymmetric arthritis involving large joints such as the hips, knees, and lower spine (sacroiliac joints). The arthritis of the spondyloarthropathy syndromes is very similar to JRA and is treated in much the same way, with medications and physical therapy. In addition, it is common for these children to develop inflammation, called *enthesopathy,* at the attachments of ligaments in areas such as the heels or around the knees, resulting in pain in these areas.

The spondyloarthropathy syndromes occur most frequently in adolescent boys. The course of these conditions is variable, ranging from remission within months to intermittent flares that may continue into adulthood.

Juvenile Spondyloarthritis

Many physicians use the term *juvenile spondyloarthritis* (also called B-27 arthritis) to describe chronic arthritis in children and enthesopathy occurring in an asymmetrical pattern in older teenaged boys. Many of these children have a positive HLA-B27 gene, but this varies from one ethnic group to another and among geographic regions. Children with this disease have chronic arthritis that looks and acts quite like JRA. Most commonly they have arthritis in two or three joints, although some children may have many joints involved. This kind of arthritis is often characterized by tremendously swollen joints. Sometimes the joints are painfree and sometimes they are acutely painful. This arthritis is treated exactly the same as JRA, with the same medications and physical therapy.

Psoriatic Arthritis

Psoriatic arthritis is diagnosed in children who have both psoriasis and chronic arthritis. *Psoriasis* is a chronic skin condition that results in a scaly, red rash that occurs commonly in the scalp or near joints. The arthritis that occurs with psoriatic arthritis is very similar to seronegative polyarticular JRA, although the joint involvement tends to be asymmetrical. Psoriatic arthritis can continue on into adulthood, and erosive disease can occur. The treatment of psoriatic arthritis is the same as the treatment for JRA.

Arthritis of Inflammatory Bowel Disease

Inflammatory bowel disease (ulcerative colitis and Crohn's disease) is a group of diseases associated with chronic inflammation of the intestines, causing diarrhea, blood in the stools, abdominal pain, weight loss, fever, and poor growth. Some children with inflammatory bowel disease develop chronic arthritis. Rarely, the arthritis develops before signs of bowel disease, and then the correct diagnosis may be elusive. This arthritis is treated the same as JRA, with medications and physical therapy. Usually the medications used to treat the bowel disease effectively eliminate the arthritis.

Reiter's Syndrome

Reiter's syndrome is a condition that results in inflammation in three different places: the joints (*arthritis*), the urethra (*urethritis*), and the eyes (*conjunctivitis*). This condition usually occurs following an intestinal or urinary tract infection. Many people have only one episode of Reiter's syndrome, after which it goes away and doesn't return. Some people do have repeated occurrences of Reiter's. The arthritis of Reiter's syndrome usually affects only a few joints. Reiter's syndrome is rare in childhood.

Reactive Arthritis

Reactive arthritis is an episode of arthritis that occurs immediately after an infection. The arthritis is usually acute and short-lived, lasting a few months at most. Reactive arthritis is common in childhood; children who have strep infections, gastrointestinal infections, or viral infections of any kind sometimes develop reactive arthritis.

Ankylosing Spondylitis

Ankylosing spondylitis is a type of arthritis that primarily affects the spine and hips. Ankylosing spondylitis may begin at the base of the spine in the sacroiliac joints, or it may begin in the hips. Hip and low back pain with stiffness are common early symptoms. As the inflammation progresses upward in the spine, the mobility of the spine is gradually reduced. Ankylosing spondylitis is difficult to diagnose in childhood, since it takes years (often more than 10) for X-ray evidence of spinal arthritis to appear. Eventually, the bones of the spine may fuse together, causing a permanent flexed posture.

Exercise is very important to maintain the mobility of the back, and children with ankylosing spondylitis must maintain good posture. Good posture can mean the difference between having the spine fuse in a forward, flexed position or in an upright, functional position.

Systemic Lupus Erythematosus

SLE is a disease that causes inflammation in many different parts of the body. The inflammation can occur in nearly any organ system. Frequently affected areas include the skin (causing a rash), the joints (causing arthritis), the heart, the blood, the kidneys, the lungs, and the nervous system. Problems can occur in any of the organ systems affected by the inflammation. Children usually do not die from SLE, but it is a serious disease that can be life threatening without proper medical care.

Who Gets SLE?

SLE occurs most often in girls, and it is somewhat more common in African-Americans, Asians, and Hispanics. SLE can develop at any time throughout life. About 20 percent of people with SLE develop it before they reach the age of 16. Although it is rarely seen in children under the age of 6, children as young as 4 or 5 years old have developed SLE.

There is an inherited genetic tendency to develop SLE in some families, in which several family members will have the disease, for example a mother and daughter. In some families, a rare inherited abnormality of a part of the immune system, called the *complement system,* can predispose family members to develop an SLE-like disease. However, there are many families in which only one person has the disease. If your child is diagnosed with SLE, it is very unlikely that your other children will also develop it.

What Causes SLE?

As with the other rheumatic diseases, the cause of SLE is unknown. A flare of SLE can be triggered by an infection, exposure to sun, or medications. Some people develop SLE initially after such an exposure, although there is no evidence that any of these factors alone cause SLE. More likely, the exposure helps to trigger the illness in someone already susceptible to it, who would have gotten it anyway.

How Is SLE Diagnosed?

Most children are quite ill at the time they are diagnosed with SLE, although some children may feel well and have only mild symptoms. Specific signs of SLE include:

- *Malar rash.* This is a butterfly-shaped rash over the cheeks and across the bridge of the nose.
- *Photosensitivity.* Exposure to ultraviolet light, such as sunlight, a tanning booth, or even fluorescent light bulbs, can cause a bad rash or can trigger a flare of SLE.
- *Mouth sores.* People with SLE sometimes have sores on the tongue and inside the mouth or nose.
- *Arthritis.* Pain, stiffness, and swelling in the joints are symptoms of SLE.
- *Serositis.* Inflammation of the lining around the heart or lungs may cause fluid to develop in these areas.
- *Kidney problems.* Inflammation may cause damage to the kidneys that may (without treatment) result in kidney failure. Swelling of the feet and ankles, or fatigue, are signs of kidney problems. About half of all people with SLE develop kidney problems.
- *Central nervous system problems.* Inflammation in the brain can cause seizures, memory loss, disorientation, mood swings, hallucinations, headaches, fatigue, and dizziness.
- *Blood problems.* Children with SLE often have a positive ANA blood test. In addition, they may have a low red blood cell count (anemia), a low white blood cell count, and a low platelet count. These blood problems may cause the child to bruise easily, to be tired, or to catch infections more easily.

The symptoms of SLE can be very different from child to child. Some children may have severe kidney problems but never have arthritis, some children may have arthritis and rashes only, and some children may have serious involvement of many organ systems. The course of the disease in an individual child can be extremely unpredictable, as well. A child who initially has fever, rash, mouth sores, and arthritis may develop kidney problems 5 years later.

The diagnosis of SLE is made according to criteria developed by the American College of Rheumatology (of the eleven criteria, four must be present before a physician can make the diagnosis of SLE):

- Skin and mucous membrane lesions, such as:
  - Malar rash (butterfly rash on the face)
  - Discoid rash (thick plaque of rash)
  - Photosensitivity
  - Ulcers in the mouth or nose
- Arthritis
- Inflammation of body cavities, including inflammation and/or fluid around the heart, and inflammation and/or fluid around the lungs
- Kidney disease (increased protein or cellular inflammation [casts] in the urine)
- Nervous system disease, including seizures and psychosis (serious psychiatric disturbance)
- Hematologic abnormalities, such as hemolytic anemia, low white blood cell count, and low platelet count
- Positive test for ANA
- Other autoantibodies associated with SLE (such as anti-DNA)

SOURCE: Revised from Tan et al. *JAMA* 248:622, 1982.

Diagnostic Tests for SLE

As the preceding list indicates, before a diagnosis of SLE can be made, there must be evidence that the patient has certain specific medical problems. Laboratory tests are very important in providing this evidence as well as in providing useful information about the extent of the disease and its activity. When the physician suspects that a child has SLE, the physician will order laboratory tests to investigate every organ system in the child.

A diagnostic investigation on this scale involves a complete laboratory screening of blood, kidneys, liver, and, often, other organs such as the thyroid gland. Laboratory tests looking for the presence of particular antibodies, such as ANA and antibodies to cell components such as DNA, will be done. Laboratory tests of a blood system called the *complement system* will give an indication of how active the disease is; the results of this test will generally improve as treatment causes the inflammatory process to quiet down.

If the kidneys appear to be involved, a biopsy of the kidney may be very helpful in making the diagnosis and guiding future therapy. This test is usually done by a pediatric kidney specialist (nephrologist) while the child is under sedation; the child may need to stay in the hospital overnight. Tests to look at the lungs (chest X ray and pulmonary function testing) and heart (electrocardiogram and echocardiogram) may be done to determine whether inflammation is present and to provide a baseline for the future. The physician may decide to order specialized testing of the nervous system, such as scans of the brain and an electroencephalogram or specific psychological tests. Other tests are sometimes ordered if the physical examination or symptoms indicate that the child has other problems.

Treating SLE

After diagnosis, active SLE is generally brought under control with high doses of steroids (prednisone). During this period, most children experience some of the side effects of steroid treatment (described in chapter 3). The steroids are slowly tapered once the disease has come under control. While the steroids are tapered, the doctor will pay careful attention to the child to be certain that the inflammation does not flare up. This is usually accomplished by regular blood and urine tests, which are generally done monthly.

If SLE cannot be adequately controlled with steroids, or if the steroid dose required for disease control is too high, other immunosuppressive medications such as azathioprine or cyclophosphamide may be added. Many children with SLE take hydroxychloroquine, an antimalarial drug, in addition to prednisone, for control of the disease. Other medications, such as NSAIDs or antihypertensive drugs, may also be necessary to control organ system problems of SLE such as arthritis or high blood pressure.

Sun protection is an important part of the treatment plan. Sunlight can make SLE worse or can trigger a flare. It is very important for children with SLE to protect themselves from the sun to keep the disease under control.

The child should avoid the sun entirely if possible during the peak hours of ten o'clock in the morning to two o'clock in the afternoon. This is the period when the sun's rays are the brightest. When the child is in the sun, he'll need to wear long sleeves, slacks, and a hat with a wide brim. It's as important for him to be protected from the sun on hazy or cloudy days as on sunny days.

Children with SLE should wear a sunscreen *every day*. Either lotion or gel form is fine; what's important is that the sunscreen have a sun protection factor (SPF) of 15 or higher. The sunscreen should be applied immediately after bathing or showering, and it should be applied to all areas that might be exposed to the sun, such as the face, lips, neck, chest, arms, and legs. After applying sunscreen, the child should wait 20 to 30 minutes before using makeup, getting wet, or going in the sun. This gives the sunscreen time to "bind" to the skin. Since one application of sunscreen lasts about 4 hours, it should be reapplied every 4 hours while the child is in the sun.

Children with SLE must get plenty of rest. SLE can cause the child to feel very tired; in addition, excessive fatigue can be a sign that the SLE is flaring up. Getting plenty of rest helps the child fight the disease and deal with the fatigue.

Because of the complex and unpredictable nature of SLE and the need for the child to take medications that have many side effects, children and their parents must work closely with other members of the health care team. Children and their parents must be well informed about the illness and possible medication side effects, for example. Frequent communication between families and the doctor is essential to ensure the best care for the child with SLE.

QUESTIONS AND ANSWERS ABOUT SLE

Is discoid lupus erythematosus the same thing as systemic lupus erythematosus (SLE)? If a child has discoid lupus, will he develop SLE in the future?

> Discoid lupus is *not* the same disease as SLE. Discoid lupus affects only the skin, not the other organ systems. Discoid lupus causes scaly, red, disk-shaped sores on the face, neck, and chest. Sores may also appear on the trunk, arms, legs, scalp, or inside the mouth, but this is rare. Children with discoid lupus almost never develop SLE.

Dermatomyositis

Dermatomyositis is a condition involving inflammation in the skin and muscle tissues. The main symptoms of dermatomyositis are:

- *Rash.* The dermatomyositis rash consists of red or purple discoloration of the eyelids, sometimes with swelling around the eyes, and red, thick, scaly patches over the knuckles, elbows, and knees.

- *Weakness.* Weakness occurs in all the muscles, but it is most significant in the muscles of the neck, stomach, shoulders, and hips. The muscles used for swallowing and breathing may also become weak. The muscle weakness usually develops gradually. At first the child may have trouble climbing stairs or getting up from a chair or the floor when playing. As the weakness becomes worse, even simple activities may become difficult. If weakness becomes severe, the muscles of the gastrointestinal tract can become involved, causing difficulty in swallowing or a nasal-sounding voice. In rare cases, bleeding or perforation of the gastrointestinal tract can occur.

Diagnosing Dermatomyositis

This disease usually develops gradually, over a period of months. The diagnosis of this disease is based on a physical examination that includes a detailed assessment of the child's strength and laboratory tests measuring the level of muscle enzymes in his blood. The laboratory tests show elevation of proteins generally found inside muscle cells that have leaked out of the inflamed cells. An electromyogram and a muscle biopsy may also be needed to confirm the diagnosis.

It is important to be absolutely certain of the diagnosis before starting treatment. Therefore, when the physician suspects that a child may have dermatomyositis, the physician will order a number of tests to measure the presence of inflammation in muscle tissue. Laboratory tests will be done to measure whether there is any elevation of muscle enzyme levels (creatinine phosphokinase [CPK], aldolase, serum glutamic oxaloacetic transaminase [SGOT], serum glutamic pyruvic transaminase [SGPT], and lactic dehydrogenase [LDH]), which is an indication that these proteins, which are generally found inside muscle cells, have leaked out of the inflamed cells into the bloodstream.

Additional tests that may be ordered to help diagnose dermatomyositis include an electromyogram and a muscle biopsy. The electromyogram is a test that measures the electrical activity of the muscles; it is performed by inserting a small needle into the muscle to be tested, and then stimulating the muscle and recording its response. This test can show whether muscle alone is inflamed or if nerves are involved as well. In a muscle biopsy, a small piece of muscle is removed through a needle or a small surgical incision. In younger children this is done under general anesthesia; in older children sedation alone may be adequate. The piece of muscle is examined under a microscope to determine whether the characteristic changes of dermatomyositis are present. This is the best way to exclude any other muscle diseases that may mimic dermatomyositis.

Treating Dermatomyositis

Dermatomyositis is treated with a combination of medications and physical therapy. The child may need to be hospitalized if he is very weak. The initial treatment is to give high doses of steroids either orally (in pill form) or by intravenous infusion. Steroids put the disease into remission in nearly all cases. Physical therapy is performed initially to prevent stiffness, and later to help the child regain normal strength. The rash of dermatomyositis can be made worse by sunlight, so the child should wear sunscreen. Unlike the case with SLE, sunlight does not trigger a flare of the entire disease process, but it does make the rash of dermatomyositis worse.

The pediatric rheumatologist will monitor the child's response to treatment at regular intervals. The initial treatment period will be intense. The child may need to see the doctor as often as once a week at the start of the disease, but the visits will gradually become more spaced out. At each visit, the child's muscle strength will be carefully measured and blood tests will be performed.

As the child recovers, his strength and the level of muscle enzymes in his blood will gradually return to normal. Most children begin to regain normal muscle strength within 3 to 5 months of beginning treatment. Continued weakness is *not* an acceptable outcome for dermatomyositis. Once the blood tests are normal and strength is returning, the steroid medication is slowly tapered off. If remission cannot be achieved with steroids alone, or if a flare occurs while the steroids are being tapered, other medications (such as methotrexate) may be added.

Course of Treatment for Dermatomyositis

Although different pediatric rheumatologists follow different treatment schedules, full treatment for one episode of dermatomyositis usually lasts 2 years. The majority of children with dermatomyositis recover completely, without any complications. Unpredictable disease flares occur in approximately one-third of children. A small percentage of children with dermatomyositis have severe disease that goes on for many years and is difficult to treat even with high doses of prednisone and other medications.

Some children with dermatomyositis may develop calcium deposits under the skin, called *calcinosis,* several years after treatment. These deposits feel like small rocks under the skin, and they may even break through the skin and come out. The calcium deposits can occur in any area, and they can be tiny or large; large deposits may make it difficult for the child to move around.

There is currently no accepted therapy that causes these calcium deposits to disappear. In most cases, they are slowly reabsorbed over time, but occasionally they can be extensive and persistent. This appears to happen more frequently if treatment for dermatomyositis is delayed in the early stages of the illness. Calcinosis occurs as a result of the disease and is not due to an excess of calcium in the child's diet. It is important not to restrict your child's calcium intake.

Scleroderma

People with scleroderma develop thickened skin that feels hard to the touch (*scleroderma* means "hard skin"). The skin thickening is due to an abnormal excess buildup of collagen, an important component of normal tissues. Although scleroderma is relatively rare in children, there are two types of scleroderma that affect children:

- Localized scleroderma
- Systemic scleroderma

Both types affect boys and girls equally often and can occur at any age. Each has a different disease course and outcome.

Localized Scleroderma

Localized scleroderma affects only the skin. It causes areas of skin to become hardened and tough, and the skin may become stuck to the underlying connective tissues. Initially, there may be only a small discolored area of skin (called a *lesion*) which appears swollen or thick. As the lesion progresses, it becomes pale white or yellow, and tightly bound to the underlying tissues. The underlying area of muscle and bone can occasionally become involved in the process of scleroderma, resulting in inflammation or abnormal growth. In general, there is little or no pain involved with localized scleroderma lesions, and children with localized scleroderma are otherwise entirely well.

Localized scleroderma can be present in two forms, distinguished by the shape of the lesions and how much skin they involve. Scleroderma that occurs in round spots is called *morphea*. Lesions that occur in a linelike pattern over an arm or leg are called *linear scleroderma*.

If the skin lesions occur over a joint, the mobility of the joint may be limited. Linear scleroderma can cause localized growth problems. The lesions cause the involved arm or leg to grow slowly, and it may become smaller than the other arm or leg, both in length and in width.

Treating Localized Scleroderma

Whether or not medical therapy will lead to improvement of localized scleroderma lesions is currently controversial. In some cases, good results have been reported using methotrexate in children with large or extensive lesions. It is important to monitor the motion of the joints and the growth of the affected limb, and to begin physical and occupational therapy to restore joint mobility if motion becomes restricted. A shoe lift may be needed if a difference in leg length occurs that is significant enough to cause changes in posture or gait. The child may require two different sizes of shoes if only one foot is involved.

Both kinds of linear scleroderma tend to become bigger and spread during the early phase of the disease. There may be just one lesion, or there may be several. After several years they stabilize in size, and eventually they become smaller. Differences in the size and shape of the limbs may continue throughout life.

Systemic Scleroderma

Systemic scleroderma is a serious condition in which the thickening of tissues occurs in other body systems as well as in the skin. Systemic scleroderma may occur in the lungs, kidneys, blood vessels, or gastrointestinal tract. This disorder is very rare in childhood. Symptoms may develop gradually over months, and it may take a long time for the diagnosis to be clear. Early signs of the disease may include swelling and thickening of the skin on the hands, cold fingers, and heartburn. Symptoms of systemic scleroderma include:

- *Raynaud's phenomenon.* This is a condition in which the blood vessels in the fingers and toes constrict when exposed to cold or stress. Raynaud's phenomenon causes the fingers and toes to turn blue, white, and then red when exposed to cold.
- *Skin changes.* The skin may become shiny, and usual skin creases may disappear. This may be most noticeable in the face, arms, and hands.
- *Problems with the fingertips.* Small sores or calcium deposits may develop in the fingertips.
- *Limitation in joint motion.* As the skin becomes tight around the joint, it may become hard for the child to move the joint through its full range of motion.
- *Gastrointestinal problems.* Swallowing problems, heartburn, and bowel involvement may occur.
- *Lung problems.* Difficulty in breathing or shortness of breath may occur.

Laboratory tests are helpful in making the diagnosis of systemic scleroderma, but it is often necessary to biopsy the skin in order to be certain. Investigations of the lungs (with an X ray of the chest and tests of lung function), the heart (an electrocardiogram and echocardiogram), and the gastrointestinal tract (with X-ray studies or endoscopy) are often indicated to help determine the scope of the problems.

Treating Systemic Scleroderma

There are no medications that cure systemic scleroderma; there are only medications that slow the progression of disease. Physical and occupational therapy are critical to maintain joint mobility. Contractures can be postponed or prevented by performing range of motion exercises faithfully every day. Children with scleroderma usually need the advice and support that can only be provided through an interdisciplinary treatment team including a pediatric rheumatologist, physical and occupational therapists, a social worker or psychologist, and other pediatric subspecialty doctors.

What Is the Usual Course of the Disease?

Systemic scleroderma is a slowly progressive disease. Many children develop an increasing number of symptoms and problems over the first three to five years of illness. Severe contractures of the finger joints can cause difficulties in functioning at home and at school. Gastrointestinal problems can lead to ulcers, problems absorbing food properly, and difficulty in maintaining weight. Lung, kidney, or heart problems can develop at any time over the course of disease. In many children, the disease activity will slow down after rapid progression in the first years of illness, and some children may be relatively stable for many years. Systemic scleroderma is a potentially life-threatening disorder, making it essential that the child receive proper and ongoing medical care.

Vasculitis

Vasculitis refers to a group of different conditions that cause inflammation in the blood vessels. The different types of vasculitis are generally distinguished by the size of the blood vessels that are inflamed. Children often have disease characteristics that do not exactly fit into one of the known vasculitis disorders, causing some confusion in diagnosis. These types of vasculitis can affect children:

- Polyarteritis nodosa
- Cutaneous polyarteritis
- Hypersensitivity vasculitis, including serum sickness, Henoch-Schönlein purpura, and allergic angiitis
- Kawasaki disease
- Wegener's granulomatosis
- Takayasu's arteritis
- Behçet's syndrome

Most children with a vasculitis have a skin rash, although skin rash is more common in some types of vasculitis than in others. Some of the more common diseases are discussed below.

Cutaneous Polyarteritis

Episodes of cutaneous polyarteritis may be triggered by an infection such as streptococcal throat infection (strep throat). Children with cutaneous polyarteritis develop reddish purple skin lumps, usually along with fever and joint pain or actual arthritis. Blood tests will indicate inflammation (such as anemia and high ESR). Often, a biopsy of the skin rash is needed to make the diagnosis, and further investigations may be necessary to determine whether internal organs are involved. Treatment with steroids may be necessary during a disease flare, and if the disease was triggered by a streptococcal infection, it may be a good idea for the child to take penicillin to prevent further such infections. Some children with this disorder may have multiple flares, but it generally is a mild condition.

Kawasaki Disease

Kawasaki disease is one of the most common vasculitis diseases of childhood, usually occurring in young children (average age about 2 years). The features of the disease are continuous high fever for at least 5 days; a pink or red rash that eventually leads to skin peeling (especially on the fingers and in the groin area); red, irritated eyes; cracked, swollen lips; swollen hands and feet; enlarged lymph nodes, especially in the neck; and arthritis. Children with Kawasaki disease are very irritable and cranky.

If this disease is suspected, a specialized test to look at the blood vessels surrounding the heart will be done, because some children with Kawasaki disease develop enlargements of these blood vessels. Treatment of children with Kawasaki disease with infusions of antibodies (called immunoglobulin) is very helpful in preventing the development of these blood vessel enlargements. With careful treatment and follow-up, most children with Kawasaki disease recover completely and do well in the future. This disease does not relapse or flare up.

Henoch-Schönlein Purpura

Henoch-Schönlein purpura (known as HSP) is another common vasculitis seen in childhood. Children with this disorder develop a rash consisting of tiny purple spots on the lower legs or buttocks that can enlarge to bigger, dark purple spots. They also have stomach pain and cramping (sometimes with bleeding into the bowel movements), blood in their urine, and arthritis.

Not every child with Henoch-Schönlein purpura has every one of these symptoms, and the symptoms don't generally show up at the same time. Some children have a mild course and others (less commonly) develop severe problems, with bleeding into the stomach and gut or kidney problems. In most cases, pediatricians can diagnose this problem. Most children with Henoch-Schönlein purpura do not need any special treatment, as the disease resolves on its own; careful follow-up is all that is required. It's not uncommon for children with Henoch-Schönlein purpura to have one or two flares over 6 months, but eventually the disease goes away.

Laboratory Tests and Procedures

Many (if not most) children with rheumatic diseases undergo a variety of testing procedures. Testing is initially done to assist in determining the correct diagnosis, whereas later testing is done to monitor the effects of the disease over time and the response of the disease to medical therapy.

The doctor determines which tests to order for your child based on your child's symptoms, the range of possible diagnoses under consideration, and the medications that your child is taking. This section describes the types of tests that are performed and what they tell us about your child's illness.

Diagnostic Testing

The most important point to remember about diagnostic laboratory tests is that *there is no one test that can definitely diagnose any of the rheumatic diseases.* Certain laboratory findings may be helpful in suggesting a diagnosis, in determining the extent of disease activity, or in ruling out other causes of the child's symptoms. But the rheumatic diseases are diagnosed *based on the combination of a number of clinical findings.* A single laboratory test cannot form the basis of a diagnosis of a specific rheumatic disease.

A general set of screening laboratory tests may be done at the time of diagnosis and at follow-up visits. These tests include a complete blood count, ESR, liver function tests, kidney function tests, and a urine test. Initially, the results of these tests may help provide clues for diagnosis and indicate the extent of the disease process. Lab tests may also be used to establish a normal baseline before starting medications with potential side effects that will need to be monitored regularly. These routine tests are discussed in the next section.

Rheumatoid factor (RF) and antinuclear antibodies (ANA) are two examples of *autoantibodies* associated with rheumatic diseases. Normally, a person's immune system manufactures antibodies that prevent and fight off diseases by attacking foreign substances like viruses and bacteria. *Autoantibody* is a general term used to describe antibodies that react with an individual's own body components, such as red or white blood cells, cell products, or cell components. The immune systems of patients with autoimmune diseases produce autoantibodies. It is not known what triggers this process, and in most cases, it is also not known how these autoantibodies cause disease. However, the association between certain antibodies and diseases is known, and this information can be helpful in diagnosing and assessing disease activity.

Rheumatoid factor. Rf is an autoantibody that reacts with a person's own normal antibodies. RFs are commonly found in adults who have rheumatoid arthritis, but they are only rarely found in children with JRA. Few children who have polyarticular JRA have a positive RF, and positive Rf is even more uncommon in children with other subtypes of JRA. In addition, Rf is not "specific" for rheumatic diseases, meaning that it can be found in the blood of patients with a variety of infections or other inflammatory conditions. A study done at Children's Hospital of Philadelphia reviewing all Rf testing done at that hospital for 1 year concluded that in no case was an Rf test helpful in establishing or ruling out a diagnosis of JRA. Rf testing, therefore, is helpful in determining the subtype of JRA to which a child belongs, but it is not a specific test to diagnose arthritis or rheumatic disease.

Antinuclear antibodies. ANA bind to a part of the cell called the nucleus. To detect the presence of ANA, the patient's blood is added to a slide to which other cells are fixed to determine whether antibodies from the patient's blood react with the nuclear portion of the cells. When the slide is stained, a variety of patterns can be seen, and these patterns are useful in the test's interpretation. ANA test results may differ when done in different labs, depending on the type of material used to perform the test and how much experience the lab personnel have in interpreting test results.

A positive ANA test is not specific for rheumatic disease; ANAs are seen in the blood of patients with a variety of disorders, including infection, malignancy, and autoimmune diseases. In addition, 3 to 5 percent of healthy children have a positive ANA that is not associated with any illness. ANAs are seen in all patients who have SLE. Between 40 and 60 percent of children with JRA will have a positive ANA test. ANAs are more frequently found in young children with pauciarticular JRA, with the highest prevalence among young children who have pauciarticular JRA and eye inflammation (iritis). Therefore, a positive ANA in a young child who has pauciarticular JRA suggests a higher risk of developing iritis. Once the ANA is positive, it usually remains positive, and monitoring the level of ANA through further testing is generally not useful in predicting disease activity or flares.

Arthrocentesis. Removal of joint fluid from a swollen joint, in a procedure called *arthrocentesis,* is sometimes necessary to diagnose a child's arthritis. It may not be possible to exclude infection without examining the joint fluid, and it is extremely important not to miss an infection, which may require speedy treatment with antibiotics. Examination of the joint fluid will also rule out bleeding into the joint from trauma. Arthrocentesis is a brief outpatient procedure, generally done in the clinic or office under mild sedation in young children.

Radiologic tests. Radiologic tests are often required in the diagnosis and follow-up of children with arthritis. Plain X rays of bones and joints are frequently done at the time of diagnosis and at regular intervals to detect any signs of destruction. Ultrasound studies of the joints are done to look for joint fluid or swelling, particularly in joints such as the hip which may be difficult to examine clinically. A bone scan, with injection of a radioactive dye that can be detected at areas of inflammation, may also be recommended during the diagnostic evaluation. Some children may need to have more extensive radiologic studies, including ultrasound studies, computed tomographic (CT) scans, and magnetic resonance imaging (MRI), to examine internal organs.

Testing to Monitor Disease Activity and Medication Effects

Throughout the course of a child's treatment for a rheumatic disease, additional tests are done to evaluate the effectiveness of treatment and to monitor for medication side effects. Which tests are done, and how frequently they are repeated, depends on the level of disease activity and the specific medications the child is taking.

Complete blood count. The CBC includes a red blood cell count (usually called *hemoglobin* and *hematocrit*), a white blood cell count, and a platelet count. In addition, the white blood cell count is usually broken down to give the counts of the different types of white blood cells (called a *differential*).

A decreased red blood cell count can indicate anemia or blood loss. Anemia is a common problem in childhood which is usually caused by a deficiency of iron in the diet. Some children with JRA who take NSAIDs, however, develop stomach irritation and continually or intermittently lose small amounts of blood from the gastrointestinal tract. This can result in a low red blood cell count in a blood test. If anemia unexplained by iron deficiency or blood loss is found in a child with JRA, it is called the anemia of chronic disease. This anemia is difficult to correct unless the underlying disease is better controlled.

The white blood cell count is increased when there is infection, and also in some children with active JRA. JRA can also increase the number of platelets. Both disease activity and medications can affect the CBC results. Therefore, the CBC provides information that is useful in determining appropriate treatment.

Erythrocyte sedimentation rate. The ESR is a nonspecific measure of the level of inflammatory activity in the body. The ESR is elevated in most infections as well as in the entire spectrum of inflammatory disorders. A high ESR only provides a clue that inflammation is present; it does not help to identify the cause of that inflammation. In addition, a very high ESR may take a long time to return to normal, and therefore a high ESR may not accurately reflect the child's clinical response to treatment.

Urinalysis. Urinalysis includes evaluation for blood, sugar, and other chemical substances in the urine, as well as microscopic analysis for the presence of cells, crystals, or bacteria. The normal urine is clear of cells, sugar, and protein. Rarely, NSAIDs are associated with the development of kidney problems, and the rheumatologist will check the urine periodically while a child is taking such medications. Children taking steroids often have their urine checked for sugar because steroids can cause a diabetes-like condition in some individuals while they are taking these medications.

SGOT, SGPT. Aspirin and other NSAIDs (such as naproxen, tolmetin sodium, and ibuprofen) cause reversible liver toxicity, in the form of mild liver inflammation, in some patients. Rheumatologists routinely monitor for this damage with liver function tests. Liver function tests measure the blood levels of enzymes (chemicals that help the body break down other substances) that are present in high concentrations in liver cells. It is normal for a small amount of these enzymes to be present in the blood. However, when there is damage to liver cells, their enzymes are released and the level of these liver enzymes in the blood increases.

The most commonly measured enzymes are SGOT and SGPT. Normal results vary from lab to lab, but are usually considered to be around 30 units or less. As with any test, a minor elevation (such as levels around 40 or 50) may only bear watching, through repeated lab tests in several weeks. A higher level, of 300 for example, may mean that the child must stop taking the medication and be retested soon afterward. The proper medical management of a child with a high level of SGOT and SGPT will vary from case to case.

The type of liver damage caused by aspirin and other NSAIDs is nearly always reversible. This is because the liver has a very high potential to regenerate itself. It is, therefore, very unlikely that a child will suffer any permanent liver damage from the NSAIDs used in the treatment of rheumatic diseases.

BUN, creatinine. The blood urea nitrogen (BUN) and creatinine are blood tests that check kidney function. These tests may be done when a child is taking NSAIDs.

Salicylate level. The salicylate level is useful in determining the correct dosage of aspirin (or aspirin-containing medication such as Disalcid or Trilisate). Aspirin must be given in much larger doses to control inflammation than are used to control pain. A therapeutic dose—one that controls inflammation with minimal side effects—usually results in salicylate levels between 20 and 30 mg/dl. Different people absorb aspirin very differently, so the physician needs to know the salicylate level in the child's blood in order to determine whether the child is receiving a therapeutic dose. That is, by measuring the salicylate level, the rheumatologist can determine the correct dose of aspirin to prescribe for a particular child. It is not possible to measure blood levels of other NSAIDs such as tolmetin sodium or naproxen.

X rays. X rays identify problems such as erosion of bone, fusion of bones, poor alignment of bones, and decrease in the spaces between bones. These are serious problems that require aggressive therapy because they can lead to permanent joint dysfunction. X rays are done to identify these problems early, so measures can be taken to prevent or limit joint damage.

Pulmonary function tests. Pulmonary function tests are done to detect any changes in lung function that may occur in children taking methotrexate. This series of tests is done before methotrexate is begun to establish baseline values and is repeated annually throughout the course of treatment with methotrexate. Pulmonary function tests are done by having the child breathe into a piece of equipment that measures lung volume, air flow rates, and gas exchange.

　　Laboratory tests and procedures, differential diagnoses, and treatment—all of these are managed and performed by various health care professionals with whom you and your child will come into contact and, in some cases, form long-term relationships. These professionals and their roles are described in the next chapter.

Chapter 2

Options for Medical Care
Health Care Professionals and
Health Care Settings

There are many kinds of health care professionals who help provide care for children with rheumatic disease. The purpose of this chapter is to familiarize you with the different health care providers you and your child may encounter, and to let you know what to expect from these various individuals.

As a parent, you are responsible for choosing who will provide health care for your child. Choosing medical care can be a stressful process. For one thing, you may be limited in your options because of restrictions in your health care plan. Or you may feel uncomfortable being put in the position of having to judge the qualifications of a medical professional. Remember, however, that as a parent, you are in the best position to evaluate whether or not the health care your child is receiving is both appropriate and high in quality. If you feel uncomfortable with a health care provider or with his or her recommendations, you may very well wish to obtain another opinion regarding your child's care. Don't be afraid to trust your own judgment!

Choosing a Specialty Care Physician

When a child is suspected of having, or is diagnosed with, a rheumatic illness, the primary care provider (the pediatrician or family physician) will usually refer the child to a specialist who has a knowledge of the natural history of the disease and who has greater experience with the appropriate medications and other modes of therapy. After being seen and being treated by a specialist, the child will probably continue to see the primary care provider for continuing care, such as periodic checkups, immunizations, and diagnosis and treatment of routine childhood illnesses such as ear infections. Nevertheless, all children with rheumatic diseases should be evaluated periodically by a specialist in rheumatic diseases. The specialist will serve as the overall team leader for the child's rheumatic illness, and will direct and oversee all of the child's rheumatology care.

You should use care in selecting your child's specialty care provider. The quality of care your child receives and her eventual health outcome will depend largely on the care she receives from the specialty provider. Several types of physicians may be qualified to serve as your child's specialty care provider. By working with your primary care provider, you will be able to determine which kind of doctor best meets your child's needs. Your choice may be influenced by the availability of specialty care within your geographic region, limitations imposed by your health insurance plan, or other factors. In the long run, however, it may well be worth traveling a long distance or negotiating with your health insurance provider in order to obtain the best health care and the best health outcome for your child.

The Pediatric Rheumatologist

The pediatric rheumatologist is a physician who specializes in providing care to children with rheumatic diseases. A pediatric rheumatologist is a fully trained pediatrician who has gone on to participate in a formal training program to become an expert in caring for children with rheumatic diseases. Such a physician generally limits his or her practice to children with rheumatic diseases, and does not provide care to children with other kinds of disorders.

The pediatric rheumatologist is the physician who is best qualified to serve as your child's specialty care provider. If a pediatric rheumatologist is available in your area, he or she is your best choice. The pediatric rheumatologist has the following qualifications:

- Has graduated from medical school and is licensed to practice medicine.
- Has graduated from a 3-year training program at an accredited facility to become a general pediatrician.
- Has passed the board examination to become a board-certified pediatrician.
- Has completed a 3-year fellowship training program in caring for childhood rheumatic diseases.
- Has passed the board examination to become a board-certified pediatric rheumatologist, or is eligible to take the exam to become board certified.

Pediatric rheumatology is a relatively new subspecialty within the specialty practice of pediatrics. Although pediatric rheumatology training programs have been offered since the early 1960s, the board examination that physicians can take to become certified was not offered until 1992. Consequently, pediatric rheumatologists may be either *board eligible* or *board certified*. A board-certified pediatric rheumatologist has successfully completed the board examinations given by the American Academy of Pediatrics to ensure that the physician designated as "board-certified" has complete knowledge and understanding of the current content of the sub-specialty. In most cases, a board-eligible pediatric rheumatologist is as qualified as one who is board certified.

Your health insurance plan may limit your choice of specialty care providers. It is possible that your health insurance plan does not have a pediatric rheumatologist on the list of physicians whose services it will cover. (You could take your child to see a pediatric rheumatologist anyway, but your insurance would not cover any of the fees involved.) As an alternative to seeing a pediatric rheumatologist, the health insurance plan may refer you to an adult rheumatologist or an orthopedist for your child's care.

As a parent, you are in a position to protest this recommendation (or any other recommendation from your health insurance carrier that you believe interferes with your child's ability to get the best possible health care). Because your child has been diagnosed with a rheumatic disease, you should insist that she receive care provided by a physician who is *board certified or board eligible in pediatric rheumatology by the American Academy of Pediatrics.* If the health plan does not provide access to a physician with these credentials within its service area, you should request a referral to a physician who is accredited in this field. Most health plans provide coverage for appropriate specialty care. In the case of a childhood rheumatic illness, a pediatric rheumatologist *is* the *appropriate* care provider. Your child's pediatrician is in the best position to assist you in pressing your health insurance plan to provide this benefit.

Most pediatric rheumatologists work in large teaching hospitals, within centers that specialize in caring for children with rheumatic illnesses. Unfortunately, relatively few pediatric rheumatology centers exist, and in some areas of the country there aren't any pediatric rheumatologists in practice. If there isn't a pediatric rheumatologist available in your area, your child may need to be cared for by another specialist: a rheumatologist, an orthopedist, or a pediatrician. If this is the case, you may want to seek a consultation from a pediatric rheumatologist on an intermittent basis, even if only once a year. Pediatric rheumatologists often help manage rheumatic disease for children who live in remote areas. He or she will make recommendations to the local specialist about managing the child's disease between visits to the specialty care center.

The Pediatrician

A pediatrician is a physician who specializes in caring for children. A licensed pediatrician has the following qualifications:

- Has graduated from medical school and is licensed to practice medicine.
- Has graduated from a 3-year training program at an accredited facility to become a general pediatrician.
- Has passed the board examination to become a board-certified pediatrician.

The benefit of getting medical care for a child from a pediatrician is that the pediatrician is a specialist in providing overall care to children. However, a general pediatrician may have little experience in caring for children with rheumatic diseases. Most pediatricians do not have formal training in caring for children with rheumatic diseases beyond a 1-month rotation on a pediatric rheumatology service.

The Rheumatologist

A rheumatologist is a physician who specializes in caring for *adults* with rheumatic diseases. A board-certified rheumatologist has the following qualifications:

- Has graduated from medical school and is licensed to practice medicine.
- Has graduated from a 3-year training program at an accredited facility to become an internist (a physician who specializes in providing medical care to adults).
- Has passed the board examination to become a board-certified internist.
- Has completed a 2-year fellowship training program in caring for adults with rheumatic diseases.
- Has passed the board examination to become a board-certified rheumatologist.

The benefit of getting care from a rheumatologist is that he or she is well qualified to care for rheumatic diseases. The drawback for a child with rheumatic disease is that the rheumatologist has limited experience in caring for children.

A rheumatologist may not be aware of developmental issues, school concerns, and other matters that are unique to children. Also, although a rheumatologist is informed about the medications used to treat rheumatic diseases in adults, he or she may not be knowledgeable about which drugs are approved for use in children, or about the alterations in dosages needed.

If your child is being cared for by an adult rheumatologist, it is important for the rheumatologist to work closely with your child's pediatrician, to be certain that all of your child's needs are addressed. Keep in mind that if your child is cared for by an adult rheumatologist, you may have to make an extra effort to meet families with children who have similar illnesses. Also, the physician's waiting room may not be child-friendly, so bring along toys or books to occupy your child.

The Orthopedic Surgeon

An orthopedic surgeon or orthopedist is a physician who specializes in caring for people with problems of the musculoskeletal system (bones and joints). A board-certified orthopedist has the following qualifications:

- Has graduated from medical school and is licensed to practice medicine.
- Has graduated from a 3-year training program at an accredited facility to become an orthopedist.
- Has passed the board examination to become a board-certified orthopedist.

The training for orthopedists usually includes some formal instruction in caring for the orthopedic problems of children. Some orthopedists have taken additional training in pediatric orthopedics, and limit their practice to children.

Frequently, an orthopedist is consulted about the care of children with rheumatic diseases when surgical procedures are needed or are being considered. In some cases, an orthopedist may primarily manage the care of a child with a rheumatic disease. The drawback of having an orthopedist as a primary care specialist is that the orthopedist may not have significant experience with the medications used to treat the rheumatic diseases.

Locating a Specialist

The following guidelines may be useful in locating an appropriate health care professional for your child:

- Call the American Academy of Pediatrics (see Appendix 2 at the end of this book) to request a list of board-certified pediatric rheumatologists, or to find out if your physician is board certified in pediatric rheumatology.
- Call or write to the American Juvenile Arthritis Organization for the names of specialists located nearest to you. If you live in a rural area, it may be necessary to travel some distance. In the long run, this may still be less expensive and less time-consuming than using a local physician who is less knowledgeable about the treatment of rheumatic diseases.
- A list of physicians specializing in the care of children with rheumatic diseases may be available from your local chapter of the Arthritis Foundation (look under "Arthritis" in the white pages *business* listings of your phone book). Such lists do not make specific recommendations, nor do they delineate the physician's qualifications. For example, an Arthritis Foundation referral list will indicate whether the physician sees children, but it will not state whether the

physician is a board-certified pediatric rheumatologist, a rheumatologist, or an orthopedist.

- Ask what credentials the doctor has that qualify him or her to be called a "specialist" in caring for children with rheumatic diseases. Be aware that many physicians list credentials such as "Fellow of the American College of Rheumatology," "Fellow of the American Academy of Pediatrics," or "Fellow of the American College of Orthopedic Surgeons"; these designations mean that the physician is a member of that professional organization. Although such membership indicates that the physician has an interest in a specific area of medicine, membership is open to all physicians and thus provides no evidence about the individual physician's qualifications. Board certification (which *is* a meaningful credential) is often not required for membership in these organizations.

- Don't hesitate to call the physician's office in advance to ask questions that will help you to evaluate the physician's credentials prior to your child's first visit.

- Find out how childhood rheumatic diseases are managed within the practice. Ideally there will be an interdisciplinary team approach, with close communication among all providers on the team, and a philosophy that includes parents as equal caregiving partners.

- Finally, as a parent, you need to be well read and curious about your child's illness. Most doctors today recognize that a well-informed parent is a valuable partner in rheumatic disease investigation and treatment for an individual child. The parent who is well informed can work closely with a doctor who welcomes the helpful discussion that a good parent-doctor partnership will foster.

The Specialty Care Center

Most pediatric rheumatologists practice in a specialty care center devoted to providing high-quality, comprehensive health care to children with rheumatic disease using an interdisciplinary team approach. Although different centers are structured in slightly different ways, the similarities among specialty centers are more notable than the differences.

In specialty care centers designed to treat children with rheumatic disease, the core health team generally consists of a pediatric rheumatologist, clinical nurse specialist, physical therapist, occupational therapist, social worker, and dietician. A pediatric ophthalmologist and orthopedist may also be available on site; complete support services are available for laboratory testing. (It is important to state that the child with a rheumatic disease just starting out may not need all of these facilities, but you should know that they exist and that they can be used to provide treatment and management for your child for any condition beyond what's covered in most routine testing and treatment.)

In this section we have described what goes on in an "ideal" specialty care center. We hope that the experiences of most parents and children are close to this ideal, though we must all take into account that sometimes things (and people) don't go exactly as we want them to. In that case we can overlook the problem (if it is a small one) or, if the problem is significant, we can try to bring about a change by calmly but firmly bringing the problem to the attention of someone who is in a position to do something about it.

The History of Specialty Care Centers

Childhood arthritis was not recognized as a unique entity until the late 1960s. At that time, few centers in the country offered specialized care for children with arthritis and related rheumatic diseases. During the 1970s, the Arthritis Foundation, the American Rheumatism Association (now known as the American College of Rheumatology), and a group of parents of children with arthritis collaborated to obtain funding for organized systems of care, research, and training in pediatric rheumatology. In 1980, the Maternal and Child Health (MCH) division of the U.S. Department of Health and Human Services recognized that children with rheumatic diseases were not served well by existing health systems. Within a year, MCH funded three specialty care centers in pediatric rheumatology; eleven centers had been established by 1985. All served as model programs with the mandate to provide comprehensive and coordinated care to children with rheumatic diseases. The number of specialty care centers for children with rheumatic diseases has increased steadily over the years. Presently, pediatric rheumatology centers are located in most geographic regions throughout the country.

Benefits of the Specialty Care Center

The benefits of having your child receive her health care at a specialty care center include the following:

- *High-quality care.* Specialty care centers are devoted solely to the care of children with rheumatic diseases. The professionals who staff these centers are experts in pediatric rheumatology care and research. They can provide your child with the highest quality care. They keep abreast of all new developments in pediatric rheumatology so they can offer your child the most current and scientifically proven treatments.

- *Comprehensive care.* The members of the interdisciplinary health care team work together to develop a comprehensive plan that addresses all of your child's needs, including areas that are frequently overlooked, such as school needs and parent-to-parent support.
- *Coordinated care.* The interdisciplinary team approach allows your child to have consultation from all providers and receive all needed laboratory and X-ray testing in one place on the same day. This convenience reduces the number of visits you must make to the center.
- *Communication among providers.* Because the members of the team are located all in one place, those caring for your child are better able to share their thoughts and findings with one another. Most center teams hold patient care conferences regularly. During these conferences, the status of each patient is reviewed by the team, and goals as well as problems are discussed. Finally, individual members of the health care team are better able to maintain contact with your community-based health providers. For example, the clinic-based therapist can discuss your child's case with her local therapist on a regular basis.

Specialty care centers do have a few limitations, though we believe that they are far outweighed by the benefits of this approach. Some of the drawbacks of specialty care centers are as follows:

- *Distance from home to the specialty care center.* The specialty care center may be located a significant distance from your home, resulting in significant travel time. This drawback may be outweighed by the benefits of improved quality of care and centralization of services so that your child can see all needed providers in one setting in one day. Also, the specialty care staff is experienced in consulting with your local health care providers to minimize trips to the specialty care center.
- *Waiting time.* Because your child will be seeing several providers in one day, the time spent waiting may be significant. This problem is shared by all pediatric rheumatology centers. Plan ahead to allow plenty of time for your child's visit, and bring some toys and books to keep the children occupied and snacks to deal with hunger.

Visiting the Specialty Care Center: What to Expect

At each visit to the specialty care center, your child will undergo a full evaluation followed by the development of a care plan. The components of the evaluation will vary, depending on your child's condition and the resources of the clinic. A detailed interim history will be taken, in which the parent and child can share information about significant health problems or other problems or milestones that have occurred since the last visit. This history taking will be followed by a complete general physical examination.

Each team member will evaluate your child's status, identify problem areas, and formulate a list of possible goals and interventions. The musculoskeletal examination will include a thorough assessment of joint range of motion, muscle strength, functional ability, and growth and development. Your child's performance in school and social interactions with friends and family will be carefully considered. Blood, radiologic, and other testing will be conducted as needed to determine the extent of the illness and assess tolerance of medication.

After each evaluation, the team will discuss their findings with you and your child. They will make recommendations for further care and treatment, and will work with you to develop a plan for the interval between examinations. Your concerns, needs, and expectations as parents will be fully addressed. You and your child will be encouraged to participate in the decision-making process, long-term planning, and goal setting. Attention will be focused on maximizing the child's overall functioning in her home, community, and school. Support and counseling services, job training for adolescents, and nutrition will be recommended as needed, and plans will be made to initiate referrals with community-based professionals.

Family education will usually be extensive, because it is important that you and your child understand the basic facts about the illness, medications, and rationale for treatments. The specialty care center team will work with you to ensure that an effective school program is established for your child, and will advise you about your child's educational rights and entitlements.

Following each visit, a detailed summary of the findings and recommendations will be sent to your child's primary care physician. Laboratory test results will be communicated to the parents, either by telephone or by letter.

Here are some tips to help you make the most of your visits to the specialty care center:

- *Prepare for each visit.* The team relies on your information and observations to make accurate assessments of your child's needs. Be prepared to be as specific as possible when reporting information. Know the names and dosages of the medications your child is taking (keeping a written list or log of medications is helpful). Be prepared to provide a summary of your child's status since her last clinic visit. Keep the health team aware of changes in your child's health and family life.
- *Ask questions.* Always ask for explanations if you don't fully understand, and don't hesitate to repeat questions if you don't get an answer the first time. Don't worry

about sounding stupid, and keep in mind that no question is trivial when it relates to your child. Write down any questions you have for members of the team before you come to the clinic so that you don't forget to ask them during the visit.

- *Encourage your child to participate in the visit.* If your child has questions, encourage her to ask them directly and encourage her to take part in reporting the interim history.

Care in a Teaching Hospital

The majority of specialty care pediatric rheumatology centers are at teaching hospitals. Teaching hospitals often provide the best-quality pediatric care to children and their families. They are also devoted to providing education and training to medical professionals. Students of medicine, nursing, and physical and occupational therapy rotate through these clinics to learn about children with rheumatic diseases. By allowing students to participate in your child's care, you are providing them with valuable education. Before your child sees the pediatric rheumatologist, she will often be seen by a physician who is training in the clinic. You are likely to come in contact with some of the following types of physicians who are training:

Medical students. Medical students have a college degree and are enrolled in a 4-year medical school to become medical doctors (M.D.). A medical student must have completed at least 2 years of medical school prior to coming to the hospital to learn to care for patients at the bedside and in the clinic. Most medical students spend 1 month in the specialty care center.

Pediatric residents. Pediatric residents have graduated from medical school and are licensed to practice medicine. They are participating in a 3-year training program to become general pediatricians. Residents usually spend 1 month in the pediatric rheumatology clinic.

Adult rheumatology fellows. Rheumatology fellows are internists (they care for medical problems in adults) who are participating in a special 2- to 3-year training program to become adult rheumatologists. Although their practice will deal primarily with adults, they often come to the pediatric specialty care center to obtain some experience in caring for children with rheumatic diseases.

Pediatric rheumatology fellows. Pediatric rheumatology fellows are pediatricians who are participating in a special training program to become pediatric rheumatologists.

Pediatric rheumatology training programs are 3 years long; fellows spend time taking care of patients as well as performing laboratory or clinical research in pediatric rheumatology. At the end of the training program, fellows are eligible to take the examination to become board-certified pediatric rheumatologists.

During a clinic visit, the fellow (or medical student or resident) may take a history and do a complete physical examination. You should provide this person with any information that might help him or her evaluate your child. Information about current symptoms and related past history, evaluations, and test results is particularly important. After completing the examination, the fellow, resident, or medical student will present the findings in detail to the pediatric rheumatologist. The pediatric rheumatologist will then come in to examine your child. The pediatric rheumatologist will often verify the history reported by the fellow, resident, or medical student and repeat the physical examination. The pediatric rheumatologist and fellow, resident, or medical student will discuss the findings with you and your family at length. They will work together with you to formulate a plan for diagnosis and treatment.

You have the right to refuse that your child be seen by a person who is training in a specialty care center. Your refusal to allow your child to be seen by a physician in training will have no impact on the care your child receives in the clinic or by the physicians and staff.

The Interdisciplinary Health Care Team

Caring for a child with a rheumatic illness takes teamwork; many specialists will contribute their expertise to provide the best care for your child. One of your roles as a parent is to encourage communication between the health care providers at the specialty care center and those in your local community. Make certain that they all have current information regarding your child's condition.

For the team approach to work, team members must understand each other's roles and communicate effectively with each other. Because so many health care specialists may be involved in your child's care, this section provides a "job description" for each team member who may take part in developing your child's care plan. Your child may not need to see all of these health professionals; still, it is a good idea to be aware of the resources available to you, the role of each professional, and how everyone works together as a health care team. We believe very strongly that you are the most important members of your child's health care team, and so we have included a job description for you, as well.

The Family

One role of the family is obvious: to implement the health care plan after it has been developed. You administer the medications, carry out the home therapy program, and take your child for further medical visits, lab work, and other tests. Family members are the only members of the team who can directly observe the day-to-day effects of the various treatments on the child, and the impact of the whole treatment program on the family. You will be the first to notice when your child's condition improves in response to therapy, and the first to see side effects from medication. Other members of the team rely on your observations to help them do their jobs. So, a second role for family members is to be good observers and reporters.

Your most important contribution to the team effort comes during the development of the treatment plan, however, and not after all the decisions have been made. Your suggestions, based on your intimate knowledge of your child and her situation, are essential in choosing among the various possible treatment approaches.

There is no single approach to treatment for rheumatic illness that works best for every child, and often, even after a treatment has been chosen, adjustments will have to be made. For example, perhaps it is difficult for your child to take medications in school. If you let the team members know this, they may be able to prescribe a medication that can be taken just once or twice a day, at home. Or you may find that your child does not have enough time to complete homework assignments because the home therapy program takes too much time. Maybe there is a way to combine therapy with recreational activities, or to do fewer exercises with acceptable results. Or you may have read or heard about a new or experimental therapy and wonder if it would help, so you ask the team about it. It takes input from *all* of the experts to develop the best plan to treat your child's illness. Because you, as parents, are the experts on your own child and family, your concerns and suggestions are vitally important.

The Primary Care Provider

All children, whether they have a rheumatic disease or not, should have a primary care provider. For most children this will be their pediatrician, but the primary care provider may also be a family practitioner or a nurse practitioner. The primary care provider sees the child for annual well-child visits, treats intermittent illnesses like colds, flu, and ear infections, and provides immunizations.

Your child's primary care provider will most likely be the first person who sees your child when she first develops symptoms of a rheumatic illness. He or she will direct the early diagnostic workup and may refer your child to a specialist to confirm the suspected diagnosis. Once the diagnosis of the rheumatic illness is confirmed, the primary care provider will continue to provide ongoing care for your child's rheumatic illness in your local community.

The primary care provider will work in partnership with you and the specialist to make sure that all of your child's needs are addressed. The primary care provider will assist you in caring for your child's illness in many ways, throughout your child's illness. The role of the primary care provider is as follows:

- To provide general pediatric care for your child throughout the illness, including the usual periodic well-child visits, immunizations, anticipatory guidance, care of acute medical complaints such as viral illnesses, and school or camp physicals as needed.
- To assist in providing medical care for your child's rheumatic disease by obtaining laboratory tests, monitoring your child for medication side effects, and administering medications as recommended by the pediatric rheumatologist.
- To have current knowledge of your child's condition and its treatment.
- To serve as your community liaison on the rheumatology team, and to assist you in locating the health care providers your child needs in your local community, such as a physical or occupational therapist.

Pediatric rheumatologists try very hard to keep in touch with a child's primary care provider, because they believe that the primary care provider plays a critically important role in the comprehensive care of children with rheumatic disease. The pediatrician knew the child before the pediatric rheumatologist did and will continue to follow her throughout her childhood. If the child has an infection or allergy, needs a school physical, or has a behavior problem, it is the pediatrician who is best equipped to help her.

Often, children with chronic diseases see various specialists, and this can be confusing. Your child's pediatrician is the person who will help you to sort through all the recommendations and choose the best overall plan. The pediatrician is often the one with the broadest perspective about what's best for your child and your family. Pediatricians are also familiar with the local schools and other support systems available in the community. Regular letters from the specialist keep the primary care provider informed about your child's current medications and the status of her condition, so that the primary care provider can tailor his or her recommendations appropriately.

The Pediatric Rheumatologist

The pediatric rheumatologist is a pediatrician who has completed a 3-year fellow-ship training program in caring for childhood rheumatic diseases and is eligible to take the exam to become board certified. The pediatric rheumatologist is the leader of the health care team at the specialty care center and is responsible for directing the care your child receives for her rheumatic disease. The pediatric rheumatologist will determine your child's diagnosis and will work with you and other team members to develop a care plan.

The pediatric rheumatologist evaluates your child by taking a complete history and doing a careful physical examination, and he or she may order laboratory tests or X rays to help with the diagnosis. Once the diagnosis is determined, the pediatric rheumatologist will consider the need for medication, physical and occupational therapy, and other services, and will prescribe these things as necessary. On follow-up visits to the clinic, the pediatric rheumatologist will review your child's progress and make changes in the treatment as needed.

The pediatric rheumatologist will communicate with your child's pediatrician after each clinic visit, either by letter or by phone. This keeps the pediatrician informed about the care plan, as well as any need for follow-up in his or her office. If necessary, the pediatric rheumatologist may also communicate with people at your child's school to help educate school personnel and provide suggestions for modifications to your child's school program.

Turn to your child's pediatric rheumatologist for information about the diagnosis and prognosis, as well as for answers to any general questions you may have. The pediatric rheumatologist should answer your questions about medications, such as potential side effects, and other treatment options. In general, the pediatric rheumatologist is the coordinator of the health care team, and is the person best able to field questions about any aspect of your child's illness and treatment.

In summary, the role of the pediatric rheumatologist is as follows:

- To determine the correct rheumatologic diagnosis.
- To serve as the leader of the health care team at the specialty care center and to direct your child's rheumatology care.
- To prescribe medications.
- To assess your child's functional disability and recommend appropriate therapy.
- To include the parents as equal partners in all aspects of evaluation and decision making.
- To assess psychosocial disability and recommend appropriate therapy.

- To educate the family and child about the disease and its treatments and prognosis; health care financing issues; and effects of the disease on development, peer and family relationships, sexual identity, and vocational plans.
- To communicate with the primary care provider and provide him or her with updated information regarding your child's arthritis.

The Pediatric Rheumatology Fellow

Pediatric rheumatology fellows are very important members of the clinic team. As pediatric rheumatologists-in-training, they fulfill the role of the pediatric rheumatologist while under the supervision of the pediatric rheumatologist. They also coordinate all inpatient hospital care and are integrally involved in the outpatient care of most children. The pediatric rheumatology fellow is likely to be the physician with whom you will have the most contact.

The Physical Therapist

The physical therapist is a licensed professional who assists your child with mobility. The physical therapist examines your child's neck, back, and legs for mobility and strength, as well as signs of arthritis. The physical therapist also examines your child's overall functional abilities, such as how well she walks, whether she can go up and down stairs, and whether she has difficulty moving around.

The physical therapist usually prescribes exercises or other therapy to improve your child's mobility. The physical therapist may also prescribe leg splints, special shoes, or other assistive devices. Your child may see two different physical therapists, one during visits to the specialty care center (for consultation) and another in your local community (for treatment).

The physical therapist is well prepared to answer your questions regarding sports and recreation, mobility issues (walking, running, etc.), joint contractures, deformities, exercises, and splints. The physical therapist can help you educate people in your community about your child's arthritis. It is often helpful if the physical therapist at the pediatric rheumatology center speaks with your local physical therapist or with people at your child's school (classroom teacher, gym teacher, coach) regarding mobility issues.

The Occupational Therapist

The occupational therapist is a licensed professional who assists your child to improve her hand and arm function. The occupational therapist examines your child's hands and arms for signs of arthritis, joint range of motion, and strength. The occupational therapist also examines your child's hand function in daily living skills, such as how well she writes, how well she manipulates a hairbrush, fork, or pencil, and how well she can tie her shoes. The occupational therapist also evaluates whether your child can bathe and dress independently or perform chores around the house.

By prescribing exercises, therapy, or compensatory techniques, the occupational therapist can improve your child's hand and arm function. The occupational therapist may also prescribe wrist splints or other assistive devices. Your child may see two different occupational therapists, one during visits to the specialty care clinic (for evaluation), and another in your local community (for treatment).

The occupational therapist can answer your questions about your child's handwriting, school work, daily living skills (dressing, bathing, cooking, etc.), and other skills involving the hand. The occupational therapist can help you educate the people in your community about your child's arthritis. It is often helpful if the occupational therapist speaks with your local therapist or with people at your child's school regarding her hand skills.

The Registered Nurse

The registered nurse is a licensed professional who will assist the physician in carrying out the treatment plan for your child. The nurse will teach you how to administer medications, and will explain the side effects and what to do if they occur. Every time you come to the clinic the nurse will ask you about the medications your child takes (including the dosage and frequency). The nurse will also ask about any problems that your child is experiencing. It may also be necessary for the nurse to teach you how to collect urine or stool specimens at home.

The nurse is a good resource for any questions you may have about your child's growth and development, school problems, nutrition, and more. Don't ever feel that any question is too silly or strange to ask the nurse. The nurse may not know all the answers, but he or she does know how to find them.

The Social Worker

The clinical social worker is a licensed professional who functions in two roles in the clinic: providing families with support to help them adjust emotionally to the child's illness, and assisting families with practical matters such as transportation and financing. The social worker helps the child and the family explore the many feelings and emotions that arise at the time of diagnosis and during the course of treatment. The social worker also assists the family with practical issues such as finances, health insurance, transportation, parking, and lodging. The social worker is familiar with the resources in the hospital and in the community, and can help the family approach various agencies (such as Social Security) to obtain assistance.

The social worker will assess your family's unique needs and help you to determine if your child would benefit from more in-depth counseling. If needed, the social worker will provide individual, family, and group counseling or help you locate outside mental health services. You can ask the social worker any questions you have about coping with a chronic illness, struggles between the child and her parents or siblings, finances, transportation, and similar issues.

The Dietician

The dietician assesses growth, teaches nutrition and meal planning, and prescribes special diets as needed.

The Parent Consultant

In some centers, there is a parent of a child with a rheumatic disease on staff whose role is to promote active family involvement in the health care process. This parent, often called the parent consultant, educates families concerning school issues, health insurance, billing problems, and negotiating the health care system. The parent consultant also offers support to families, helping them cope with the day-to-day problems that arise from childhood chronic illness. The parent consultant distributes relevant reading material to parents and maintains a resource library for families. The parent consultant also acts as a liaison with health care providers and serves as an advocate for children and their families, both within the hospital and in the community. In centers where there is no specific parent consultant, there may be an informal network of parents who are available for you to contact. Ask your team social worker or nurse if he or she can help arrange for you to contact another parent for support.

The Nurse's Aide

The nurse's aide works under the direction of a licensed nurse or physician. The nurse's aide will bring your child to an examination room and measure her blood pressure. The nurse's aide will also measure your child's height and weight at each clinic visit.

The Clinic Secretary

The clinic secretary at the specialty care center schedules rheumatology appointments, passes messages on to other team members, schedules appointments with other departments, and schedules appointments for tests. The clinic secretary tries to consolidate all of your child's appointments so that they all take place during a single day. It is important to inform the clinic secretary of any change in your address, phone number, or health insurance status.

The Ophthalmologist

The ophthalmologist is a physician who specializes in caring for the eyes. The ophthalmologist will check your child's eyes for problems and treat eye disease. All children with JRA need to be evaluated regularly by an ophthalmologist (every 3 months for pauciarticular JRA and every 6 months for other subtypes of JRA) because of the risk of chronic iridocyclitis (see chapter 5 for more information about the eyes).

The Orthopedic Surgeon

The orthopedic surgeon (orthopedist) is a physician who specializes in diagnosing and treating diseases of the bones and joints and who performs orthopedic surgery when it is needed. An orthopedist may be consulted because of the possibility of joint deformity or the need for reconstructive surgery or orthotics (shoe inserts).

The Dentist, Orthodontist, or Oral Surgeon

These specialists provide dental care and can help your child if arthritis in the temporomandibular joint results in a small jaw with crowding or deformation of the teeth.

The Pharmacist

Your pharmacist will fill all of your child's prescriptions at your local pharmacy. The pharmacist will answer questions about medications, including their side effects and cost.

The Psychologist or Psychiatrist

The psychologist or psychiatrist counsels you and your child and helps you deal with emotional difficulties resulting from the rheumatic disease. The psychologist or psychiatrist may also give your child specialized testing and help your child with pain control or behavior problems.

Your Child's Rights and Yours in the Doctor-Patient Relationship

Children and their parents have well-defined rights when they deal with their health care providers. Being aware of these rights is important in establishing good communication and cooperation between family members and health care professionals.

This is especially so for families of children with rheumatic illness, since, whereas the healthy child sees a pediatrician once a year for a well-child visit, the child with a rheumatic disease may see her doctor once a month or even more often, depending on the severity of the illness. In addition, the doctor visits may be lengthy, due to the number of providers involved, and the examinations can be painful. Knowing your rights can help you avoid some problems and can help you resolve others.

You and your child have the right to expect the following from a concerned health care provider:

- To be seen on time or to be given an indication of the approximate waiting time.
- To be treated respectfully, to be called by your proper names, and to have all interviewing and record taking done in privacy.
- To be talked to in language you fully understand. Some physicians routinely talk "over their patients' heads." If this happens, tell the doctor that you don't understand and ask the doctor to use simpler language. If you speak another language, you have a right to have an interpreter present. (This service is available at most large medical centers; be sure to request an interpreter when you make an appointment.)
- To have everything explained to you and your child before it happens. The doctor should explain the reason for the procedure, whether it will hurt, any possible side effects, and the expected results.
- To know the name and dosage of any medication given to your child and to know the reason for any blood, urine, or tissue specimens taken from your child. You have a right to know what tests are performed on your child and the results, when known.
- To change doctors if you feel that doing so is necessary to get the level of care your child requires. You have the right to obtain a summary of your child's record and all pertinent X rays or studies being forwarded to your new doctor at your written request. If you are leaving a doctor for a specific reason, future patients will benefit if you inform the doctor of your reason and suggest ways in which the doctor might improve his or her practice.
- To know the cost of any procedure and whether it is covered by insurance.
- To review your child's medical record.
- To request a second opinion. Any good doctor will encourage you to seek a second opinion if you so desire. The doctor providing the second opinion may give you additional information or recommendations regarding your child's care, but sometimes this person cannot offer any information that you are not already aware of. In these latter cases, the opinion is still useful, because it helps

you to feel confident in your doctor's abilities and to know that you have done everything you can to help your child.

- To be informed of any research studies to be performed, or of any students being assigned to your child's care. You have the right to have full information on what's involved in both, and you have the right to refuse either or both.
- To be given a full explanation, in terms you can understand, of any tests, evaluations, and treatments to be performed, including the consequences of refusing such treatments for your child.

The Clinic Guide

Many pediatric rheumatology clinics have written guides describing the services they offer and how to obtain access to them. If your center does not have a clinic guide, you may find it helpful to create your own directory following the instructions in chapter 6. You may wish to include the following information:

- How to contact the physicians and other members of the health care team.
- How to obtain test results and prescription refills.
- What to do in an emergency. Find out whom to call and where to go in the event of an emergency. You may want to ask your child's pediatric rheumatologist what the usual procedure is for handling emergencies at night and on weekends, so you know what to expect.
- How the clinic operates, including what the normal hours of operation are, who the members of the health care team are, and what to expect during a clinic visit.
- Where and how to obtain specialized testing such as laboratory tests, X rays, and eye exams. Be sure to find out the location as well as the hours of operation.
- What the procedures are for clinic and hospital billing. Understanding the billing procedures and fees beforehand can help you prevent problems with insurance coverage. Insurance companies sometimes require referrals, and as the parent you are responsible for obtaining such referrals.
- What the range of fees is for a clinic visit. Be aware that fees vary depending on the type of visit, and that initial evaluations are usually more expensive than follow-up care. Find out if there are additional fees for tests, special procedures, or services such as physical therapy, occupational therapy, or dietary counseling. If so, check with your insurance carrier to see if separate referrals are required for each individual provider. Find out who on the team can provide assistance with billing problems.

- What other services may be available to you, such as care coordination services, library materials, translator services, family support programs, and parking assistance.

A sample clinic guide, from the center at the Floating Hospital for Children, has been included in Appendix 1. This guide will give you an idea of the kind of information generally included in such guides, as well as the kind of information you will want to pull together if you are going to compile a guide to the center where your child receives care. Chapter 6 contains blank forms that can be useful in preparing such a guide, too. (Please note that because telephone numbers are subject to frequent change, we have not used real telephone numbers in the sample guide.)

QUESTIONS AND ANSWERS ABOUT HEALTH CARE

My daughter's rheumatologist asked if we wanted to speak with a social worker. What can the social worker do for my daughter, who has SLE?

Social workers are part of the interdisciplinary team in rheumatology and can help children and families in many different ways. They can help children and their family members deal with a range of expected feelings associated with having a newly diagnosed disease. This, of course, is a particularly stressful time for all family members. Additionally, social workers can assist in the coordination of services in the school and community and make sure that care in the hospital is meeting everyone's needs in the best way possible.

At the time of diagnosis, the social worker will meet with your family to determine any immediate concerns and will continue to be available to other family members according to their needs. Depending on the individual needs and wishes of the family, the social worker may encourage parent and family meetings, individual play sessions with children and siblings, or group meetings. Since the social worker wants to be responsive to what works best for you, you should let him or her know about any ideas or suggestions you may have.

Chapter 3

•

The Range of Available Medications

A wide variety of medications are available to treat the childhood rheumatic diseases. The primary goal in using medications for children with rheumatic disease is to reduce inflammation, although many of the drugs used to reduce inflammation also help to relieve pain. The most frequently used medications are described in this chapter. Because many of them are marketed under a number of different *brand* names, we have chosen to refer to the medications by their common chemical names (called the *generic* names). The most common brand names of the medications are provided within parentheses at the beginning of each section.

The medications used to treat the childhood rheumatic diseases are broadly classified as follows:

- Nonsteroidal anti-inflammatory drugs (NSAIDs), such as aspirin, ibuprofen, tolmetin sodium, indomethacin, and sulindac.
- Slow-acting antirheumatic drugs (SAARDs) such as sulfasalazine, injectable and oral gold, hydroxychloroquine, and d-penicillamine.
- Immunosuppressive agents such as methotrexate, cyclophosphamide, and azathioprine.
- Corticosteroids, such as prednisone.

In selecting a medication, the physician will take into account your child's specific diagnosis, the severity of his symptoms, and the course of his disease. Several medications may be used at the same time. The pediatric rheumatologist can give you copies of medication fact sheets or Arthritis Foundation brochures that provide detailed information about each medication your child is taking. Remember that your child's medications are prescribed according to his weight and disease activity; the dosage must *not* be changed without the doctor's instructions.

Nonsteroidal Anti-inflammatory Drugs

NSAIDs are effective and relatively safe in reducing the inflammation of the childhood rheumatic diseases. There are many types of NSAIDs, some of them available

TABLE 1. MEDICATIONS COMMONLY USED TO TREAT THE CHILDHOOD
RHEUMATIC DISEASES

Category	Generic Name(s)	Brand Name
Nonsteroidal anti-inflammatory drugs (NSAIDs)	Aspirin (acetylsalicylic acid)	Bayer, Bufferin, St. Joseph's, etc.
	Nonacetylated salicylic acid	Disalcid, Trilisate
	Ibuprofen	Advil, Motrin, Nuprin, Rufen
	Naproxen	Naprosyn, Aleve
	Tolmetin sodium	Tolectin
	Diclofenac	Voltaren
	Nabumetone	Relafen
	Piroxicam	Feldene
Slow-acting antirheumatic drugs (SAARDs)	Injectable gold	Myochrysine, Solganol
	Auranofin (oral gold)	Ridaura
	Hydroxychloroquine sulfate	Plaquenil
	d-Penicillamine, penicillamine	Cuprimine, Depen
	Sulfasalazine	Azulfidine
Immunosuppressives	Azathioprine	Imuran
	Cyclophosphamide	Cytoxan
	Methotrexate tablets	Rheumatrex
	Injectable methotrexate	Methotrexate sodium, Folex, Mexate
Corticosteroids	Prednisone, methylprednisolone, prednisolone	Deltasone, Orasone, Medrol, Delta-Cortef
Miscellaneous	Acetaminophen	Tylenol
	Cimetidine	Tagamet
	Ranitidine	Zantac
	Misoprostol	Cytotec

without prescription. The NSAIDs for which prescriptions are required are not necessarily more effective or "stronger" than the nonprescription NSAIDs.

Of all the NSAIDs, only aspirin, naproxen, tolmetin sodium, and ibuprofen are approved by the U.S. Food and Drug Administration (FDA) for use in children. The FDA approval process requires years of experimental studies on large numbers of patients and is difficult to accomplish in children with rare conditions. There is a large body of experience in the use of different NSAIDs in children with rheumatic diseases, however, and pediatric rheumatologists commonly prescribe unapproved

TABLE 2. NONSTEROIDAL ANTI-INFLAMMATORY DRUGS

Generic Name	Brand Name(s)	Use in Children	Prescription Status
Aspirin	Bayer, Bufferin, St. Joseph's, etc.	FDA approved	Nonprescription
Nonacetylated salicylic acid	Disalcid, Trilisate	FDA approved	Prescription required
Ibuprofen	Motrin, Advil, Nuprin, Rufen	FDA approved	Nonprescription
Naproxen	Naprosyn, Aleve	FDA approved	Nonprescription
Tolmetin sodium	Tolectin	FDA approved	Prescription required
Sulindac	Clinoril	Not approved	Prescription required
Diflunisal	Dolobid	Not approved	Prescription required
Piroxicam	Feldene	Not approved	Prescription required
Indomethacin	Indocin	Not approved	Prescription required
Diclofenac	Voltaren	Not approved	Prescription required
Nabumetone	Relafen	Not approved	Prescription required

drugs if the approved medications do not effectively control the symptoms of an individual child.

NSAIDs have both anti-inflammatory and pain-relieving effects. These medications do not cure arthritis, but they do help to control symptoms. They reduce swelling, pain, stiffness, and warmth in the joints, and they reduce fever, as well. The medications can bring about improvement within 2 weeks of starting them, but another 6 weeks of therapy may be required to see the full benefits. You can expect gradual rather than rapid improvement in your child's symptoms after he starts taking an NSAID.

Different children respond differently to the different NSAIDs. It may be necessary to try a variety of these medications, one after the other, to determine which one will be most effective in reducing inflammation for your child. Your child's doctor may prescribe more than one NSAID at a time to try to control your child's symptoms.

General Instructions for Taking NSAIDs

Each dose of an NSAID must be taken right after a snack or a meal, to help prevent stomach upset and ulcers. It need not be a large meal; a glass of milk or juice and crackers is sufficient. Your child's doctor will determine the optimal dose of medication based on your child's weight; do not give your child more than the doctor recommends. If your child takes less medication than recommended, the medication is unlikely to have any effect.

Possible Side Effects of NSAIDs

NSAIDs are relatively safe medications, but they can produce side effects, including the following:

- *Gastrointestinal effects.* NSAIDs can irritate the stomach lining, causing mild irritation (called *gastritis*) which can progress to bleeding or even an ulcer. Watch your child for signs of stomach pain, nausea, poor appetite, vomiting, or changes in the stools (dark or black bowel movements).
- *Liver effects.* Reversible liver irritation can occur. Your child's doctor will monitor for this by doing blood tests regularly.
- *Skin effects.* Rarely, children may develop allergic skin rashes, such as hives or itching.
- *Blood effects.* These medications cause the blood to clot less easily than usual. Platelets are the part of the blood that sticks together to cause clots. Blood clots are important because they stop your child from bleeding if he is injured. NSAIDs do not "thin the blood," but they do cause the platelets to be less sticky than usual. This is not dangerous and does not mean your child will bleed excessively from minor trauma; it does mean that NSAIDs should be stopped well before your child has surgery or dental work that may involve tooth extraction. Some children taking NSAIDs may bruise easily or have more nosebleeds than usual.

Aspirin

Aspirin is the least expensive NSAID and has been used for many years to treat children with rheumatic diseases such as arthritis. Aspirin is one form of a group of chemical compounds called salicylates. Some of these preparations are available over the counter and others require a doctor's prescription.

To achieve an anti-inflammatory effect, aspirin must be taken in much larger doses than the doses used to control common ailments like colds or fever. There is considerable variation among children in how well their bodies absorb aspirin. Forms of aspirin that are "coated" to protect the stomach (called *enteric coated*) generally are not reliably absorbed by children. The amount of aspirin in the blood (called the *salicylate level*) can be measured by a blood test, and your child's doctor can use the results of this test along with other clinical findings to determine the most effective dose.

In general, children should not take aspirin to alleviate the symptoms of an acute illness, because the use of aspirin by children with flu or chicken pox has been associated with a rare neurologic disorder called *Reye's syndrome*. The incidence of Reye's syndrome has been very low in children taking aspirin on a long-term basis for arthritis. Nonetheless, if your child is taking aspirin to treat his arthritis, it should be discontinued temporarily whenever your child has the symptoms of the flu (influenza) or chicken pox. Children taking aspirin should receive a flu vaccination in October of each year, as long as they continue to take aspirin. Here are two additional tips for children taking aspirin:

- Children who chew their aspirin should brush their teeth after each dose because aspirin causes tooth decay if it stays in contact with teeth for a long time.
- Consult your pharmacist before giving your child any nonprescription drugs, such as cold and cough remedies, because many over-the-counter drugs contain aspirin. Combining drugs could cause aspirin toxicity.

In some children, toxic side effects from aspirin occur even with small doses and a low salicylate level. Therefore, your child's doctor will monitor your child regularly, and you should report any of the following symptoms to the doctor:

- Ringing in the ears or temporary hearing loss
- Breathing fast, deep breathing, or sighing often
- Behavior changes, either hyperactivity or fatigue

Naproxen (Naprosyn, Aleve)

Naproxen is frequently prescribed for children with rheumatic diseases because of two important convenience features. Naproxen is available in a liquid preparation, which is useful with young children, and it only needs to be given twice a day.

Naproxen can have an unusual side effect, called *pseudoporphyria,* which involves the skin. This condition is relatively common in children taking naproxen who have fair skin, blond or reddish hair, and blue eyes, namely those children who usually burn easily in the sun. These children may develop unusual scratches or blisters, with scarring of the skin after minor injuries. The scratches or blisters take a long time to heal. A superficial scar remains once the initial scratch resolves, but the scar may fade after a few months. The most common place for these scars is in sun-exposed areas of the skin, usually the face and sometimes the hands. The combination of a particular skin type, the medication, and the sun increases the fragility of the skin, causing the superficial layer to separate from the deeper layers below. This complication may not occur immediately; it has developed in some children months or even years after the medication was started. The recommended treatment is to discontinue the naproxen. Do not discontinue the drug until your child has been looked at by his doctor to be certain that the diagnosis is correct. This complication appears to be unique to children who use naproxen.

Ibuprofen (Advil, Motrin, Nuprin, Rufen)

Ibuprofen is used increasingly to treat the symptoms brought on by common childhood problems such as fever and the flu. The dose used to treat childhood rheumatic disease is several times higher than that used to treat fever or flu. Ibuprofen appears to have an improved safety profile compared with other NSAIDs (it has a lower rate of stomach problems), but it may be somewhat less effective for arthritis. It comes in liquid and chewable forms that may be easier to administer to young children.

Indomethacin (Indocin)

Indomethacin is a potent NSAID. In addition to the same general side effects seen with all NSAIDs, headache is somewhat more common. If it occurs, the headache may resolve within a few days to a week after first starting the medication. There is a slightly increased risk of gastrointestinal complications reported with this medication.

Sulindac (Clinoril)

Sulindac is taken only twice a day. It is reported to have less kidney toxicity than the other NSAIDs, but it has never been extensively studied in children.

QUESTIONS AND ANSWERS ABOUT NSAIDs

My daughter has taken many different medications for JRA. They seem to quit working after a while. Do drugs used to treat rheumatic diseases in children become less effective after prolonged use?

There are several reasons why medications may appear to lose effectiveness. If there is a change in the underlying condition leading to a flare of the disease, then a previously effective drug may not be adequate to deal with the new situation. This would give the impression that the drug is no longer effective, but in reality it reflects the variable nature of the disease itself.

Second, sometimes drugs do change their potency. For example, aspirin, after prolonged use, may induce changes in the body's metabolism such that the drug level in the body is lowered. Thus, monitoring of blood aspirin level over time is necessary to ensure continued adequate dosage of aspirin. Other medications may also influence drug levels. For example, the use of antihistamines or phenobarbital may decrease the blood level of aspirin or similar drugs. It may be necessary for your child's doctor to adjust the dosage of the drug, again, guided by the blood drug level.

Finally, changes in general health can influence the effectiveness of drugs. A change in the digestive system, for example, can adversely affect the absorption of the drugs that are taken by mouth. Different kinds of change in health may influence the processing of the drug in the body and can lead to side effects, even though the child has had no problems taking the drug previously.

Naproxen works well in controlling my child's arthritis, but lately she has been complaining of ringing in her ears. I'm afraid if we lower the dose the arthritis will get worse. What should we do?

Many of the NSAIDs, most notably aspirin, can cause ringing in the ears when the level of the drug is peaking in the bloodstream. This problem is not necessarily indicative of too much medicine, but children who report this problem should be evaluated for other signs of drug toxicity, such as elevated liver enzymes.

If the drug is not causing other side effects, then it becomes a matter of how disturbing the ringing is. Does it interfere with proper hearing or concentration? Is it there all the time, or only 1 or 2 hours after the last dose? If the ringing occurs only after the drug is taken, then the medication could be given more frequently at a smaller dose. However, if the ringing is present all day and interferes with normal function, then another medication may need to be tried.

Slow-Acting Antirheumatic Drugs

SAARDs are a more aggressive form of drug therapy than NSAIDS, and they are used to control aggressive inflammation that does not respond adequately to NSAIDs. These agents slowly accumulate in the body, and the effects of taking them are generally not apparent for 3 to 6 months. NSAIDs are frequently given in conjunction with SAARDs. The SAARDs include sulfasalazine, injectable and oral gold, hydroxychloroquine, and d-penicillamine.

The slow-acting drugs have a potential for serious side effects, for which your child must be monitored frequently by the pediatric rheumatologist. Blood and urine tests must be done at regular intervals. Specific side effects depend on which drug is used; the liver, kidneys, eyes, bone marrow, and central nervous system can be affected. Gastrointestinal irritation, rashes, itching, mouth sores, and headaches can also occur. Despite this, most children tolerate these medications well and many have significant improvement of their rheumatic complaints.

Sulfasalazine (Azulfidine)

Sulfasalazine is a medication that combines an aspirin compound and a sulfa antibiotic. No one understands the mechanism by which this medication works in the treatment of arthritis. The aspirin preparation in this compound is poorly absorbed, so anti-inflammatory levels of aspirin are not reached in the blood. Some have speculated that the sulfa antibiotic treats an as yet unknown bacterial cause of arthritis, but there is no evidence to support this theory. Sulfasalazine has been used safely in children for the treatment of inflammatory bowel disease for many years, and recently it has been used more frequently for children who have JRA. It appears particularly effective for children with spondyloarthropathy syndromes. Children with systemic JRA have an increased incidence of severe side effects when taking this drug, so these children should be monitored closely. *Sulfasalazine should not be used if your child has a known allergy to sulfa drugs* (such as Bactrim).

Instructions for taking sulfasalazine. Sulfasalazine is usually started at a low dose of one or two pills per day. The dose is gradually increased over 1 to 2 weeks to decrease the incidence of gastrointestinal upset. It is generally taken twice a day. It can be taken with or without food, and with any other medications your child may be taking. Laboratory tests should be done soon after starting this medication and at regular intervals as prescribed by your physician.

Possible side effects of sulfasalazine. Sulfasalazine is generally well tolerated. It has less potential for long-term safety problems than some of the other long-acting medications. Rarely, dramatic allergic reactions can occur, causing liver inflammation, severe rash, and decreased blood counts. The following list includes some of the more common side effects of sulfasalazine. Contact your child's doctor if any of these symptoms, or other symptoms, occur:

- Rash
- Bruising
- Stomach upset, including nausea, diarrhea, or vomiting

Injectable Gold (Myochrysine, Solganol)

Gold injections have been used for more than 50 years as a treatment for arthritis. It is unclear exactly how gold works, but we know that it slows down the inflammatory process. It takes 10 to 15 weeks before any benefits of gold can be noticed, and improvements in symptoms can take up to 6 months to be evident. NSAIDs are usually prescribed along with gold therapy.

Instructions for taking injectable gold. Gold salts are given by intramuscular injection, usually in the buttock. The physician or nurse may want your child to rest for 20 to 30 minutes after the injection to prevent dizziness and flushing. The shots are given weekly for approximately 20 weeks, and then the dosage schedule is gradually tapered to a maintenance level of monthly injections. The injections may be temporarily or permanently discontinued if any side effects are seen.

Possible side effects of injectable gold. There are many side effects that can occur with injectable gold treatment, both mild and serious. Side effects are extremely common and are reported to occur in one-third of all children who begin the medication. The medication often needs to be discontinued because of a side effect. It is critically important that blood and urine tests be monitored before every gold injection to check for any signs of toxic reactions. This means a weekly blood test, with the results checked by the nurse or doctor before the injection is administered. These tests screen for damage to the liver or kidney, or a decrease in the numbers of blood cells or platelets. If problems are detected, they are generally reversible by discontinuing the drug. Gold may make the skin more sensitive to sunlight. A maximum-protection sun block should be worn when outdoors.

The following list includes some of the most common side effects of gold injections. If these or other symptoms occur, call your child's doctor:

- Skin rash, itching
- Mouth sores
- Metallic taste in the mouth
- Paleness, easy bruising, frequent infections
- Diarrhea

Auranofin (Ridaura)

Auranofin is an oral gold compound. It is unclear exactly how it works to treat arthritis, but it appears to control inflammation in some children. At this time, auranofin is not commonly used to treat JRA, as controlled studies have failed to show significant effectiveness. Some children, however, may benefit from this drug. Children who have responded well to injectable gold may not have the same response to treatment with oral gold. With oral gold as with the injectable form, improvements in joint pain, swelling, and stiffness may take 3 to 6 months to become apparent. NSAIDs are usually prescribed along with auranofin. This drug has not yet been approved by the FDA for use in children.

Instructions for taking auranofin. Auranofin is usually taken once a day, either morning or night. Regular blood and urine tests are necessary to determine if the gold is causing any problem; test results are usually checked weekly at the beginning of auranofin therapy and then monthly. These tests screen for damage to the liver or kidney, or decreases in the number of blood cells and platelets.

Possible side effects of auranofin. Most children tolerate auranofin extremely well. The most common side effects are listed below. If these or any other symptoms develop, call your child's doctor:

- Gastrointestinal upset, such as diarrhea
- Skin rash
- Bruising easily, bleeding gums
- Mouth sores
- Tiredness, paleness

Hydroxychloroquine Sulfate (Plaquenil)

Hydroxychloroquine is an antimalarial drug that has been used for many years to treat adult arthritis and that is sometimes used for JRA. The mechanism of action is not known. Studies of children with JRA taking Plaquenil have not shown impressive benefit, although the medication may be helpful for individual children. Hydroxychloroquine is often used to treat the rashes and joint problems of children with SLE. Improvement may be slow under hydroxychloroquine. It may take 6 weeks before any benefits are seen and another 6 weeks for the full benefits. Children who are taking hydroxychloroquine may take an NSAID as well.

Instructions for taking hydroxychloroquine. Generally hydroxychloroquine is given once or twice a day. It is usually very well tolerated by children. Taking the medication after a snack or a meal may help to prevent stomach upset, which is fairly rare. Hydroxychloroquine can make the skin more sensitive to sunlight; a maximum-protection sun block should be used when outdoors.

Possible side effects of hydroxychloroquine. Hydroxychloroquine is a safe drug with few serious side effects. The principal concern is the potential for eye problems consisting of deposits in the retina and some loss of vision. The risk of eye toxicity is very low with the doses of hydroxychloroquine used to treat arthritis and SLE. However, the child should see an ophthalmologist every 6 months while taking the medication.

The following is a list of the most common side effects caused by hydroxychloroquine. If these or any other unusual symptoms occur, call your child's doctor:

- Blurred vision, light sensitivity, blind spots
- Stomachache, nausea, vomiting
- Skin rash and itching, sun sensitivity
- Nervousness, headache, easy bruising, frequent infections

d-Penicillamine (Cuprimine, Depen)

d-Penicillamine is a drug used to control the inflammation of arthritis; it is frequently used in adults with rheumatoid arthritis but only rarely in children with JRA. Although "penicillamine" sounds like "penicillin," it is not an antibiotic. d-Penicillamine can be taken even by people who are allergic to penicillin. It may be taken for many months before there is improvement in symptoms. It is usually given in conjunction with NSAIDs.

Instructions for taking d-penicillamine. d-Penicillamine is usually taken once daily in the morning on an empty stomach, or 1 hour before meals. There may be interactions with other common medications such as iron supplements or antacids when they are taken with d-penicillamine. Ask your child's doctor if you need to give your child these medications at different times to avoid problems. Regular checkups, including blood and urine tests to detect side effects, are important while your child is taking d-penicillamine.

Possible side effects of d-penicillamine. d-Penicillamine can cause problems with gastrointestinal upset, decrease in red blood cells or white blood cells, and kidney problems. Here is a list of some side effects to watch out for. If these or other symptoms develop, call your child's doctor:

- Stomach pain, nausea, vomiting, diarrhea
- Loss of taste sensation, appetite loss, mouth sores
- Rash
- Blood in the urine
- Ringing in the ears
- Tiredness, paleness, easy bruising

My 7-year-old son has had arthritis for several years and began taking gold 4 months ago. He has always been well behaved at home and attentive at school. His behavior has recently taken a turn for the worse. His teacher says he is having trouble paying attention in class and is occasionally disruptive. He has been picking fights with his brothers and has stopped listening to us. Could this be a side effect of the medication? What should I do?

You should relax—this could be good news! Gold is not known to have side effects related directly to behavior. Slow-acting drugs, such as methotrexate or gold, take months to have a noticeable impact on a child's arthritis. The initial changes can be subtle. Swelling and joint contractures may seem unchanged, and the doctor may not see any difference when joints are examined. How do we know if the medication is working? A change in a child's attitude or behavior is often one of the first signs. Activity increases as pain subsides. Parents report less morning stiffness. Children feel better and are able to do things they were previously incapable of doing. Many children start misbehaving!

Arthritis pain saps energy, and children with significant disease are often well behaved because they don't have the energy to act out. As they start feeling better, they may begin to break rules at home or in school. Although a permanent change in behavior is undesirable, a change in attitude may indicate that the child is responding to the medicine and beginning to improve. So, if your child is starting to act out, consider it a good sign, especially if it is associated with an increase in physical activity. He may be acting like a regular kid for the first time in a long time.

Immunosuppressive Drugs

Immunosuppressive drugs such as methotrexate, cyclophosphamide, and azathio-prine work by suppressing the functioning of the immune system. Similar to SAARDs, they are very potent medications with serious potential side effects. They are used to treat active disease that does not respond to less aggressive therapy. These drugs decrease the functioning of various elements of the immune system that may be hyperactive and may lead to the inflammation present in a rheumatic disease. However, they also decrease the ability of the immune system to fight off the usual body infections with viruses and bacteria, leading to a risk of potentially serious infections. Methotrexate is less potent in its effects on the immune system than other drugs in this class; cyclophosphamide is very potent in its effects.

Methotrexate (Rheumatrex)

Methotrexate is used to treat aggressive JRA and dermatomyositis with good results in many children. Methotrexate has been used in high doses to treat childhood cancer for many years. More recently, it was found to be effective in much smaller doses ($1/100$ of the cancer-fighting dose) for the treatment of rheumatoid arthritis. Although this drug has not yet been approved by the FDA for use in treating arthritis in children, a large multi-institutional study conducted in the United States and Russia has shown methotrexate to be safe and effective in the treatment of childhood arthritis. Overall, nearly two-thirds of the children who took methotrexate in this study had a good to excellent response.

Although we do not yet completely understand its effects, methotrexate is believed to be helpful in treating children with rheumatic disease because of its effects on the immune system. Methotrexate works on cells that are proliferating rapidly, including cells that function in the immune system. Probably by decreasing the overgrowth and overactivity of the immune system's cells, methotrexate results in decreased inflammation and improvement in clinical symptoms of rheumatic illnesses.

Methotrexate does not cure arthritis or other rheumatic diseases. Since it is possible for the disease to flare severely if the methotrexate is discontinued, some children need to take this medication over a long period of time. There are now reports of safe use of methotrexate for as long as 10 and 15 years in adults. Long-term follow-up studies in children have not yet been done.

Instructions for taking methotrexate. Methotrexate is given *once a week* either by mouth (in pill form) or by injection. If oral doses have not been effective or well tolerated, switching to injections may help. If your child is receiving weekly injections, you may be able to learn to give the injection yourself, thus avoiding a weekly trip to the doctor's office. Methotrexate is extremely well tolerated, even by very young children. Some children develop mild gastrointestinal upset. These children may benefit from taking the methotrexate on Friday to avoid any disruption in their school schedule. Occasionally children will complain about the taste of the tablets.

Careful, regular follow-up with the pediatric rheumatologist is essential when your child is taking methotrexate. Blood and urine tests should be done regularly, usually once a month, to screen for side effects. Your child's doctor may ask for a chest X ray and lung function tests once a year to screen for lung complications, although these are quite rare in children. Children should avoid taking the combination antibiotic trimethoprim and sulfamethoxazole (Bactrim) while taking methotrexate. Sulfamethoxazole and methotrexate work in similar ways in the body and the use of them together may cause a drug interaction. It is also important to avoid any alcohol consumption while taking methotrexate.

Possible side effects of methotrexate. Methotrexate can cause side effects involving several body systems. These can include:

- *Mild skin rash* or increased sensitivity to the sun
- *Mouth sores*
- *Gastrointestinal upset.* This is a fairly common but usually tolerable side effect and doesn't require stopping the medication. Some children feel nausea after the medication. Less commonly, diarrhea occurs. Some children have a poor appetite the day after taking methotrexate.
- *Liver inflammation.* Mild liver inflammation can occur while taking methotrexate. Your child's doctor will monitor your child's liver functioning with blood tests, and if abnormalities are found, he or she will usually hold back a dose or two or decrease the dosage. In most cases, the liver inflammation resolves and children are able to tolerate the methotrexate again. Very rare cases of permanent liver damage have been seen in adults taking methotrexate, but this has not been reported in children.
- *Lung inflammation.* Rarely, children taking methotrexate will get an allergic-type lung inflammation. Many doctors will screen for this with lung function testing. If your child develops a persistent cough or trouble breathing, call his doctor right away.
- *Immune suppression.* Just how much methotrexate suppresses the immune system is a controversial matter. Some doctors believe that it does not suppress the immune system at all in small doses, and others believe that it may. In either case, methotrexate has less suppressive action on the immune system than other medications such as steroids, azathioprine, or cyclophosphamide.
- *Hair loss* is listed as a potential side effect of methotrexate. In the small doses we use for children with rheumatic disease, we do not find this to be a problem.

Azathioprine (Imuran)

Azathioprine is a cytotoxic drug that suppresses the immune system and leads to decreased inflammation. Like methotrexate, it has been used as a treatment for cancer in large doses. Azathioprine is rarely used to treat children with JRA but is more commonly used in childhood SLE.

Instructions for taking azathioprine. This medication is usually taken once a day, along with NSAIDs and other medicines. Careful, regular follow-up is essential to determine if the medication is causing any problems.

Possible side effects of azathioprine. Azathioprine may decrease fertility, and it has the potential to increase the risk of malignancy later in life. The benefits of taking azathioprine must be weighed against these potential side effects. If your child is taking azathioprine and develops any of the following side effects, which are rather common, or if other symptoms occur, call your child's doctor:

- Nausea, stomachache, diarrhea
- Mouth sores
- Tiredness, paleness, easy bruising
- Increased number of infections or unusual infections

Cyclophosphamide (Cytoxan)

Cyclophosphamide is a very potent immunosuppressive drug which in rheumatology is most often used to treat organ system inflammation in people with SLE. The use of cyclophosphamide in people with serious kidney disease due to SLE, for example, has greatly improved their long-term outcome, with fewer of them developing kidney failure.

Rarely, cyclophosphamide might be used in treating unremitting severe cases of arthritis or vasculitis. Cyclophosphamide is used in cancer chemotherapy, and rheumatologists use similar doses for the treatment of rheumatic conditions as oncologists use for cancer therapy. Cyclophosphamide is generally given as an intravenous infusion once a month, but it can be taken orally as well.

Possible side effects of cyclophosphamide. Most people who take cyclophosphamide will develop at least one side effect, but this does not necessarily require discontinuing the drug. The direct effect of cyclophosphamide is usually a lowered white blood cell count, because the medication is given in doses sufficient to decrease the body's ability to form blood cells. Cyclophosphamide suppresses the immune system more than many of the other medications used to treat rheumatic diseases; therefore, people taking the drug are susceptible to infection.

Nausea and gastrointestinal upset, which can occur during cyclophosphamide infusions, can be effectively treated with medication to prevent these symptoms. Hair loss can occur with monthly infusions. Cyclophosphamide can cause serious irritation to the bladder with resultant bleeding and pain; people receiving intravenous cyclophosphamide will also receive extra fluid infusions to wash the medication safely through the bladder. Additional medication may be given to protect the bladder during infusions.

The two most serious potential side effects of cyclophosphamide are the risk of future problems with fertility and the potential for developing a malignancy. These are not universal long-term side effects, however. The risk of developing a malignancy because of taking cyclophosphamide is quite low but present. The risk of future infertility may be less in young girls who take the medication than in women. You will want to carefully discuss the risks and benefits of cyclophosphamide for your child with your child's doctor before making a decision about this form of treatment.

QUESTIONS AND ANSWERS ABOUT IMMUNOSUPPRESSIVE AGENTS

My daughter takes 10 milligrams of methotrexate a week. Is she immunosuppressed? Are there any special precautions we should take?

Because of its effect on the immune system, it is generally believed that methotrexate therapy can interfere with the body's ability to fight off infection. Therefore, your child is mildly immunosuppressed while taking methotrexate. The white blood cell count is generally measured regularly in children receiving methotrexate therapy to monitor the degree of immunosuppression. If the white blood cell count drops to unacceptably low levels, methotrexate will be discontinued until the count rises.

As long as the white cell count is normal, the degree of immunosuppression is not severe, and there are few precautions that those receiving methotrexate should take. Infections such as ear infections, strep throat, or urinary tract infections should be identified and treated promptly. Fevers should be evaluated by a pediatrician to attempt to identify a cause, and the white blood cell count should be checked at that time. Many physicians recommend a yearly influenza vaccine for children taking methotrexate for arthritis. You should contact your pediatric rheumatologist for specific recommendations for your child.

For most children receiving methotrexate, severe or recurrent infection is not a problem. Although it is prudent to evaluate children receiving methotrexate more carefully than others, with monthly monitoring and careful attention to fever or other signs of infection, most children do very well. There is no reason to restrict the activity of children receiving methotrexate. School and socialization should be encouraged, and as long as children feel well, there is no reason to set limits or to worry about an increased risk of infection.

Why do some children take methotrexate orally while others get injections?

Most children start methotrexate treatment with oral tablets. There are three reasons why children may receive their methotrexate by intramuscular injections instead. First, injectable methotrexate may be absorbed better than the oral form. Although oral methotrexate is usually absorbed nearly completely, some children may have less than ideal absorption because of subtle problems with their gastrointestinal system. For these children, the injectable form of methotrexate would deliver a higher percentage of the drug than the oral form. Children on oral methotrexate who are not responding to maximal doses are often switched to injectable methotrexate before discontinuing the drug entirely.

The second reason for switching to injectable methotrexate would be to minimize drug toxicity. If children develop painful mouth sores or significant stomach upset, switching to intramuscular methotrexate may prevent those irritating, but not serious, side effects.

Last, injectable methotrexate can be cheaper than oral methotrexate. If a family's insurance does not cover the cost of methotrexate tablets, it may cover the cost of the injection as long as it is administered in the clinic or doctor's office. Also, the injectable form of methotrexate is less expensive than methotrexate tablets, when equivalent dosages are compared. Recently we've started to give younger children the injectable methotrexate liquid by mouth, mixing it with a pleasant-tasting cherry suspension. This method makes it easier for the child to swallow methotrexate and also reduces the cost. Since injecting methotrexate introduces an additional painful and invasive procedure, this treatment decision must be made after careful consideration of your child's individual medical needs.

The nurse in my pediatrician's office refuses to give my child methotrexate injections. Does this drug expose the nurse to harmful side effects?

Methotrexate is classified as an antineoplastic (cancer chemotherapy) agent because its original use was for treating cancer. The concerns of your pediatrician's nurse relate to important general concerns about the handling of any cancer drug. Chemotherapy agents, methotrexate included, are known to cause chromosomal damage in animals, to potentially have some small risk of inducing a malignancy, and to possibly have some relationship to causing fetal loss or birth defects in women taking these medications during pregnancy. It is important to remember that the methotrexate dose for JRA is $1/100$ of the usual dose for cancer, and that therefore there is a smaller dose exposure, both to your child and to the nurse administering the drug.

The question of whether a long-term, low-dose exposure to methotrexate is a significant occupational hazard has not been completely answered. The few studies that suggest a potential risk of malignancy are poor ones, involving years of regular exposure to high-dose chemotherapy by a health care professional with minimal protective precautions. However, given the potential concerns, basic precautions should be followed by health care professionals who administer injectable methotrexate. They should be careful with the vials of methotrexate, reporting any unexpected spillage or leakage, and cleaning up with care, using gloves. Gloves are adequate skin protection when drawing up methotrexate for injection and should be used at all times. It is important to properly dispose of gloves, syringes, and needles in a hazardous waste area. A special airflow hood is not necessary when drawing up methotrexate for injection, since the medication is supplied premixed. Pregnant women or breast-feeding mothers may not want to be exposed to methotrexate.

When these basic precautions are followed, administering methotrexate injections to your child should be a safe procedure.

Does the use of methotrexate have any impact on a child's future fertility?

The prognosis seems to be excellent for normal fertility in children who have taken methotrexate. The fertility of people who have taken methotrexate has been studied in cancer patients, who have taken much higher doses of methotrexate than children with JRA. The fertility rate among women who have taken methotrexate in the past is essentially the same as for women in the general population. However, women should not attempt to get pregnant while on methotrexate, as it has been associated with an increased risk of birth defects. This risk goes away completely once the individual has been off of methotrexate for several months. There is a definite decrease in sperm production among men taking high doses of methotrexate, and men may be infertile while taking the drug. These effects are completely reversible once the methotrexate is stopped.

Corticosteroids

Corticosteroids are very powerful drugs that are most often used to treat SLE and dermatomyositis. They are only used to treat JRA if a child has severe systemic symptoms, such as fluid around the heart (called *pericarditis*), high fever, or anemia, or when severe joint inflammation is likely to cause permanent damage. Corticosteroids are potent anti-inflammatory agents with serious side effects. Nearly all children taking corticosteroids will experience some of the dangerous and unpleasant side effects caused by this medication.

Corticosteroids are usually given systemically (in a way that affects all organ systems). They are usually given by mouth, in a pill called prednisone, although some children may be hospitalized to receive corticosteroids intravenously. Corticosteroids may also be given locally, such as with eye drops to control iritis or by joint injection to control individual joints with severe arthritis. Corticosteroids given locally are not absorbed into the rest of the body in large amounts and do not cause the serious side effects of systemic steroids. Nevertheless, all corticosteroids are potent medications, and their use must be carefully monitored by a physician. This section describes the uses and effects of *systemic* corticosteroids.

Chemically, prednisone is a corticosteroid drug that is similar to chemicals naturally secreted by the adrenal glands that help control the body's response to stress. With more severe stress, such as your child's illness, the body is unable to control the disease and may need a boost from outside. When additional steroids are given, the body adjusts to these higher levels and may produce less steroid itself. Steroid doses must be tapered gradually to allow the body to resume production of sufficient corticosteroids on its own. Once corticosteroid therapy has begun, it can *never* be stopped abruptly.

You will hear *prednisone* referred to as a steroid. Remember, however, that it is a *corticosteroid,* which is quite different from the anabolic steroids which some athletes use to bulk up their bodies. Anabolic steroids have received a great deal of negative press recently for their serious and detrimental side effects. Though prednisone has its own side effects, they are different from those caused by anabolic steroids.

Instructions for taking prednisone. It is important to follow the instructions for taking prednisone carefully.

- *Never stop prednisone therapy abruptly.* Because prednisone is similar to chemicals naturally secreted by the adrenal glands, treatment with prednisone fools the body into shutting off its own corticosteroid production. These chemicals are vital and necessary to regulate normal, daily body functions. Therefore, prednisone therapy *cannot* be stopped abruptly. It *always* has to be tapered to give the body a chance to begin secreting its own corticosteroids again. The speed of the taper will depend on your child's disease activity and the length of time he has been on prednisone.

- *Do not miss even a single dose of prednisone.* If your child is vomiting or cannot keep the medicine down for any reason, it is important that you notify your child's doctor. Your child may need to go to the pediatrician or local hospital to get the medicine by injection that day. Be sure to refill your prednisone prescription long before it runs out, to avoid being unexpectedly without medication. If you accidentally forget a dose, give it as soon as you remember. If you miss more than one dose, call your child's doctor immediately.

- *Some stressful situations will require that you give extra prednisone.* Your body requires extra steroid when it is severely stressed by events such as major accidents, operations, or severe infections. If any of these things occur, your child will need extra doses of prednisone. Notify your pediatric rheumatologist so that he or she can advise you and your child's pediatrician about the necessary extra prednisone dose. Even minor surgeries, such as dental extractions, may require additional steroids. Your child should have a Medic Alert badge that, in case of an accident, will tell emergency and hospital personnel that he is on prednisone.

Possible side effects from prednisone. Generally, the more common side effects of prednisone are reversible when the dose of the drug is reduced. These side effects include the following:

- *Increased susceptibility to infection.* Prednisone works by suppressing inflammation that results from an overly active immune system. Unfortunately, prednisone doesn't just quiet down this "bad" immune response, it also suppresses the "good" response that helps fight off infection. Prednisone will make your child more susceptible to infections, and they can become serious. It is *very important* that you contact a doctor any time your child has a fever of 101 degrees or greater, and if symptoms such as a cough, sore throat, vomiting, diarrhea, or headache are anything other than very mild or if they persist for more than 2 days. If you are unsure about how serious a particular symptom is, it is always better to be safe and call your pediatrician or pediatric rheumatologist.

    One infection we worry about in particular is chicken pox. *It is very important that you call your child's doctor right away if your child breaks out with or is exposed to chicken pox.* You need not worry if your child has had chicken pox in the past, because in that case he will not get it again. However, if your child has never had chicken pox, he can get a severe infection while on corticosteroids. In a person with a suppressed immune system, the chicken pox virus can spread to almost any organ in the body and become severe. When a child is exposed to chicken pox, there is an injection he can be given to help prevent a full infection from occurring. It must be given within 4 days of exposure, and it is more effective the sooner it is given. Once your child actually breaks out, there is another medicine that can be given to decrease the severity of the illness. It may be given intravenously in the hospital or taken orally at home.

- *Increased appetite.* Prednisone will almost certainly make your child very hungry. He will gain weight quickly if his diet is not carefully controlled. Most children will gain weight to some degree despite a strict and careful diet. This tendency to gain weight decreases as the prednisone dose is lowered. Because it is very hard work to lose weight, help your child minimize weight gain while on prednisone by encouraging good food choices such as fruits and vegetables. See chapter 5 for tips on low-calorie nutrition for children on steroids.
- *Increased fluid retention.* Prednisone will make your child's body retain fluid. It is important to restrict the intake of salty foods while on prednisone because this tendency will be worsened by salt in the diet.
- *Increased blood sugar.* Prednisone may increase the level of sugar in your child's blood. Usually the increase is small, but sometimes the level can rise to the same as in a child with diabetes. It is important to restrict the intake of sweets to maintain acceptable blood sugar levels. Increased blood sugars are reversible once the steroid is decreased.
- *Increased fat and cholesterol in the blood.* Prednisone will increase the level of fats and cholesterol in your child's blood. It is important for your child to avoid foods that are high in fats and cholesterol while taking prednisone. As you might know, high levels of these substances put your child at risk of heart disease later in life.
- *Suppression of growth.* Prednisone may temporarily suppress your child's growth. His growth will resume when the steroids are stopped. It is important to remember that growth ends when puberty ends. The closer your child is to the end of puberty when the steroids are stopped, the less time there will be for his growth to catch up. Your child's growth will be monitored carefully at each clinic visit.
- *Osteoporosis.* Prednisone may cause some weakening of the bones, which can make them brittle and more likely to break. This can be partially prevented by exercise and a diet rich in calcium (such as milk and other dairy products). If weakening of the bones is severe, calcium supplements will be given to your child.
- *Avascular necrosis.* Rarely, prednisone causes the blood supply to the bone to be cut off, causing parts of certain bones to die off. This most commonly occurs in the hip bones. In some cases it must be corrected surgically.
- *Muscle weakness.* Rarely, prednisone causes muscle weakness.

- *Increased blood pressure.* Prednisone can cause an increase in blood pressure. Except when it is severe, this does not cause problems, and it is reversible when the dose of prednisone is lowered. Your child will be monitored at every clinic visit. Occasionally medication will be needed to treat the high blood pressure. Increased blood pressure, when severe, can lead to increased pressure in the brain, resulting in severe headaches, or increased pressure in the eyes (called glaucoma), which can cause headaches or changes in vision. These effects are rare, but if your child develops headaches or changes in vision, you should contact a doctor as soon as possible.
- *Cataracts.* Prednisone can cause an opaque area to develop on the lens of the eye, called a *cataract.* This usually occurs only after a long period of treatment. Cataracts resulting from prednisone are different from the cataracts older people get, and they usually do not affect vision. In the rare cases in which they do affect vision, they can be corrected easily with surgery. Your child will be evaluated for these at every checkup and should see an ophthalmologist at least yearly.
- *Stomach inflammation and ulcers.* Prednisone has been said to cause stomach inflammation (gastritis) and ulcers in adults, although controversy exists as to whether prednisone is truly the cause. We rarely see this in children, but please tell your child's doctor if your child develops indigestion, heartburn, or stomach pain.
- *Thinning of the skin.* Prednisone can cause some thinning of the skin and purplish "stretch marks" over the abdomen and other areas. These will partially resolve when steroids are stopped, but they can be permanent to some degree.
- *Mood swings.* Prednisone can make your child a little hyperactive, or it may cause mood swings. Some children also have trouble sleeping when they are on high doses of prednisone. These effects tend to go away when the dose is lowered, but they can sometimes be severe.
- *Hair growth.* Some children may experience unwanted facial and body hair growth while taking prednisone. They may also get acne, which can become severe. These effects usually only occur with high doses of prednisone and are reversible when the dose is lowered. The hair growth can be treated with usual cosmetic means. Children are generally referred to a dermatologist if a bad case of acne develops.

As long as your child is on prednisone, his diet should be low in salt, sweets, and fat. We realize that it is very difficult to keep a child from the sweets and salty, fatty "junk foods" that he loves so much, but it is very important. You and your child should consult a dietician to get further guidance regarding his diet while on prednisone. Many of the metabolic effects of prednisone are preventable with dietary measures. We must warn you, however, that some of these effects may occur to some degree, especially at high prednisone doses, despite a strict diet.

Joint Injections with Corticosteroids

Injecting steroids directly into a joint with active arthritis is sometimes very effective in calming inflammation quickly and allowing improved functioning. Your child's doctor may suggest this form of therapy if your child has only one or two affected joints and there is poor response to the usual treatment with NSAIDs or difficulty in taking them. The affected joint usually responds quickly (within a few days) with a decrease in swelling, stiffness, and pain. In some cases, the arthritis will remain quiet for many months after an injection. Once the steroids have begun to work, your child will then be able to mobilize the inflamed joint to gain back any lost range of motion or muscle strength with physical therapy.

One of the benefits of giving steroids directly into the joint is that the medication will have effects locally with little absorption in the rest of the body. There is much less risk of all of the worrisome side effects of prednisone this way. Children who have had a steroid injection into a joint do not need to be on a low salt diet or worry about cataracts, diabetes, high blood pressure, weight gain, or growth suppression. *Avascular necrosis,* a condition in which the blood supply to the bone is cut off causing part of the bone to die, is a potential side effect of steroid injections. Weakening of the ligaments of the joint with eventual tearing can also occur. For these reasons, repetitive steroid injections (more than three or four injections) into the same joint are generally not recommended for children. Whenever an injection is done, there is a small risk of bleeding or infection, although your doctor will give the injection in a clean and sterile fashion.

Although a steroid injection sounds scary, it doesn't need to be a terrible experience, even for a young child. Application of a topical anesthetic cream (numbing medication) before the procedure can decrease the discomfort of the injection. Young or anxious children should receive sedation with a short-acting oral sedative; ask your doctor about this before the procedure. The procedure lasts less than 30 minutes. Your doctor may recommend rest for the injected joint for a day. After that, your child can return to normal activities.

QUESTIONS AND ANSWERS ABOUT CORTICOSTEROIDS

My child is taking prednisone and is always scraping her knees. I'm very worried about infections. What should I do?

It is impossible to keep children who take immunosuppressive medications in an environment in which they are never exposed to infection. In fact, we would rather have children be active and participate in usual childhood activities than be overprotected and isolated. Thus, all children on these medicines will scrape a knee or get a cut, and occasionally a more serious wound. When this happens, don't panic. Wash the wound thoroughly with plenty of soap and water. The wound should be kept clean and dry. Early signs of infection include increasing redness or tenderness on or around the wound, fever, or pus. At the earliest sign of infection, parents should contact their doctor so that the wound can be evaluated and properly treated.

Other Drugs

Acetaminophen (Tylenol)

Acetaminophen is the preferred medication for treating fever associated with common childhood illnesses and flu. It is also effective in relieving pain (it has analgesic properties). Acetaminophen *does not* have any appreciable anti-inflammatory effect, however, and therefore it is not used to treat the childhood rheumatic diseases. Acetaminophen is mentioned in this section only to point out that it *is not* a substitute for NSAIDs, although it may be given along with NSAIDs for a short time to control fever or relieve pain.

Medications to Protect the Stomach

Some of the medications used to treat the childhood rheumatic diseases can cause significant gastrointestinal irritation. Small areas of bleeding from the stomach, or even ulcers, are known to occur. It is recommended that children always take their NSAID with food to help prevent this problem. All stomachaches should be reported to the pediatrician and the pediatric rheumatologist. Children who have had problems with stomach irritation may need to take medication to protect the stomach. Cimetidine, ranitidine, or misoprostol are frequently prescribed. These medications have few side effects and can be taken with NSAIDs to try to prevent stomach problems.

Immunizations

Most of the routine childhood immunizations can be given to your child as usual. These include the diphtheria-pertussis-tetanus (DPT), polio, hepatitis, and *Haemophilus influenzae* type B (HIB) vaccines that children receive in the first 2 years of life, as well as tuberculosis (TB) testing. Some immunizations will need to be changed if your child is taking an immunosuppressive drug such as prednisone. Children who are taking prednisone should not be given live virus vaccines, such as measles-mumps-rubella vaccine (MMR), which is usually given at 15 months of age. A booster MMR vaccine is often recommended for children entering middle school (grade 7), and this should also be postponed if your child is taking prednisone. Current recommendations also suggest not giving the chicken pox vaccine (varicella vaccine) to children who are immunosuppressed. It is not clear whether the vaccination schedule should be modified for children taking methotrexate. Check with your pediatric rheumatologist for specific immunization recommendations.

A yearly vaccination for influenza (flu) is recommended for all children on long-term aspirin therapy and for those who are immunosuppressed, including children who take prednisone. A suppressed immune system is not as efficient at fighting infection, and children who are immunosuppressed are at increased risk for more serious illness and complications if they contract flu. Reye's syndrome, a serious but rare illness, has been associated with aspirin use during viral illness, especially flu and chicken pox. Influenza vaccine is given to all children on long-term aspirin therapy to reduce the risk of Reye's syndrome.

Getting Your Child to Take Medications without a Fight

Even adults have trouble remembering to take their medications every day, and they understand how important it is to do so. Children, on the other hand, often cannot understand why medicine is important. If the child feels well, or at least better, it may be hard for him to see the need for the medicine. Getting your child to take medicine every day can be a real chore, especially if your child puts up a fight. So what's a parent to do? Let's look at some approaches.

- *Be clear.* The first and most important step is for the adult to be absolutely clear about the need to take the medicine. Your child must know that the medication is be taken, period!

    If there is any room for negotiation or if you have any ambivalence about the need for the medicine, your child will sense it. (You may want to speak to someone on the medical team if you find that your own fears or ambivalence about your child's medicine or its potential side effects are causing you some difficulties in this area.) If you are just as clear about this as with other safety issues (for example, your child knows that he may not *ever* run out into the street or play with matches), your child will not find any emotional room to bargain with you. This does not require parents to display anger; they need only display clarity.

Parents and children often argue about daily matters such as what to wear to school, what to watch on television, and how late to stay up at night. Medication should be put in a different category from these daily battles. You can make the doctor the bad guy, which will help to ease the struggle between you and your child. Tell your child, "The doctor said you must take your medicine every day, whether or not you want to." This makes taking medication less of an issue between you and your child.

- *Establish a routine.* Taking medications must become like brushing your teeth before bed. You just always do it. Maybe it is always before breakfast, or after cereal, or as soon as you return home from school, or when *Sesame Street* is on at 3:00, or something else fairly predictable. Pick a time and stick to it every day.
- *Offer rewards for a job well done.* Mary Poppins was right; a spoonful of sugar really does help the medicine go down. Offer your child a small reward to help him get into the medication routine. A food to eat with the medicine, a program on television after taking it, a sticker on the calendar or shirt, or any positive gesture will help. Avoid offering major rewards that can't be increased or repeated, such as gifts of major toys.
- *Practice swallowing pills.* By the age of 8 or so, most children can learn to swallow pills. Many want to learn to swallow pills to avoid the unpleasant taste of liquid medications. Learning to swallow pills can be tricky. Have your child practice by swallowing a Tic-tac or an M&M with juice or water, without chewing, while you supervise. You could also try a single raisin or Cheerio, or small pieces of food cut into the size of a pill. The trick is to use plenty of liquid. Have your child drink liquid to lubricate the throat before swallowing the pill and plenty of liquid after swallowing it.

Tips for Giving Medicine to Young Children

Unfortunately, not all medicines come in liquid form, and some that do taste horribly bitter. Giving medicine to a young child can be a challenge. Be sure to talk to your child's doctor if your child consistently refuses to take medicines. Here are a few pointers that may help:

- Most pills can be crushed for young children. It may help to put the crushed pills in something with a strong taste that your child will like, such as applesauce, ice cream, yogurt, or pudding, and feed it to him with a spoon. Use only a very small amount of the "treat," only as much as will fit on one spoon. We have had good success spoon-feeding crushed medicine mixed with a small amount of chocolate syrup.

- If the liquid medication has a strong taste, try following it with a glass of strong-tasting juice that your child likes.
- Try to make medication time a calm and accepted part of the day. If you get nervous and uptight about giving your child the medication, he will sense it and become anxious before even getting it.
- Do not dissolve pills or put liquid medication into a full glass or bottle of liquid. You will never be certain whether your child is getting the full and appropriate dose of medication.
- Try tasting the medication yourself so you can understand your child's reluctance.
- Give your child choices regarding the medication to allow him some control over the process. Allow him to choose which juice or syrup will be used to mix the medication, or allow him to choose whether to take the medicine from a spoon or from a syringe.
- Never "hide" the medication in a child's favorite food or snack and give it to him without telling him.

As always, be sure to keep all medications safely locked away and out of the reach of children. Post the phone number of your nearest poison center in a convenient place, and keep syrup of ipecac on hand for use in an emergency. When measuring medications, be sure to use a measuring spoon rather than household tableware, to ensure accurate dosage.

QUESTIONS AND ANSWERS ABOUT GIVING MEDICATIONS

What should I do if my child vomits shortly after taking the medication?

Check with your child's doctor for advice regarding vomiting. We generally instruct parents to repeat the dose of medication if the vomiting occurs within 15 minutes of taking the medication. If the vomiting occurs after more than 15 minutes, wait until the next scheduled dose.

Chapter 4

•

Physical and Occupational Therapy

Physical and occupational therapy are crucial elements of the treatment plan for children with arthritis or dermatomyositis. Therapy is as important as medications, perhaps even more so! Medications reduce pain and inflammation, but medications alone will not restore lost motion in a joint or lost strength in a muscle. Strength and motion can only be regained through exercise. Physical and occupational therapy are necessary to:

- Keep joints mobile.
- Keep muscles strong.
- Regain lost motion in a joint or strength in a muscle.
- Make everyday activities like walking or writing easier.
- Improve general fitness.
- Minimize pain.

A physical therapist or an occupational therapist—or both—will work with you to evaluate your child's needs and identify problem areas that can be addressed through exercise. The therapist will devise an individualized therapy program that is based on the problems and goals identified for your child. The therapy program might include therapeutic exercises, splints, pain reduction techniques, assistive devices, or training in physical skills such as gait or activities of daily living.

It is very important for your child to exercise every day. For the most part, this physical and occupational therapy can be performed at home, with you, the parent, as the therapist. Unfortunately, most children do not like to exercise. The exercises are boring and often hurt. Performing the daily exercises requires self-discipline and patience, two characteristics that children notably lack. Don't make the mistake of allowing your child not to exercise. Children who do not exercise are at risk for developing permanent disability. This chapter will help you understand the types of exercise that are important for your child, how to do them, and where to turn for help when you need it.

Therapeutic Exercises

Therapeutic exercises are specific exercises recommended by a physician or therapist. They are usually the most important component of the physical therapy program. Therapeutic exercises are essential to maintain joint motion and muscle strength and will make it easier for your child to walk and perform activities of daily living, like opening jars and writing. A rare child with very mild disease may get enough exercise through play and other daily activities, but most children need to perform a specially designed set of exercises.

Children should plan to spend at least 20 to 30 minutes each day exercising. The exercise program can be performed at any time of day; however, it will have the most lasting effects if done at the times of day when the child is having the least amount of pain and stiffness. Exercises should be done on both "good" and "bad" days; however, you can change your child's program to be more gentle if she is having a flare. Moist heat before exercising (a shower, bath, hot pack, or paraffin) can decrease joint stiffness and relax tense muscles, making exercise easier. Deep breathing may also help relax your child during the exercises.

Finally, there are many daily activities that incorporate the elements of stretching and strengthening. Fun activities should be encouraged throughout the day to supplement, *but not replace,* a traditional exercise program. Some ideas include baking (without the use of an electric mixer), making things with play-dough, swimming, yoga, bike riding, coloring, finger painting, or badminton. Other beneficial daily activities (that may not be fun) include washing dishes, setting the table, folding clothes, and hanging clothes on a line.

Why Exercise?

Arthritis. Arthritis causes pain, stiffness, and loss of motion in every joint it affects. In the past, people with arthritis were often advised by their doctors to avoid any strenuous exercise or activity that might aggravate their disease. In recent years, however, researchers have studied the effects of exercise on arthritis and have found that a carefully planned and well-supervised exercise program can help people with arthritis stay active and move more easily, with less pain and stiffness. The purpose of physical and occupational therapy for children with arthritis is to relieve the following problems:

- *Stiffness.* Arthritis makes it hard for a joint to move freely. This feeling of stiffness is often worse upon waking up in the morning, or after any period of inactivity. For some children, stiffness lasts all day long. Your therapist will probably ask you how long the morning stiffness lasts; this is an important barometer of how active the arthritis is. Exercise can reduce the feeling of stiffness and make it easier to move.

- *Limitation of motion.* Prolonged inflammation and stiffness often cause joints to become fixed in a bent position. For example, a knee with arthritis may be unable to straighten out all the way. This limitation of motion is called a *contracture.* The therapist will measure the amount of contracture in each joint using a tool called a *goniometer.* A contracture can only be reduced through exercise and positioning. Medication alone will not restore motion to the joint.

- *Muscle weakness.* Arthritis itself does not directly affect the muscle; however, the muscles that support an arthritic joint will lose their strength and become smaller as a result of the inflammation. This wasting away of the muscle is called *atrophy.* The therapist will measure the amount of atrophy by using a tape measure and the amount of weakness by performing a manual muscle examination. Because your child has arthritis, it is important to keep her muscles as strong as possible. The stronger the muscles, the better they will be able to support and protect the arthritic joints. Strengthening can only be achieved through active exercise. Medication alone will not build up the power or size of the muscles.

- *Pain.* If your child's joints hurt, she may not feel like exercising, but unless she exercises, her joints will become even more stiff and painful. The natural response to having a painful joint is to avoid using it, by limping, favoring the limb, or holding the limb in a bent position. This exacerbates the loss of strength and motion throughout the whole extremity. It is important to break up the pain cycle by exercising.

- *Difficulty performing activities of daily living.* Pain, weakness, and loss of joint motion make it hard for a child to perform daily activities. Tasks such as walking, going up and down stairs, dressing, or writing become difficult. Addressing the symptoms through exercise will make it easier for your child to function overall.

- *Osteoporosis.* Arthritis, lack of activity, and some medications all contribute to osteoporosis, a condition in which the bones become weak and brittle. Exercise is a proven way to strengthen bones.

Before the 1980s, many doctors thought physical activities could cause arthritis flares or worsen joint damage, but recent research indicates that moderate exercise is good for both children and adults with arthritis. Studies have shown that exercise can help improve such a person's ability to perform daily routines without becoming fatigued and weak. Researchers have also found that exercise promotes self-esteem, a happier mood, increased pain tolerance, and a more active social life. In short, exercise will help your child feel better, so she can do more.

The amount and type of exercise your child will need to perform will depend on the level of her disease activity. Joints that are *acute* or *highly inflamed* are very painful, warm, and swollen, and have significant morning stiffness. The goal of the exercise during the acute period is to prevent loss of joint motion and prevent muscle atrophy. Exercise at times of acute arthritis activity consists only of gentle range of motion and isometric strengthening. *Controlled joints* were previously inflamed but are now only mildly swollen, barely uncomfortable, and have little morning stiffness. The goal of the exercise for controlled joints is to achieve normal motion and strength. Exercises can be much more vigorous, and can include both stretching and moderate resistive exercises.

Dermatomyositis. The purpose of physical and occupational therapy for children with dermatomyositis is to relieve the following problems:

- *Muscle weakness.* Muscle weakness is the hallmark sign of dermatomyositis. Childhood dermatomyositis causes weakness in muscles throughout the body. The large muscle groups, such as the neck, stomach, shoulders, and hips are often most seriously affected. The muscles will also become smaller, a condition called *atrophy.* The therapist will measure the amount of your child's strength by performing a manual muscle examination. Strength in the muscles can only be regained through active exercise. Medications alone will not build up the power or size of the muscles.
- *Loss of endurance.* Endurance is the ability to perform an activity repetitively over a period of time, like walking through a shopping mall. Dermatomyositis limits a child's endurance, causing fatigue and making it hard for her to do any activity for a prolonged period of time. Exercise helps a child to increase endurance.
- *Loss of muscle flexibility.* Dermatomyositis causes muscles to lose their flexibility and become stiff, which may limit range of motion in the joint. Loss of flexibility is most common during the acute stages of the disease, and among children with chronic dermatomyositis who have developed *calcinosis* (calcium deposits under the skin). Loss of flexibility can occur in any muscle group, but is most common in muscles that pass over two joints, like the muscles behind the knee (hamstrings) and behind the calf (heelcords or gastrocnemius). The therapist will

measure the flexibility of the muscles using an instrument called a *goniometer.* Muscle flexibility can only be regained through exercise. Medication alone will not restore motion to a joint.

- *Difficulty performing activities of daily living.* Weakness and loss of endurance make it hard for a child to perform daily activities. Tasks such as walking, going up and down stairs, dressing, or writing become difficult. Addressing these symptoms through exercise will help your child to function better in everyday life.
- *Osteoporosis.* Prednisone, the drug used to treat dermatomyositis, causes osteoporosis, a condition in which the bones become weak and brittle. Exercise is a proven way to strengthen the bones and reduce osteoporosis.
- *Weight gain.* Prednisone also causes children to gain weight. Weight gain can be a significant problem for children who have been on prednisone for some time. One of the most important components of any weight loss program is exercise. Exercise burns calories and is an important element for controlling weight among children taking prednisone. Children often feel that they do not need to exercise once the muscle strength has returned; however, it is important for children who are overweight to exercise as long as they are taking prednisone.

The kind and amount of exercise your child does will vary depending on the activity of the disease. At first, your child will be very weak. The exercises will seem very simple, but they will be hard for her! As your child's strength increases, the exercises will become more vigorous. Your child will perform more repetitions of each exercise, and eventually weights will be added to increase resistance.

For most children with dermatomyositis, the stretching and strengthening exercises can be vigorous as long as the child is comfortable. For children who have developed calcinosis, however, stretching needs to be approached with caution. Calcinosis can cause significant limitations in muscle flexibility. Forceful stretching of muscle fibers will make the calcinosis worse. Children with calcinosis need gentle stretching combined with positioning to gain flexibility; strengthening exercises can continue to be quite vigorous.

Scleroderma. The purpose of physical and occupational therapy for children with scleroderma is to relieve the following problems:

- *Limitation of motion.* Scleroderma causes areas of skin to become hardened and tough. The involved areas of skin often become stuck to the underlying connective tissues. If the scleroderma occurs over a joint, the joint will become limited in its mobility; it may become fixed in either a bent or a straight position, called a *contracture.* If the scleroderma occurs over a muscle, the muscle will lose its flexibility, which may limit range of motion in nearby joints. The therapist will measure the range of motion of the joints and the flexibility of the muscles using an instrument called a *goniometer.* It is very important for children with scleroderma to perform exercises to prevent joints or muscles from losing range of motion and flexibility. It can be very hard to regain lost motion once a contracture occurs.

- *Muscle weakness.* Scleroderma causes weakness in the muscles that underlie the areas of skin affected by the scleroderma. These muscles will become smaller, a condition called *atrophy.* If the scleroderma affects one leg and not the other, you will probably notice that the girth of the involved leg is smaller. The therapist will measure the amount of atrophy by using a tape measure and the amount of weakness by performing a manual muscle examination. The size and strength of the muscles can only be increased through active exercises. Medications alone will not build up the power or size of the muscles.
- *Arthritis.* Children with scleroderma can develop arthritis. Those who do should understand the reasons to exercise outlined previously in this chapter.
- *Difficulty performing activities of daily living.* Limitation of motion, muscle weakness, and lack of flexibility make it hard for a child to perform daily activities. Tasks such as walking, going up and down stairs, dressing, or writing become difficult. Addressing the symptoms through exercise will make it easier for your child to function overall.

Systemic lupus erythematosus. The purpose of physical and occupational therapy for children with SLE is to relieve the following problems:

- *Arthritis.* Children with SLE can develop arthritis. Those who do should understand the reasons to exercise outlined previously in this chapter.
- *Osteoporosis.* Prednisone, the drug used to treat SLE, causes osteoporosis, a condition in which the bones become weak and brittle. Exercise is a proven way to strengthen the bones and reduce osteoporosis.
- *Weight gain.* Taking prednisone causes people to gain weight. Weight gain can be a significant problem for children who have been on prednisone for some time. One of the most important components of any weight loss program is exercise. Exercise burns calories, and it is an important element for controlling weight among children taking prednisone. It is important for children who are overweight to exercise as long as they are taking prednisone.

Types of Exercises

Many different types of exercises can be performed to achieve the goals of the therapy program. These exercises may be very gentle, or they may be quite vigorous. The intensity of the therapy program will depend on the amount of inflammation your child has. Children who are having an acute flare of arthritis may worsen their condition by engaging in exercises that are too vigorous, whereas children who are recovering from dermatomyositis may need to perform an exercise program that is very vigorous. Your child should follow the exercise program that is specifically designed for her by a physical therapist.

Range-of-motion exercises. Range of motion is the amount of movement a joint has in each direction. Range-of-motion exercises involve moving a joint as far as it can go through each movement it can make. The purpose of range-of-motion exercises is to keep joints moving freely and easily. They can prevent a joint from losing motion or help to regain motion that has been lost. Range-of-motion exercises also reduce stiffness. Range-of-motion exercises are especially important for children with arthritis.

One advantage of range-of-motion exercises is that you can perform them for your child. Your child does not need to actively participate, she only needs to cooperate. Your child's physical and occupational therapists will teach you a variety of exercises designed to move each involved joint through all of its possible motions. These exercises must be done at least once, and often several times, every day. Performing some range-of-motion exercises first thing in the morning can help to relieve morning stiffness. Range-of-motion exercises to increase joint motion should be performed later in the day, when the stiffness has passed. A sample range-of-motion exercise program can be found at the end of this chapter.

Stretching exercises. Stretching refers to moving a joint or muscle through its available range of motion and then applying gentle or firm pressure to help it move farther. By applying pressure where movement is restricted, tissues are stretched and their flexibility is increased. Stretching exercises are important for children with dermatomyositis who have lost flexibility and whose muscles have become tight. They are also important for children with arthritis who have lost motion in a joint or whose joints have become fixed in a contracture. When stretching, the joint is moved just past the point of beginning pain. The child should feel pressure but not excessive pain. The stretch should always be held *steady* for 5 to 10 seconds; the muscle should never be "bounced."

Strengthening exercises. Strength, or power, is the ability of a muscle to generate force—the force needed to lift a heavy object, for example. Strengthening exercises build muscles, making them larger and more powerful. Strengthening exercises are the key component of an exercise program for children with dermatomyositis. Strengthening exercises are also important for children with arthritis, because strong muscles protect the joints and improve joint stability. Muscles must work hard to get stronger. A burning sensation often can be felt in the muscle during a strengthening exercise.

Strengthening exercises must be performed actively by the child; you *cannot* perform strengthening exercises for your child. Children under 3 are generally too young to perform specific strengthening exercises. (Tips for improving strength in young children are provided later in this chapter.) There are three categories of strengthening exercises: isometric, isotonic, and resistive:

- *Isometric exercises* strengthen the muscle without moving the joint. Isometric exercises are often prescribed for children with arthritis, because strengthening exercises that move the joint can aggravate arthritis. The benefit of isometric exercise is that the muscles get stronger, but since the joints are not moving, the joints are protected from increased stress. Isometric strengthening is done by contracting the muscle as much as possible and holding it that way for 10 seconds at a time. An example of an isometric exercise is standing with your arm against a wall and pushing against the wall with your arm, without moving your arm. Isometric exercises are often performed with elastic bands that stretch only slightly.
- *Isotonic exercises* strengthen the muscle by moving the joint. Isotonic exercises are done by actively moving the joint through its range of motion. Examples include lifting a leg or arm up and down against the pull of gravity.
- *Resistive exercises* strengthen the muscle by moving the joint against resistance. Examples include lifting weights or working with a firm putty to strengthen the fingers. Isotonic and resistive exercises are important for children with dermatomyositis to restore strength in the weakened muscles. Although they are occasionally recommended for children with arthritis, resistive exercises can be stressful to inflamed joints, so you should always consult with your child's therapist or doctor before embarking on this kind of an exercise program. Resistive exercises should not be performed during flares of arthritis.

Endurance exercises. Endurance is the ability to perform an activity repetitively over a period of time, like walking for 20 minutes, running distances, or climbing several flights of stairs. Endurance exercises improve fitness as well as endurance; they strengthen the cardiovascular system as well as the muscles. The terms *endurance exercise, aerobic exercise,* and *conditioning exercise* are often used interchangeably. Children who have arthritis or dermatomyositis may not have enough endurance to engage in much running and play activity. As a result, they may fatigue easily and become short of breath during vigorous activity.

Your child's physical therapist can suggest appropriate endurance exercises and activities to increase your child's level of fitness. Endurance activities can include a number of activities that your child will enjoy. Walking briskly, bike riding, and swimming are excellent examples. To achieve an aerobic benefit, the exercise must be performed continuously for at least 20 minutes without taking a break and repeated at least three times per week. If your child becomes tired, decrease the intensity of the exercise (that is, walk more slowly) but try to continue to do it for 20 minutes at a time. Endurance exercises are very important for children who are exercising to control their weight or reduce osteoporosis. For these children, teen fitness classes, offered at local YMCAs, can be very helpful. To prevent osteoporosis, endurance exercises must be performed in an upright position. Good activities include walking, jogging, and jumping rope. Swimming will not reduce osteoporosis.

Therapy through Play for Infants and Toddlers

Strengthening exercises can be problematic for young children. Infants and toddlers are too young to effectively participate in a formal strengthening program. At this age, general activity is often the best therapy. Encourage your child to walk and run and generally just to use her muscles and joints the way nature intended. Walking and performing activities of daily living cause the joints to move (increasing motion) and the muscles to contract (increasing strength). In many ways, this is nature's way of achieving the therapy goals.

Try to think of fun games and activities that can incorporate the therapy goals. "Simon says reach for the ceiling!" is a good example. Or set up an obstacle course that requires the child to pull a wagon from one spot to another, push big blocks out of the path, climb up and down on climbing structures, and more. Any toy or activity that involves gripping or moving against resistance (pushing, pulling apart, picking up) will increase strength when used repeatedly. Toys and activities that are especially useful for stretching and strengthening include the following:

- *For hands. Toys:* Hammering sets and other carpentry tools. Climbing equipment. Pop-beads and other interlocking toys that can be pulled apart and pushed together. Squeeze toys (such as frogs that hop when a connected bulb is squeezed). Play-dough,* modeling clay, silly putty. Templates and textured surfaces for scribbling on, paper for ripping and crumpling. Shovels and digging toys. Jars with screw-on lids. Foam toys (such as Nerf balls). Peg boards, puzzles, grip-handle squirt guns, construction kits with large nuts and bolts. *Activities:* Drawing, finger painting, coloring, making cookies (stir, knead, and roll cookie dough, and use cookie cutters, or cut cookies off the roll with a plastic knife).

*You can make your own nontoxic play-dough using this recipe:

HOME-MADE PLAY-DOUGH

1 cup white flour	*1 cup water*
1/4 cup salt	*2 teaspoons food coloring*
2 tablespoons cream of tartar	*1 tablespoon cooking oil*

Mix flour, salt, and cream of tartar in a medium-sized pan. Add water, food coloring, and oil. Cook and stir over medium heat for 3 to 5 minutes. The mixture will appear to be a glop of muck. You will be sure this is not going to work, but it will! When it forms a ball in the center of the pot, turn it out and knead on a lightly floured surface. When stored in an airtight container, this play-dough will last several months.

- *For arms.* Most of the activities listed under hand strengthening also increase arm strength. Other ideas include playing with push-and-pull toys, pushing swings, and throwing balls. Wagons and wheelbarrows can be loaded or unloaded to modify the amount of weight to be pulled. Ask the child to pull the wagon to a designated place. Increase the distance and add more weight (throw in another teddy bear) as the child's strength increases.
- *For legs.* Pedal toys (such as tricycles and Big Wheels) and ride-on toys. Kicking balls, climbing structures, climbing ladders, "pumping" on swings, marching in place, kicking in water, and games involving walking or running (like tag or red-light, green-light).
- *For feet and ankles.* Walking on heels and toes with assistance, walking in sand, jumping on a trampoline, and hopping and jumping games.

Encouraging Children to Exercise

Why do children hate to do their exercises? Because doing exercises is like doing homework. It is boring and repetitive and, even worse, it often hurts. Even adults, who fully understand the benefits of exercise, often have difficulty establishing an exercise routine. Is it any wonder that children have trouble, too? Children need help and encouragement to get through this daily chore. The following tips may help you to encourage your child.

Children of all ages. Although an exercise program is as important as medication in treating your child's arthritis, incorporating a daily program into a family's busy schedule is never easy. The following suggestions may help you in establishing an exercise routine.

- Most people prefer to exercise with someone else; maybe that's why exercise classes and health clubs are popular. We recommend that you exercise with your child. Exercising will be a lot more fun if you do it together, and the exercises will benefit you, too! Exercising with your child can be a wonderful way to make certain that your child has your undivided attention for a certain period of time each day. Use the time to talk about your child's day and the things she is interested in. For her, the benefit of your company will outweigh the pitfalls of exercising. You may develop a whole new level of understanding when you discover that the exercises really are boring and repetitive, and you don't like them either! Finally, it is important for you to be available to assist or coach your child through the program because the exercises may hurt.
- Make exercise part of your daily routine. Schedule exercises for a specific time each day, and stick to it. For school-aged children, after school is a good time to do the exercises, in conjunction with homework.
- Set a good example by exercising regularly yourself. You can demonstrate the self-discipline needed to exercise regularly by doing so yourself.
- Give your child lots of encouragement and praise your child for a job well done. Offer modest rewards, such as stickers or treats to reward her for reaching her goals.
- Treat exercises like homework. Since exercises are not optional for children with rheumatic diseases, an exercise program should be treated like homework. What limits do you set to ensure that homework is done each night? No television until the homework is complete? The same rules should apply to the exercise program.
- Give the child some control over the exercise program. Although completing the exercise program is not negotiable, there are ways to give your child a feeling of control. Let her choose the order of the exercises or pick the room in which she wants to do her exercising.

- Make the exercises a family affair when possible. Ride bikes, go for walks, and exercise as a family. This way, everyone shares an activity that can otherwise be very isolating.
- If the exercises are a big problem, ask the therapist for ideas to make the therapy more fun and less time-consuming.

Infants and preschoolers. Infants and preschoolers are too young to do the exercises themselves; they need to have their parents do the exercises for them. This puts the parent in control, and means that the exercises are more likely to be accomplished. The following tips may help you if your child fights the exercises.

- Break the exercises up over the course of the day. The short attention span of a toddler makes it impossible to do 20 to 30 minutes of exercise in one sitting. Try to do a few repetitions of each exercise at various points throughout the day. Say, for example, the therapist has instructed you to perform knee range of motion with end-range stretching, 30 repetitions, with 5-second holds for each stretch. Rather than trying to accomplish 30 repetitions in one sitting, do 5 repetitions at a time, in 6 sittings over the course of the day. Your child will not get as bored, and you will probably be able to sneak them in before your child even knows you are doing them. Diaper changes are a good time to sneak in a few exercises for infants.
- Do the exercises in the bathtub. Many young children will allow you to do the exercises during their bath time, even if they fight it at other times of the day. The water makes them feel more comfortable, making the exercises less painful. Children like to play in water and the water often distracts them from the exercises you are trying to accomplish.
- Distract her! Take her attention away from the exercises you are doing by giving her a favorite toy to play with, or try to get in a few exercises while a family member or a friend is talking.
- Sneak the exercises in while she sleeps. If your child is a very sound sleeper, you may be able to get in a few stretches at night before you go to bed. This technique only works in children under 18 months of age, as older children are likely to wake up.
- Teach your day-care provider to do the exercises. She or he can supplement the exercise you are doing during nonwork hours. Make sure that she keeps a log, so you can be sure the exercises are getting done.

School-aged children. School-aged children are too busy to exercise! The following ideas may help you schedule the exercises into a busy day.

- Provide help and support. This age group of children thrives on parent participation. Do not expect your child to be responsible enough to do the exercises
  independently and without prompting. Most children need frequent reminders
  and close supervision to do exercises correctly and routinely.
- Develop a monitoring system. A monitoring system can help you and your
  child keep track of whether the exercises were done. It will also provide your
  child with an incentive to do them. Some children need to record only whether
  the exercises were done that day. Others need to record whether each individual
  exercise was done, to illustrate that the exercise program was completed in its
  entirety. Still others need to record the amount of time they spent exercising to
  demonstrate that they did the exercises properly and did not "rush" through
  them.
- Offer modest rewards for a job well done. Some children will be satisfied with a
  hug and praise, while others want a sticker, a book, or a special privilege. Start
  with the simplest rewards, and save the more elaborate rewards for when they
  are really needed. Don't underestimate the value of simple rewards like hugs,
  praise, or personal attention. Many children crave these things more than any
  others, and they will respond best to a chance to earn such a reward. Rewards
  other than hugs, kisses, and praise should be cumulative in nature, and not
  offered on a daily basis. The child should complete the exercises 5 days in a row,
  for example, before she "earns" the reward. Have your child help in deciding
  what the rewards should be; the more she likes the reward, the more likely she
  is to comply with the exercises. Here are some suggestions of rewards for
  school-aged children:

PRAISE	"You are so wonderful for doing your exercises." "I'm so proud of you."
PERSONAL ATTENTION	Hugs and kisses A special outing, like a fishing trip A special task, like baking cookies
SPECIAL TREATS	Stickers Inexpensive books Inexpensive toys Coloring books Crayons or markers
SPECIAL PRIVILEGES	Earn an extra half-hour of television or Nintendo time Have a friend sleep over Take a trip to the library Get a cone at the ice cream store Bedtime delayed for half an hour

Work with your child to establish a system of monitoring the exercises and offering "rewards" for a job well done. The following methods of monitoring achievement work very well:

- Post a large piece of white paper on the refrigerator and title it with your child's name. Each day your child exercises, draw a big happy face on the paper, continuing across in a row. When your child gets five consecutive happy faces, give her a reward. If she resists the exercise, draw a big sad face and start a new row the next day, like this:

Jennifer's Exercises

☺ ☺ ☺ ☺ ☺   (Give reward)

☺ ☺ ☹   (Start a new row)

☺ ☺ ☺ ☺ ☺   (Give reward)

- Mount a calendar in a prominent place in your household. The calendar can be ready-made, or you and your child can make one together. Have your child help you pick out colorful stickers that she likes. Each day after she exercises, let her choose a sticker to place on the calendar. If necessary, give her a reward for each week of the calendar that has a sticker on every day.
- Make a large, colorful exercise chart with a list of each exercise in the first column. Write the days of the week in the remaining columns and have your child check off each exercise as it is done. Stickers can be used in place of checks, or she can write in the number of exercises she did and the corresponding amounts of weight she used for resistance. Here is an example of an exercise chart:

Barbara's Exercises							
Name of Exercise	M	T	W	T	F	S	S
Straight leg raise, 10 times	✓						
Knee range of motion, 10 times	✓						
Therapy putty, 10 minutes	✓						

The other children in your household may get jealous of the rewards and privileges offered to the child with a rheumatic disease. If so, give each child a list of *extra* chores and institute a similar policy for the extra chores completed. The rewards should only be offered for extra, out-of-the-ordinary chores. If you offer rewards for routine chores, the child with the rheumatic disease may feel cheated that she only gets rewards when she exercises, and not when she does her chores.

Teenagers. Teenagers are old enough to do most of the exercises themselves, without assistance from a parent. Parents should set a good example by exercising themselves and exercising together with the teen if possible. Try these techniques to improve compliance:

- Tell your child the exercises will make her look better! Teens really care about their appearance. One way to get teens to *want* to exercise is to convince them that exercising will make them look better, which it will. Exercises can make legs look straighter, can make muscles symmetric from side to side (so that the right thigh is no longer bigger than the left, for example), and can make her look "less different" from her peers. Exercises will also help the teen to perform better athletically.
- Exercise to music. Have the teen put on her favorite music when she exercises. If it helps, turn it up loud.
- Keep a log. Have the teen keep a log of the exercises she does, how often, when, and how many. This will help you stay on top of whether the exercises are being done as recommended.
- Join an exercise class. Many local YMCAs now have exercise classes designed and run strictly for teens. The exercise classes may achieve the therapy goals in an atmosphere that is more fun. Ask your child's therapist if such classes might be a useful alternative for your child.

Getting Help

Some children require outside assistance with the therapy program. You should consider getting outside assistance for your child if her contractures don't improve, if she refuses to exercise, or if your family is unable to carry out the home program effectively. In these instances, your child's doctor may suggest that your child see a physical therapist in your local community for a formal exercise program several times a week. If your child's doctor recommends local therapy, here is what you need to do:

- Obtain appropriate referrals. Your child's pediatric rheumatologist will write a prescription giving the therapist specific instructions about the type of therapy program your child should have. If your insurance is provided through a health maintenance organization, you may also need a separate referral from your child's primary care provider in order for the therapy to be covered by insurance.
- Call your health insurance carrier. Find out exactly how much insurance coverage your child has available for therapy. The number of visits may be limited, or you may be required to contribute toward the cost of the therapy. The insurer may require that you see a specific therapist with whom they have a contract.
- Locate a therapist in your community. Community-based therapists can be identified by calling the school (if the therapy is necessary for your child to benefit from school), a local hospital, a private therapy office, or a home care agency. Your child's rheumatologist will help you determine what type of therapist or agency your child should see for therapy, based on your child's needs. Most pediatric rheumatologists see children from a wide geographic area, however, and are not familiar with the resources in individual communities. Therefore, you'll probably need to call your child's pediatrician and ask whether he or she can identify qualified therapists in your area. Your choices may be limited by your health insurance policy.
- Once you identify a therapist, make an appointment for an initial evaluation. Bring the appropriate referrals with you to the first visit.

Because childhood rheumatic diseases are rare, there are not many therapists in the community who have a great deal of experience in treating them. A therapist who knows a lot about arthritis may have no experience with children. Similarly, a pediatric therapist may have little experience with arthritis. In either instance, however, it is still possible to get therapy that is of high quality. The referral from the pediatric rheumatologist will provide the therapist with specific guidelines regarding your child's care. A well-qualified therapist will then seek out additional knowledge by reading available publications and contacting your child's doctor or clinic-based therapist. As a parent, you can further promote high-quality care by taking the following steps:

- Encourage your child's therapist and her other health care providers to talk with each other. Encourage the local therapist to contact the clinic-based therapist. A phone call or a note can help provide the therapist with direction regarding your child's care. Encourage the local therapist to send progress reports to the pediatric rheumatologist at each clinic visit.

- Understand the goals and recommended treatment plan for your child's therapy. If you understand the goals of the therapy, you can check your child's progress toward the goals as a way of monitoring the effectiveness of therapy. Similarly, if you understand what should be done, you can assess the quality of the service you are receiving. Finally, once the goals are achieved, the outpatient therapy can be discontinued.
- Switch therapists when needed. There may be times when you feel you might be better off with a different therapist. If this happens, don't be afraid to make a change. If your child is no longer making progress, the therapist may be just as happy to turn her over to another therapist.

QUESTIONS AND ANSWERS ABOUT THERAPEUTIC EXERCISES

My son's therapy takes 1 hour each day. We do it every night before bedtime, the only time we have free. We never go anywhere or do anything spontaneously because "we still have therapy to do." Is it safe to skip this therapy once in a while?

Enjoying new experiences and social activities is an important part of any child's social and emotional development. Certainly this is so for a child with rheumatic disease. Provided your child does his exercises regularly, an occasional missed session will not result in long-term motion or strength losses. The benefits to his other developmental needs will more than make up for any temporary losses that may occur. Keep in mind that there are times when therapy is particularly important, depending on whether the disease is in an active or a quiet stage. Your son's therapist or doctor can help you identify these critical times and plan accordingly.

My 7-year-old daughter has arthritis in many joints. A therapist has given her exercises that she should perform daily, but she finds them boring and repetitious. She has developed an interest in ballet, and would like to take classes rather than suffer through the daily exercises. Is this appropriate?

Although ballet classes are beneficial, they cannot substitute for your child's therapeutic exercises. The classes may help develop strength, balance, and coordination, but they will not provide the specific stretching and strengthening that are necessary to maintain or improve arthritic joints. The therapy exercises will help your daughter to perform better at ballet, but the ballet is not an appropriate substitute for therapy. You may wish to ask your daughter's therapist to review the exercise program to find ways to make it more fun and less time-consuming for your daughter.

Splints, Crutches, and Other Devices

Splints

Splints are used to keep joints in a good position and to relieve pain. For some children, exercise alone is not enough to keep joints mobile. If a joint becomes fixed in a contracture, a splint may be used to gradually stretch that joint back to its normal position.

Splints are usually worn only at night, while the child is sleeping, since it is important for the child to move her joints and use her muscles during the day. These nighttime splints are called *resting* splints. Sometimes a child will also wear a daytime splint, called a *functional* splint, to make activities of daily living easier for her. Splints are custom-made for each individual child and are adjusted as the child grows or as the joint position changes.

Arm and hand splints are made of plastic and are fabricated by an occupational therapist. Wrist extension splints are commonly recommended for children whose wrist extension measures 45 degrees or less. Leg splints are made of cast material and are fabricated by an orthopedic technician. *Bivalve casts* are frequently recommended for children who have a flexion contracture of 15 degrees or more of their knees. Splints made of cast material are molded to your child's leg when wet, then split and lined when dry. This type of splint is generally inexpensive and more effective than expensive plastic and metal braces. The cast saw used to split the dry cast is very loud, and the noise often terrifies young children. It is helpful to prepare your child for the noise and bring headphones to mask the noise.

Splints need to be adjusted regularly as your child grows or as the joint changes position. All splints should be comfortable. If your child is uncomfortable wearing a splint, the splint needs to be adjusted. Inspect the skin under the splint each time the splint is removed. Any reddened areas should turn white (blanch) when pressed and should disappear completely within 20 minutes of removing the splint. Reddened areas that do not blanch or disappear in 20 minutes indicate that the splint fits poorly, is creating excess pressure, and needs to be adjusted.

Footwear and Shoe Modifications

Appropriate footwear can help a child with arthritis walk for longer distances with less pain. Shoes with rigid soles or high heels should be avoided. Desirable features include flat heels, flexible soles, a wide toe box, and plenty of cushion. Well-built athletic shoes are usually the best choice, because they have all of these features plus certain biomechanical advantages. High-top athletic shoes may provide more support to a child with ankle arthritis. Price is often (but not always) an indication of quality. Ask your physical therapist if there are specific features you should look for in shoes.

Special shoe modifications may be recommended for your child. A *shoe lift* will be recommended if one leg is longer than the other. A *metatarsal bar* can be placed on the sole of your child's shoe to decrease pain in the ball of the foot when walking. A *heel cup* can be inserted into the shoe to reduce heel pain when walking. *Orthotics* are custom-made shoe inserts that may be recommended if other approaches fail to relieve foot pain.

Crutches and Braces

Crutches and braces are usually avoided, because they promote leg weakness, loss of joint motion, and osteoporosis. It is important for a child to bear full weight on her legs and to move her legs normally when walking, in order to avoid these same problems. When a child needs to use crutches or braces, it is important for the child to use them according to the therapist's instructions. Children should learn to use the crutches to assist normal walking. One common mistake is to allow the child to "swing through" the crutches. It is important instead for her to take normal steps and not swing through with the feet together. Children who use braces or crutches must perform special exercises to keep muscles strong and joints moving. Braces, like splints, need to be adjusted as the child grows.

Wheelchairs

Children with arthritis suffer a great deal of pain. Their pain makes many activities, such as walking or running, difficult or even impossible. Wheelchairs may seem like a perfect solution. In a wheelchair, a child with arthritis is able to keep up with her friends, shop in the mall, visit museums, and do other things that may not be possible otherwise. Yet, we don't see very many children with arthritis in wheelchairs. Why not?

Children who have other disabling childhood disorders (such as spina bifida or cerebral palsy) use wheelchairs if they are not capable of keeping up with their peers. It is important for children to do all the things their friends do. If wheelchairs make this possible, then they are the best choice for the child. Unfortunately, wheelchairs are the *worst* choice for children with arthritis. For them, wheelchairs contribute to crippling and should be the last resort. The most important way to prevent disability in children with arthritis is to keep joints moving and muscles strong. When a wheelchair is used, joints develop contractures and muscles weaken, no matter what else is done to prevent this.

A child's legs are bent all day when she sits in a wheelchair. As a result, her hips and knees become more and more difficult to straighten. Eventually they become "stuck" in a bent position. Because it is impossible to walk without straightening the hips and knees as much as possible, even range-of-motion exercises can't substitute for the stretch provided by walking. Muscles are similarly affected. A person sitting in a wheelchair doesn't use her muscles at all. Even strengthening exercises can't substitute for the benefits provided by standing up and walking. Finally, weight-bearing is important for keeping bones strong. In the absence of weight-bearing, osteoporosis (a thinning of the bones) occurs. Children who use wheelchairs regularly are at greater risk of breaking bones because their bones are weakened by osteoporosis.

The loss of strength and mobility that occurs with wheelchair use is worsened as children become dependent on the chair. The more the child uses the wheelchair, the more she comes to believe that she must use it. When a child with arthritis uses a wheelchair, it doesn't hurt the child to get around anymore. Mobility becomes much easier. Because it's easier to get around, the child will want to use the wheelchair more and more. Eventually, it becomes impossible to get along without it. This puts parents in a very difficult position. Most children who receive wheelchairs are supposed to use them only occasionally—to get to school, for example. When a child becomes mentally dependent on a wheelchair, parents have to be the "bad guys" and make the child walk. Since walking hurts, this is hard for parents to do.

There will be times when a child wants to go somewhere that she cannot go without a wheelchair. Perhaps she will not be able to go to the mall with her friends if she doesn't use the wheelchair. Isn't it better that she use the wheelchair? Probably not. Even in the strictest of families, a child will become more and more dependent on the wheelchair. In time, parents will lose their perception of what the child is capable of, and will allow the child to use the wheelchair more often. Eventually, most such children end up in the wheelchair permanently. It is a lot harder to get a child out of a wheelchair than to keep her from getting into it in the first place.

Alternatives to using a wheelchair. Work with your child's health care team to maximize your child's comfort with medications and maximize function through exercise. If your child has trouble getting to and around school in the morning without a wheelchair, you might consider arranging for her to arrive late for school, or allow extra time for her to navigate between classes. If necessary, she might borrow the school's wheelchair to use only in the morning, until the morning stiffness has passed.

Children with arthritis can't do as much as other children, and this may put a damper on the activities of the entire family. A child with arthritis may not be able to walk around a museum or a mall. The entire family may have to miss out on the trip. Or, if you go anyway, the amount of walking needs to be restricted, with plenty of rests. Many places where long-distance walking is required have wheelchairs available to rent or borrow during your visit. Disney World, for example, loans wheelchairs free of charge. When a wheelchair is used just for the day, your child will not have the opportunity to develop a dependency. She may beg you for one when you get home, but it is much easier to say no to a purchase than to say no to the chair in the closet.

When your child really needs a wheelchair. For some children, using a wheelchair is inevitable. If your child needs one, you shouldn't feel as if you have failed. If a child is absolutely unable to attend school without a wheelchair, then a wheelchair is a must.

If your child needs a wheelchair, she should be evaluated by a physical therapist with special expertise in wheelchair prescriptions. The therapist will prescribe the chair that is most appropriate for your child's needs. When buying a wheelchair, consider whether your child is still growing. If she is, then the chair needs to be able to accommodate growth. For children who have stopped growing, the chair should be as small as possible to allow for maneuverability.

Children with arthritis usually use lightweight, sports model wheelchairs because these chairs are easier to propel. The wheelchair seat is often set lower than usual so that the child can use her feet in addition to her arms to propel the chair. Keep in mind that when your child is using a wheelchair, her arms substitute for her legs as a means of locomotion. Since children often have arthritis in their hands as well as their legs, propelling the chair can be difficult.

The electric wheelchair. A child's first wheelchair will be a manual wheelchair, because the child can use her arms and legs to propel the chair, it is lightweight, and it can be transported without a special van. As the wheelchair-bound child enters adolescence, it is time to consider powered mobility. An electric wheelchair should only be considered for a child who has little hope of regaining the ability to walk much of the time, who has been using a manual wheelchair for some time, and who is unable to propel the wheelchair with her arms.

The electric wheelchair allows the adolescent to move about independently, without relying on assistance from another person to propel the chair. She can move from class to class in school, and get out of the house to interact with peers, without adult supervision. The drawbacks of electric wheelchairs include the following:

- The child is able to achieve mobility without using the arms or legs in any way.
- They are expensive, usually costing $5,000 or more. Most insurance policies will subsidize a portion of the purchase price, but the parent must bear the majority of the expense.
- They require a special van to transport.
- Home modifications will be required for the child to be able to maneuver the wheelchair in the home.

Sample Range-of-Motion Exercise Program

Range of motion is the type of exercise that is most frequently prescribed for children with any type of arthritis. The following pages illustrate several range-of-motion exercises that your child can perform to maintain joint mobility.

Check with your child's doctor before having your child perform any exercises, and consult with your child's physical therapist for instructions regarding these and other exercises that your child should perform.

We suggest that children with arthritis perform range-of-motion exercises to any affected joint once a day. Each stretch should be held for 5 seconds, and each exercise should be repeated 10 times.

Neck Exercises

1. *Neck extension and flexion.* Sit up tall in a chair. Look up at the ceiling, stretching your head back as far as you can, then look down at the floor. Try not to move your shoulders, only your head.

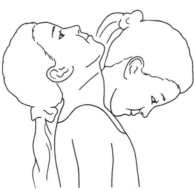

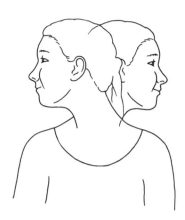

2. *Neck rotation.* Sit up tall in a chair. Turn your head and try to look over your shoulder as far as you can, then turn and look over the other shoulder. Try not to move your shoulders.

3. *Head tilts.* Try to touch your ear to your shoulder without shrugging your shoulder. Repeat on the other side.

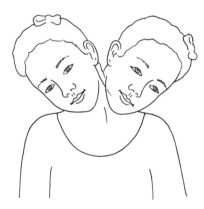

Back Exercises

1. *Knee-to-chest.* Lie on your back with your legs extended. Bend one leg up, grab your knee with your hands, and try to pull the knee into your chest. Be sure to keep the opposite leg straight.

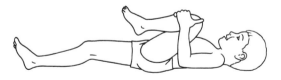

2. *Double knee-to-chest.* Lie on your back with your knees bent. Flex your legs, grab your knees with your hands, and pull both knees into your chest.

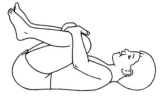

Shoulder Exercises

1. *Shoulder flexion.* Lie on your back on a firm surface. Start with your arms down at your sides. Raise your arms up and over your head until your arms cannot reach any farther.

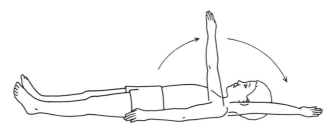

2. *Shoulder rotation.* Lie on your back on a firm surface. Place your arms straight out from the shoulder, bent at the elbow with your fingers pointing straight up. Rotate your arm forward and back, touching your hand to the ground in each direction.

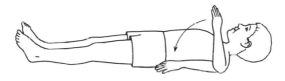

3. *Elbow wings.* Lie on your back with your hands clasped overhead. Bend your elbows, sliding your hands behind your head. Slowly lower elbows to flatten against the bed, then touch your elbows together in front of your face.

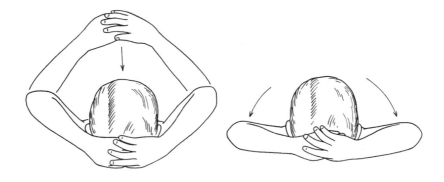

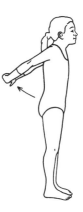

4. *Shoulder extension.* Clasp your hands behind your back. Push your hands away from your body.

5. *Shoulder abduction.* Lie on your back with your arms at your sides. Move your arms away from your body, bringing your arms out to the side and then up to your ear, like the hands on a clock.

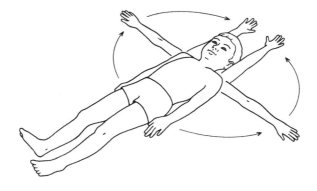

Elbow Exercises

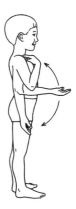

1. *Elbow flexion and extension.* Starting with your palm facing upward, bend the elbow to touch the fingers to your shoulder on that same side; then straighten.

2. *Supination and pronation.* Start with your elbow bent by your side. Turn your palm upward and then down toward the floor.

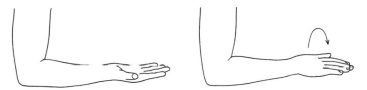

Wrist Exercises

1. *Flexion and extension.* Lift your hand at the wrist with your fingers relaxed. Then lower your hand. Using the other hand, gently push your wrist up and then down.

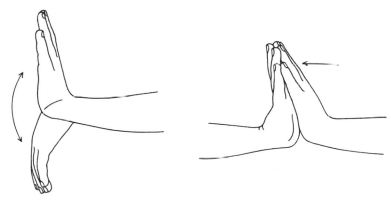

2. *Extension stretch.* Place your hand on a flat surface and raise your arm until deep wrinkles appear at your wrist.

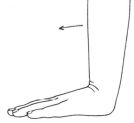

3. *Lateral deviation.* Hold your hand in a straight position and move it from side to side.

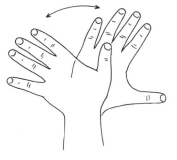

Finger Exercises

1. *Finger flexion and extension.* Bend your fingers to make a tight fist; release and straighten.

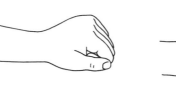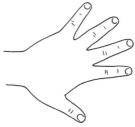

2. *Finger extension.* Place your hand flat on the table with your palm facing down. Use your other hand to push the top of your fingers to straighten them.

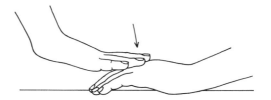

3. *Finger flexion.* Make a fist with one hand. Close your other hand over the fist and squeeze to make the fist close tighter.

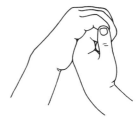

Hip Exercises

1. *Knee-to-chest.* Lie on your back with your legs straight. Flex one hip and knee, bending your knee into your chest. Grab the leg with your hands and gently pull the knee to your chest.

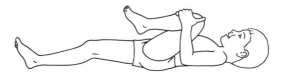

2. *Leg spread.* Lie on your back with both legs extended. Spread your legs apart as far as you can, then pull them together.

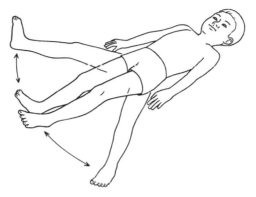

3. *Leg rolls.* Lie on your back with both legs extended. Roll your legs in and out as far as you can.

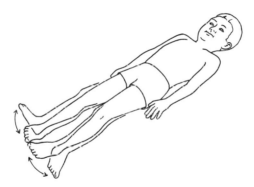

4. *Straddle stretch.* Sit on the floor with legs spread apart and knees extended. Reach out in front of you with both hands, stretching forward.

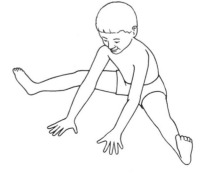

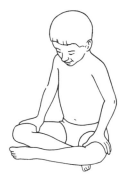

5. *Indian stretch.* Sit with legs crossed "Indian style." Place your hands on your knees and gently press them down to the floor.

Knee Exercises

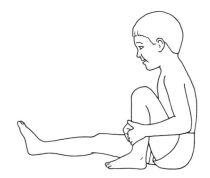

1. *Range of motion.* Lie on your back or sit, whichever is more comfortable. Bend your knee, grab your lower leg with your hands, and try to pull your heel to your buttock.

2. *End-range extension stretching.* Sit up tall with the knee extended. Place your hands with one above your kneecap and the other below. Gently but firmly press down, stretching the knee as straight as it will go. (A note to parents: If you are stretching your child's knee, place one hand above the knee as indicated. Place the second hand beneath the leg at the top of the calf. Gently press up with the bottom hand as you press down with the top hand. The stretch should be firm but not forceful. The child should feel a stretch, but not pain.)

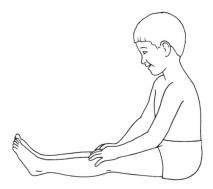

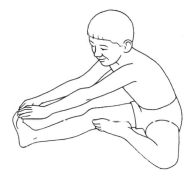

3. *Hamstring stretching.* Sit up tall with one leg straight and the opposite leg bent. Stretch toward the toes of the straight leg with both hands. Hold for 5 seconds, then relax. Be sure to keep the knee straight!

Foot and Ankle Exercises

1. *Ankle pumps.* Pump your feet up and down alternately as hard as you can. Be sure to stretch each foot as far as you can in each direction each time.

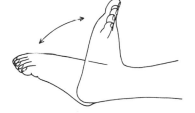

2. *Ankle circles.* With your legs extended, circle your feet around, making the largest circle you can. Try to keep your legs still and only move your feet. Repeat in each direction.

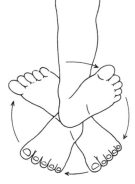

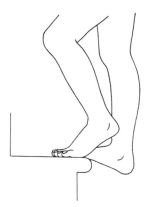

3. *Heel cord stretch.* Stand on a stair with the balls of your feet on the edge of the stair and the heels over the edge. Bend one knee slightly, keep the other knee straight. Drop the heel of the straight leg down toward the step below; you should feel a stretch behind the calf.

4. *Ankle stretch.* Sit on a flat surface with your legs extended in front of you. Have a helper press the ball of your foot up toward you until you feel a good stretch behind the calf.

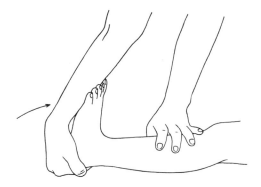

Chapter 5

•

Other Treatments for Children with Rheumatic Disease

Many children with a rheumatic disease feel better after taking medications and following a program of physical therapy. Other treatments are likely to be needed to help your child be more comfortable and to ensure that he grows and develops properly. In this chapter we discuss some of these treatments, as well as what to expect if your child is hospitalized or is scheduled for surgery. We'll also help you decide what to do about unproven remedies that may be recommended to you by friends, relatives, the media, or salespeople. In this chapter we'll describe:

- How to help your child manage the pain of arthritis
- How to care for your child's eyes
- How to make sure that your child receives adequate nutrition
- What to expect during a hospitalization or surgery
- What to make of unproven remedies

Managing Arthritis Pain

Children with arthritis learn to live with pain every day: arthritis hurts. Despite being in constant pain, children with JRA have a positive attitude, and they don't let the pain get in the way of their trying new things. Their resilience is impressive. Even so, as a parent, you want to do whatever is possible to help relieve your child's pain. This section provides practical suggestions for helping him feel better. These methods of pain relief are meant only to *supplement* medications and exercise; they cannot be used *in place o%-9f* medications and exercise.

The pain of arthritis is most often caused by inflammation in the joints. Medications are the most important therapeutic approach used to decrease both inflammation and pain. If your child continues to have significant pain on a daily basis, this may mean that he needs to have his medications changed or the doses adjusted. Contact your child's doctor for advice. You should be aware that an *increase* in pain may signal a disease flare, in which case, too, the physician needs to be contacted.

You are the best monitor of your child's pain because you are with him every day. It is very important that you keep the doctor informed about the amount of pain your child is having. The doctor will assess your child's pain at each clinic visit by asking questions about pain intensity, stiffness, and functional abilities such as:

- What joints are hurting the most? How severe is the pain? Have you noticed any change in the pain since last visit?
- How long does your child's morning stiffness last? Is he less able to function during this period of morning stiffness? For example, does he have trouble dressing or walking in the morning? Does stiffness occur at other times of the day? Have you noticed any change in stiffness since the last visit?
- Does your child's pain limit his functional abilities? For example, does pain limit how far he can walk? Have you noticed any change in your child's functional abilities since the last visit?

In addition to inflammation, arthritis pain can be caused by muscle strain, overuse of muscles, joint wear and tear, or damage to joint tissues. Exercises and splints are used to relieve these types of pain. If your child continues to have significant pain due to causes other than inflammation, he may benefit from a different regime of exercises. Be sure to give your child's therapist an accurate picture of the pattern and intensity of your child's pain; this will help the therapist devise an appropriate physical therapy plan.

In addition to giving him his medications and encouraging him in physical therapy, you can try the following techniques to improve your child's comfort throughout the day:

- Have your child take frequent *activity breaks* to prevent stiffness when doing quiet activities such as reading, watching television, or sitting at his desk in school. Have him stand, stretch, and walk around to break up the inactivity.
- Have your child take frequent *rest breaks* during prolonged activity, to prevent discomfort from overuse.
- Be sure he gets plenty of sleep. A child with arthritis may need more sleep than other children his age.

Heat and Cold Treatments

Applying heat or cold to sore joints is a good way to provide temporary relief from pain and stiffness. Most children prefer the feeling of warmth to the feeling of cold, but either one is effective. Often, applying heat or cold to stiff or painful joints before the child begins his therapeutic exercise program makes the exercises go easier. Heat and cold treatments should be applied to the sore area for 15 to 20 minutes at a time. Try the following:

- *Warm baths*
- *Hot packs or hydrocollator packs.* Make sure that the packs are not hot enough to burn the skin. If the packs feel too warm, use extra layers of toweling between the skin and the pack.
- *Paraffin baths.* Paraffin baths are hot wax treatments for small parts of the body. They are an effective way to relieve pain and stiffness for children who have arthritis in their hands. Small, portable units costing between $70 and $100 may be purchased for use at home or school. The paraffin unit melts the wax and keeps it at a safe temperature that will not burn the skin. The hand is dipped repeatedly into the wax until a thick layer is formed over the skin. The hand is then wrapped in plastic and covered with a towel for about 20 minutes. After 20 minutes, the wax is peeled from the skin and replaced in the unit for future use. The paraffin is very soft and does not stick to the skin or cause pain when it is peeled off. Children with significant hand stiffness may benefit from using a paraffin unit when they arrive at school in the morning, to decrease hand stiffness in preparation for a day of writing.
- *Ice packs.* A bag of frozen peas can be used as an ice pack. It conforms well to joints and is reusable.

Children whose pain is not relieved after local heat and cold treatments may benefit from relaxation techniques, biofeedback, or other methods of pain control. Your child's therapist can explain these techniques and teach them to you and your child.

Morning Stiffness Relief

The fluid in an inflamed joint "gels" after any period of prolonged inactivity, causing stiffness. As a result, many children experience a period of stiffness when they wake up each morning. The length of time a child is stiff in the morning can be an important barometer of disease activity. Usually, the more active the disease, the longer the period of morning stiffness. Your child may also notice stiffness after taking a long car ride, sitting at his desk in school, or sitting through a movie.

The duration of your child's morning stiffness can be shortened by applying heat and performing gentle range-of-motion exercises. To decrease morning stiffness, try these suggestions:

- Have your child sleep on a heated water bed. Many children find that this relieves morning stiffness tremendously. The benefit probably comes from a combination of the heated water and the motion of the mattress. The water bed moves all night, so the joints have less chance to get stiff. When buying a water bed, *do not* buy a motionless mattress. Water beds should not be used by children who have had total hip replacements, because these beds increase the risk that the surgically replaced hip joint will become dislocated.

• Keep your child warm at night. Have him sleep in a sleeping bag or with a down comforter. Put extra warm clothes on the joints that are the most troublesome; use leg warmers for knees, knee socks for feet and ankles, and mittens for hands.

• Have him take a hot bath or shower first thing in the morning.

• Have him perform gentle range-of-motion exercises upon waking. Some children benefit from doing these exercises in a warm bath or shower, while others prefer to do them before they get out of bed.

• Soak his hands in a paraffin bath.

• Apply a cold pack (a plastic bag filled with ice or a pack of frozen vegetables both work well).

QUESTIONS AND ANSWERS ABOUT PAIN MANAGEMENT

My daughter has arthritis, and her joints get stiff during cold winter days. Family members have suggested moving to a warmer climate such as Arizona to help my daughter feel better. Moving to Arizona would be impossible for us, but should I keep my daughter out of the cold weather during the winter?

All people experience stiff joints when they are cold, and children with arthritis are no exception. Most children with arthritis find that their joints feel stiffer in the cold and more limber in the warm weather. Cold weather, however, does not make arthritis worse and it will not result in any long-term changes in your daughter's condition.

If your daughter likes to play outdoors during the winter, you should not prevent her from doing so just because she has arthritis. Rather, try to keep her as warm as possible by dressing her in appropriate clothes. Down mittens and jackets offer the best protection from cold weather. Boots should be warm and waterproof. Have her wear wool socks inside boots or skates. Numerous layers of thin clothing offer the most warmth. You may also want to consider wool hats, snow pants, and warm tights. After being in the cold, a warm bath and range-of-motion exercises can help to reduce the stiffness.

It is fine to keep your daughter inside if she dislikes the cold and would prefer indoor activities. If she stays indoors, try to compensate for the lack of outdoor physical activity by planning appropriate indoor activities. Some children feel generally stiffer in the winter, whether or not they go outside in the cold. These children can benefit from having extra blankets on their beds at night, using a down blanket, or sleeping on a water bed. Wearing warm pajamas, leg warmers, or mittens to bed can also help reduce stiffness.

My 4-year-old recently developed arthritis, and he wants me to carry him a lot. How do I know whether he is in pain or is using the arthritis as an excuse so I'll carry him?

This is a difficult problem that most parents of young children with rheumatic disease must confront at some time or another. It is important to remember that walking is good therapy for arthritis, and that too much carrying may be detrimental. It is important for children with arthritis to walk to keep the muscles and bones strong and to keep their joints moving. Carrying a youngster for extended periods may also be unhealthy for his emotional and social development.

Most healthy young children exhibit regressive behavior (behavior that is more appropriate for a child of a younger age) when they become acutely ill with a cold, flu, or earache. This is not a problem, because they get well relatively quickly and return to their previous age-appropriate behavior. Children with chronic rheumatic diseases, however, do not get better quickly. They have pain or discomfort for extended periods of time. The regressed behavior patterns that can develop at the early stages of the disease may get reinforced and last throughout the illness. Giving in to this behavior now may promote regressive behavior throughout the illness. Finally, if you frequently carry your child you will place yourself at risk for developing a significant back injury.

Considering all of this, we recommend that you encourage your child to walk independently whenever possible, whether or not he is uncomfortable. Establish a slow pace, and take frequent rests when walking distances. Everything you do will now take longer, so it will help to allow extra time. Encourage and reward independent behavior, and teach him other ways to cope with stresses and pain. Carry your child only for short distances or in special circumstances, just as you did before he developed arthritis.

Through a consistent, concerted effort made by both parents, your child's requests to be carried can be decreased over about 4 to 8 weeks. If this does not occur, contact your pediatrician or another member of the health care team for additional recommendations. Of course, there will still be times when you are in a hurry and cannot take the extra time for a slow stroll with frequent breaks. At other times, your child may need the comfort of being in your arms. The important thing is for you to encourage your child to walk, for your child to develop independence appropriate for his age, and for both of you to learn to slow things down.

Caring for Your Child's Eyes

Children with rheumatic diseases sometimes develop problems with their eyes, either directly related to the disease itself, or as a result of drug therapy. Eye problems can become severe enough to cause permanent visual loss if they are not detected and treated early, so your child's eye care may be as important as his rheumatologic care. Some children are at risk for developing eye problems and require specialized ophthalmologic care. They are:

- Children with JRA, especially those with pauciarticular JRA
- Children taking prednisone
- Children taking hydroxychloroquine

This section will help you understand how the eyes are affected and what you need to do to protect your child's vision.

Juvenile Rheumatoid Arthritis

JRA can produce inflammation in the eyes just as it does in the joints. The eye inflammation is frequently referred to as *iritis,* although the more accurate term is *iridocyclitis.* (We will use the shorter term in this section.) Iritis is inflammation in the front portion of the eye. The cause of the inflammation is unknown, although it may be that the eyes and joints share a microscopic structure that is attacked by the immune system in certain children with JRA. Serious visual problems and, rarely, blindness can develop if iritis is not treated.

Early detection and treatment are the best way to preserve normal vision. Iritis is not easy to detect, and because it almost never causes symptoms—such as eye pain, redness, or blurred vision—until it is very far advanced, there's no way that you or your child can monitor the eyes on your own.

Because iritis seldom causes symptoms and can only be seen with specialized ophthalmologic equipment, your pediatric rheumatologist will ask that you take your child to visit an *ophthalmologist* (a physician who specializes in eye care) frequently. The diagnosis of iritis is made by the ophthalmologist using an instrument called a slit lamp. A slit lamp is a microscope with a narrow light that allows the eye doctor to detect inflammation in the eye. The slit-lamp examination is easy to perform, and even young children can cooperate. (It is best to have young children examined by a *pediatric* ophthalmologist, since he or she will have more experience getting young children to cooperate with the exam.)

Your child's first visit to the ophthalmologist will be for a complete eye examination and will include the use of eye drops to dilate the pupils. Follow-up exams usually take only a few minutes.

Who gets iritis? Not all children with JRA are at equal risk of developing iritis. Children with systemic or polyarticular JRA rarely develop iritis. Children with spondyloarthropathy can develop an acute form of iritis that is associated with eye pain and redness; these children may also suffer from recurrent conjunctivitis. Children who have both pauciarticular JRA and a positive antinuclear antibody (ANA) blood test are most likely to develop iritis; about 40 percent of these children will get iritis at some point. Iritis can develop at any time, even if it is not present when the arthritis begins. Iritis can even develop a few years after the arthritis is in remission.

Treatment. The standard treatment for iritis is steroid eye drops. Drops to dilate the pupil may be added as well, to prevent scars from forming inside the eye. It is often necessary to administer the steroid drops several times a day when the iritis is active. When the inflammation subsides, the eye doctor will slowly decrease the frequency of the drops while watching to make sure the inflammation does not flare up.

Steroid eye drops are not absorbed by the body in significant amounts; therefore, the risk of systemic complications from steroid eye drops is low. If the drops are used for long periods of time, however, cataracts (clouding of the cornea) or glaucoma (high pressure inside the eye) can develop, leading to loss of vision. The eye doctor will monitor your child for these side effects.

Course. The severity of the iritis may not correspond to the severity of the arthritis. There may be no iritis when the joints are severely affected, and there may be severe iritis when the joints are normal. Once it develops, iritis usually improves over time. Your child may have a cyclic course with flares and remissions, or he may have a single episode. In rare cases, iritis can be persistent for years and become difficult to treat. Vision is usually preserved, even in these circumstances, if good ophthalmologic care is provided.

Guidelines for follow-up care. Children at risk for iritis should be seen by an ophthalmologist four times per year for a slit-lamp examination. All children with pauciarticular JRA are considered at risk; those with a positive ANA are at highest risk. More frequent exams are required when the iritis is active. Eye examinations are usually continued for 5 years after there have been no further signs of active arthritis or iritis. These guidelines may be modified by your pediatric rheumatologist or ophthalmologist as your child's situation warrants.

Children Taking Prednisone

The side effects of prednisone may involve the eyes, so children who take steroids should be monitored for eye problems. The most common eye problem associated with prednisone use is the development of an opaque area on the lens of the eye called a *cataract*. Cataracts usually occur once a child has taken steroids for some time; however, they can occasionally form even if a child has taken steroids only briefly. The cataracts are usually very small and do not cause symptoms or interfere with vision. If they are allowed to become large (as they may with continued steroid use), they may have to be removed surgically.

Cataracts can often be detected by the pediatric rheumatologist when he or she examines your child's eyes in clinic. It is recommended that any child taking steroids have an eye examination for cataracts by an ophthalmologist twice a year, and more frequently if problems are detected. If cataracts are found, the pediatric rheumatologist may try to taper your child off steroids or consider using other medications to allow this tapering to occur.

A less common side effect of steroids is a buildup of pressure inside the eye, called *glaucoma*. If glaucoma is not detected and treated, it can damage the visual nerve and cause loss of vision. The ophthalmologist will test for glaucoma by testing the pressure in your child's eyes at each examination. If your child develops unexplained headaches or blurred vision, it's a good idea for him to have an eye examination, since these symptoms may indicate the onset of glaucoma.

Children Taking Hydroxychloroquine

The major potential side effect of hydroxychloroquine involves the eyes. As mentioned in chapter 3, hydroxychloroquine can accumulate in the retina of the eye and lead to vision loss or blindness. This complication rarely occurs today, because rheumatologists use much lower doses of hydroxychloroquine than in the past. All children being considered for hydroxychloroquine therapy should have a complete eye examination before starting treatment, and an exam every 6 months while taking the medication. The eye side effects are often reversible if the problem is detected early, when vision loss is minimal, and the medication is promptly stopped.

Nutrition

Eating a well-balanced diet is important for everyone, but it is especially important for growing children. When a child develops a rheumatic disease, proper nutrition becomes critical. This section reviews the principles of good nutrition; it will help you to understand your child's dietary needs and how to address those needs at home.

Some children with rheumatic diseases have special nutritional concerns, including:

- Children who are underweight or growing poorly. This group includes children who are small for their age, those whose gain in weight or height is less than expected, and those who are underweight for their height.
- Children who are overweight, or whose weight gain is greater than expected.
- Children taking prednisone.

You should consult your physician whenever you are concerned about the adequacy of your child's diet, his growth, or his weight (either overweight or underweight). Do not hesitate to request a referral to a registered dietician. The dietician can conduct a full nutritional assessment by reviewing your child's growth records and taking additional measurements to determine if your child is growing properly. She or he can also analyze your child's dietary intake to determine if calorie, protein, vitamin, and mineral intakes meet your child's needs.

The dietician will work with you to develop a diet plan that both meets your child's nutritional needs and takes into consideration your child's food likes and dislikes and his life-style. She or he can help you to increase or decrease calories and adjust vitamin and mineral intake as needed. A full nutritional assessment should always be done if there are not appropriate gains in height and weight.

A Guide to Good Nutrition

Like all children, your child should consume a well-balanced diet that includes a variety of foods. Meals should be planned using the U.S. Department of Agriculture's Food Guide Pyramid with serving sizes appropriate for age. The key to promoting healthy eating habits is for you to take responsibility for what your child is offered, and for your child to take responsibility for how much he eats. The following tips will foster good eating habits in your child:

- Set a good example for your child by practicing healthy eating habits yourself.

- Never fight with your child over food; you will never win the food battle. Food is one area where children can exert control, and this can be especially important to a child with a chronic illness who may feel out of control.
- Offer well-balanced meals and snacks. Use your role as the food purchaser to influence your child's food choices.
- Take your child's likes and dislikes into consideration when planning menus, but do not cater to them. Offer a variety of foods, and let your child pick and choose from what is available; don't offer substitutes.
- Serve a well-balanced family dinner every evening, if schedules allow. To keep mealtimes pleasant, use the time to share daily experiences among family members and avoid arguing or criticizing at the table.
- Insist that your child come to the dinner table and be pleasant, but do not pressure him to eat a meal. Forcing him to eat will make both of you feel bad and may result in poor food intake and poor growth.
- Take snacks seriously by planning both the food and the time.
- Unless there is a medical reason (such as a food allergy) for the child not to eat a particular food, don't forbid any food. If you forbid certain foods, your child will crave them. Moderation, rather than prohibition, is the key.
- Never use food as a reward. Don't make dessert a reward for eating dinner.

There are no known dietary supplements or dietary restrictions that have been proved to be effective in *treating* the childhood rheumatic diseases. A daily multivitamin and multimineral supplement may be appropriate for children who do not consume a well-balanced diet. Ask your doctor for recommendations before you start vitamin or mineral supplements.

Calcium. Calcium is important to keep bones and muscles strong. Children with arthritis, or those who are taking steroids, tend to develop osteoporosis (a thinning of the bones). Osteoporosis can be prevented by consuming an adequate amount of calcium and getting plenty of exercise. Infants between the ages of birth and 12 months, and youths between the ages of 9 and 17 years, have the largest calcium requirements. A well-balanced diet provides enough calcium to meet the daily requirement of most children. Many teenagers, however, especially girls, do not take in adequate calcium in their daily diet.

There are several steps you can take as a parent to make sure that your child is getting enough calcium. First, review your child's diet. He should be eating three or four servings a day of calcium-rich foods, including:

BEST SOURCES OF CALCIUM	GOOD SOURCES OF CALCIUM
Milk	Broccoli
Cheese	Dark green leafy vegetables
Yogurt	Tofu processed with calcium sulfate
Cottage cheese	Sesame seeds
Orange juice with	Almonds
added calcium	Baked beans
Other dairy products	Refried beans

If your child isn't eating enough of these foods, try these suggestions to increase his calcium intake:

- Add cheese to vegetables, casseroles, potatoes, noodles, sandwiches, and salads.
- Offer desserts made with milk, such as ice cream, custards, and pudding.
- Add nonfat dried milk powder to mashed potatoes, casseroles, hot cereals, ground meat, and sauces.

If your child has difficulty with the recommended diet, talk with your child's physician about calcium supplements. Calcium supplements may be recommended for children whose calcium intake is insufficient or for children who are taking steroids.

Remember, the combination of proper diet and exercise is important for everyone.

Iron. Children with rheumatic disease often have a low red blood cell count, called *anemia.* Children with mild or even moderate anemia may adjust to it and have no symptoms. Some children with anemia, however, experience excessive fatigue, difficulty concentrating, and trouble with exercise endurance. Severe anemia can result in serious medical complications, such as heart failure. Mild anemia is a common problem in healthy children as well, and is usually due to iron deficiency. In children with rheumatic disease, the anemia is generally related to their illness, but iron deficiency can contribute to it. Therefore, although iron-rich foods or supplements cannot completely reverse anemia in children with rheumatic disease, an adequate intake of iron *is* recommended.

Find out from your doctor whether your child is anemic. If he is, try to increase the amount of iron-rich foods in his diet for a few months. Iron-rich food sources include meat, beans (baked or refried), iron-fortified cereals, nuts, peanut butter, eggs, and dark green leafy vegetables. If diet alone does not improve the anemia, iron supplements may be needed.

Snack facts and traps. Everyone snacks, and there is nothing wrong with snacking. For children, snacks are especially important, because their stomachs are small and they usually can't eat enough in three meals to meet their energy needs or satisfy their appetites all day. Within about 3 hours after a meal, children are usually hungry. Snack time is a good time to get in nutrients they are missing from the rest of the day. Preschoolers and teens rely on snacks more for their daily nutrient intake than do people at any other age.

- *Schedule snack time.* Contrary to popular belief, snack time is not all the time. Don't let your child have unlimited access to snacks all day long. What seems to work best is to schedule a snack sometime midway between meals; this satisfies children's hunger but prevents them from filling up on snacks and losing interest in regular meals.
- *Promote good snacks.* Good snacks are those that help provide children with essential nutrients they may be missing the rest of the day. They are also substantial enough to ward off hunger until the next meal. A small glass of juice or a piece of fruit can help tide your child over when you are getting dinner ready or are on the way home from day care. A heavier snack, one containing protein, carbohydrate, and fat (such as a small sandwich of turkey, lettuce, and tomato), might be in order when your child will be waiting several hours for his next meal. Fresh fruits and vegetables and unsalted popcorn are good snack choices.
- *Avoid snack traps!* Snack traps are the foods that provide too many calories without supplying their share of nutrients. These include chips, candy, cookies, snack cakes, and soft drinks, as well as any foods that are highly processed, rich in fat, sugar, or salt, and lacking in dietary fiber. Children who are allowed to fall into "snack traps" may become overweight and have poor intake of vitamins and minerals.

    Snack traps supply lots of calories but not enough of the vitamins and minerals needed for growth. For example, both a soft drink and a glass of orange juice provide about the same number of calories, 160 per cup. But choose the juice and you'll get a full day's supply of vitamin C as well as other important vitamins and minerals. Choose the soft drink and all you'll get are the calories, along with sugar, flavorings, colorings, and possibly caffeine. Too often, these empty calorie foods fill children up so that they are no longer hungry for more nutritious foods. That's why "treats" should stay "treats" and be served only once in a while.

Children Who Are Underweight or Who Are Growing Poorly

Many children with rheumatic illnesses are underweight and grow poorly. Children do not eat well when they feel sick or are in pain. Further, some medications may cause them to lose their appetite. Both fever and chronic inflammation *increase* a child's energy needs, so the combination of poor intake along with increased caloric needs means that some children may not consume enough calories to promote normal growth.

You can monitor your child's growth by plotting his height and weight on a growth chart (see chapter 7). If you notice changes in your child's eating habits, or worry that he is not growing properly, there are some steps you can take. For example, you can keep a food diary for a few days. Record everything your child eats or drinks as well as the quantity of food he eats and the time he eats. You may find that your child is eating more than you thought. If you have questions about whether your child's diet is adequate, you can request a consultation with a dietician who can compare your child's calorie and nutrient requirements with his intake. If your child is taking in too few calories, try these ways of adding calories to his diet:

- Add cheese, gravy, and sauces to meat, potatoes, and other foods.
- Add butter or margarine (they both have the same number of calories) to vegetables, bread, potatoes, rice, casseroles, cooked cereals, and sandwiches. Use butter or margarine instead of lower-fat substitutes.
- Substitute whole milk for water in recipes for soups, cereals, instant cocoa, and puddings.
- Add cheese to vegetables, soups, casseroles, and salads.
- Make fortified milk by adding dry skim milk powder to whole milk.
- Offer high-calorie, nutrient-dense snacks, such as nuts, sunflower seeds, dried fruit, granola bars, peanut butter crackers, or crackers and cheese.
- Make high-calorie milkshakes and fruit drinks.
- Use less water than recommended when reconstituting frozen juices.
- Avoid low-fat or sugar-free foods. Be sure everything that your child eats has calories. Avoid fad diets and other food trends that may be harmful.

To help create an atmosphere in which your child will eat healthfully and well, avoid making eating an issue. Do not force your child to eat if he is not hungry, even if the clock says that it's dinner time. Also, buy foods your child likes. Before going grocery shopping, ask him if there is some special food or snack he'd like. At school, make sure your child has enough time to eat and that he has assistance during meals at school if he needs it. A midmorning snack, even at school, may help improve daily intake of calories.

Finally, review your child's growth with his doctor to determine if he is growing as expected. The doctor may be able to provide you with additional guidelines to supplement your child's diet, or he may refer you to a registered dietician for further counseling.

Children Who Are Overweight

Extra weight puts stress on the joints, heart, and lungs. Children who become overweight during childhood have a high risk of being overweight as adults. The most common reason for children with rheumatic disease to be overweight is that they are on steroid therapy (covered in greater detail in the next section). But children with rheumatic disease should not become overweight, because extra weight puts extra stress on joints.

If your child has already gained too much weight, it is important to prevent further weight gain and try to help him lose weight. Weight loss is not an easy matter for anyone, and there are no magic tricks. There are golden rules of weight loss, however, and here they are:

- Limit fat intake.
- Consume low-calorie foods.
- Limit the quantity of foods eaten.
- Get plenty of exercise.

It is especially important to reduce fat intake. One easy way to do this is to reduce the fat used in food preparation (a change that will benefit the whole family). You can decrease fat by baking, boiling, or broiling instead of frying. Sauté with nonstick pans and vegetable oil spray. Use lower-fat alternatives for ingredients that are high in fat; substitute skim milk for whole, whole milk for cream, and nonfat yogurt for sour cream. Nonfat yogurt can be successfully substituted for fat in many baking recipes; just substitute nonfat yogurt in a quantity equal to half the total volume of oil, butter, and eggs. Here are some tips to help your child follow a low-fat, low-calorie diet successfully:

- Minimize the amount of high-fat red meat you serve. Serve poultry, fish, and pasta with fresh vegetable sauces instead.
- Avoid serving fatty foods such as hamburgers, hot dogs, french fries, sausages, cold cuts, and salads made with mayonnaise.
- Avoid using butter on vegetables and potatoes; substitute a little grated parmesan cheese for flavoring.
- Avoid foods that are fried or prepared in sauces and gravies.
- Serve small portions of food and encourage your child not to take second helpings.
- Encourage your child to drink a lot of water with meals.
- Have low-fat, low-calorie snacks available and ready to eat. Good choices include fresh fruit, fruit canned in water or juice, sugar-free Jell-O, fresh vege-

tables (with low-calorie dip if needed), plain popcorn, and pretzels. Many low-fat snack products are available, but be sure to read the nutrition label on these products carefully. Low-fat does not necessarily mean low-calorie. Low-fat cookies can contain as many calories as their higher-fat counterparts.

- Avoid high-calorie drinks, like regular soda. Serve flavored seltzer or juice mixed with club soda. Serve skim or low-fat milk if your child is over 1 year of age.
- Plan meals and snacks together with your child.
- Help your child get involved in other activities during times of the day when he is most likely to want to eat.
- Keep high-calorie foods out of sight.
- Encourage your child to wait 20 minutes if he says he wants to eat shortly after a meal or snack. He may soon feel fuller, or become involved in an activity that distracts him from wanting to eat.
- Decrease the focus on food in family activities.
- Don't nag your child about diet.
- Have one place to eat. Do not allow eating in front of the television or while on the run. This rule should apply to everyone in the family.
- Cookies, candy, and ice cream are high in calories and should be used only for special treats on rare occasions.

Increasing physical activity is an important component of a weight management program. Consult your child's doctor or physical therapist for recommendations regarding appropriate physical activities for your child. You can help by promoting a life style that includes active leisure-time activities, limited time spent watching television, and increased physical activity. Finally, some children who have gained significant weight may benefit from participating in a supervised diet program such as Weight Watchers. Ask your doctor or dietician for recommendations.

Children Who Are Taking Prednisone

Children who are taking steroid medications have a number of dietary concerns. Steroids cause children to gain weight, have high blood pressure, lose calcium from their bones, and have high cholesterol. Some children taking steroids develop a diabetes-like condition. Paying careful attention to your child's diet while he is taking prednisone is very important. The best diet for children taking steroids is one that is low in fat, calories, and salt. He may need to take calcium supplements. Because this type of diet is complicated and so very important, it is helpful to consult a registered dietician for counseling as soon as your child starts steroid treatment.

Controlling weight gain. It is critical for you and your child to understand that people taking steroids develop an insatiable hunger. Children taking prednisone will often eat multiple helpings at meals and request constant snacks. We have even heard stories of young children stealing their friends' lunches at school! This increase in appetite is not your child's fault. It is difficult to control, but it will improve as the dose of steroid is decreased.

Your child will gain an unacceptable amount of weight if he eats as much as he would like, and this weight will be difficult to lose later on. Although it may not be possible for your child to lose weight while he is taking high doses of steroids, you may be able to prevent him from gaining a large amount of weight. As soon as steroids are started, begin following the tips for a low-calorie diet in the previous section.

Reducing salt. Although a high-salt diet is not good for anyone, salt intake is an even bigger concern for a child on steroids. Some of the major side effects of steroids include fluid retention, edema (puffiness of the hands, face, and ankles), and weight gain. Eating foods high in sodium makes these side effects worse. For this reason, doctors recommend a low-sodium diet so that these side effects can be minimized.

Salt is a naturally occurring compound made up of the minerals sodium and chloride. Sodium is a natural component of a variety of foods, but usually only in very low amounts. On the other hand, sodium is artificially added to food by manufacturers to preserve and add flavor to their products. Unfortunately for consumers, too much sodium is added to nearly all packaged foods. Salt is an acquired taste and can become an unhealthy habit; the more salt you eat, the more you want to eat. Most adults eat 4,000 to 9,000 milligrams of sodium per day compared to the 1,100 to 3,300 milligrams recommended by health professionals. Children's diets are often as high in sodium as adults' diets. Between salt-laden breakfast cereals, high-salt school lunches, packaged snacks, and convenience foods, a child's salt consumption can easily reach *5,000 milligrams* per day.

Because salt is used extensively in prepared foods, preparing a diet that's lower in sodium may require modifying how you cook and shop. Listed below are some tips to lower the sodium in your family's diet. Remember, everyone will benefit from these changes:

- Keep the salt shaker off the table! One teaspoon of salt contains 2,300 milligrams of sodium.
- Eliminate, or cut in half, the salt in recipes. Don't add salt to water when you boil noodles or vegetables. Most added salt is for flavor and is not needed to cook the food. Use spices that do not contain sodium to flavor food.

- Become a label reader. Nutritional labeling gives the sodium content per serving. Choose foods with the lowest amount of sodium and avoid foods that have more than 300 milligrams of sodium per serving. Look at the ingredient list for the word *salt* or *sodium;* avoid foods that have salt or sodium near the top of the ingredient list.

The following guidelines will help you make smart food choices in designing a diet that is low in salt.

	RECOMMENDED FOODS	FOODS TO AVOID
FRUITS	Fresh, canned, or frozen fruit	None
VEGETABLES	Fresh vegetables, plain frozen vegetables, low-sodium canned vegetables, salt-free tomato paste or puree, salt-free tomato juice	Regular canned vegetables, frozen vegetables in sauce, tomato juice, pickles, olives, canned baked beans, commercial soups, potato mixes, prepared salad dressings
DAIRY	Milk, yogurt, natural cheese (swiss, cheddar, mozzarella), eggs	Buttermilk, processed cheese, feta cheese
MEAT AND FISH	Fresh meat, fresh fish, fresh poultry, unsalted canned tuna	Bacon, cold cuts, corned beef, ham, sausage, hot dogs, canned meat or chicken, regular canned tuna, frozen prepared meat and poultry, frozen prepared fish (like fish sticks)
BREADS AND STARCHES	Breads (especially low-sodium); low-sodium crackers; shredded wheat cereal; cooked cereal with no salt added; pasta, rice, and potatoes if cooked without salt; salt-free pretzels	Breads with salted tops, salted crackers (Saltines, Wheat Thins, Ritz), instant cereal, commercial rice and noodle mixes, stuffing mix, seasoned bread crumbs, some cold cereals, bread and cake mixes, pancake mix, pizza, prepared spaghetti sauce, salty snack foods (pretzels, popcorn, potato chips, corn chips)

QUESTIONS AND ANSWERS ABOUT NUTRITION

My child refuses to eat any vegetables. What can I do?

Fruits and vegetables are an essential part of a well-balanced diet, and it's important for your child to eat them regularly. If your child balks at eating vegetables, try disguising them by adding grated vegetables to quick breads, muffins, spaghetti sauce, and meatloaf; add vegetables to omelets, casseroles, or other mixed dishes. Serve vegetables topped with cheese and use spices to enhance the flavor. Make soups using pureed vegetables, such as cream of broccoli, carrot, or spinach.

Keep trying different vegetables, prepared different ways. Always put some vegetables on your child's plate, but do not insist that he eat them. Your child may be more likely to eat the vegetables if he helps to prepare them, so invite him into the kitchen. Finally, fruits and fruit juices contain many of the vitamins and minerals found in vegetables. If he continues to refuse vegetables, try offering more fruits.

My two-and-a-half-year-old daughter has polyarticular JRA. She eats very little, and I am concerned that she is not eating enough.

The growth rate of toddlers is slow, much slower than that of infants, because it takes more energy to grow than to play. Thus, the energy needs of toddlers are not high. If your child is growing normally, she is getting enough to eat. Toddlers do not have adult-sized stomachs. A normal serving size for a toddler is 2 to 4 tablespoons of fruit, vegetables, rice, or pasta, half a slice of bread, and one ounce of meat. Keep portion sizes small. Put even less than you think your child will eat on her plate, and let her ask for seconds. Do not show disapproval or concern when your child doesn't eat. Offer foods only at regularly scheduled meal and snack times. You might consider involving your child in a quiet activity before mealtime, which will prepare her for the transition from play to eating.

Hospitalization and Surgery

For most children with JRA, medication and physical therapy together are effective in keeping symptoms under control. These children can function well at home, at school, and in the community, and they are not disabled by pain. Some children don't respond well to medical management, however, and some of them can only be helped by being cared for in the hospital for a time, or by having surgery.

A child with a rheumatic disease may be hospitalized to receive medical management or rehabilitative care, to have surgery, or for other reasons. No matter why the child is in the hospital, hospitalization can be a stressful and frightening experience for the child, his parents, and the entire family. This section describes what you can expect during your child's hospital stay and offers tips to make the hospital stay more constructive for your child.

Hospitalization

Before hospitalization. Children are sometimes hospitalized on short notice because of a medical emergency, but in most instances the hospitalization is planned in advance. In these cases, doing everything you can to prepare for the child's hospitalization is indispensable. The better prepared you and your child are for the hospital experience, the easier it will be for both of you.

There are several steps you can take to prepare for this experience. First, be sure that you fully understand the reason your child is being hospitalized. Find out as much as you can about what you and your child can expect. Questions to ask your doctor include:

- What are the goals of the hospitalization? What changes can I expect in my child's health at the end of the hospitalization, as a result of the treatment?
- What types of procedures will be performed on my child during the hospitalization? Will he have X rays, blood tests, or other diagnostic tests? Will he receive new medications, traction, physical therapy, or other therapeutic interventions? Will surgery be performed?
- Are there any alternatives to hospitalization? If so, how do they compare to the recommended hospitalization in terms of benefits and length of treatment?
- How long will my child be hospitalized? How long will he be out of school?
- Will the hospitalization be covered fully by my health insurance, or will I be liable for some of the cost?
- Who will be caring for my child while he is in the hospital? Will the team members in the outpatient clinic (pediatric rheumatologist, nurse, physical and occupational therapists, and social worker) be the direct care providers during the hospitalization, or will new health professionals be involved?
- What is my child's day going to be like during the hospitalization? Are toys available, or is there a playroom my child can use?
- Will I be able to stay with my child?
- Is a tutor available to help prevent my child from falling behind in schoolwork?
- Are there any written materials available from the hospital to help me prepare my child for the hospital experience?
- What resources are available to me in the hospital? Hospital resources for parents include parking vouchers, meal vouchers, kitchen privileges, lending libraries, support groups, interpreter services, long-distance phone calls, religious services, check cashing, and laundry facilities. Find out where nearby restaurants and coffee shops are located; you may want to get away from the hospital—or at least from hospital food—from time to time.

Once you have an idea of what the hospital experience is going to be like, you can prepare your child for the experience. Your child will probably be anxious about going into the hospital. You can help him to cope with his fears by answering his questions and telling him in simple language what is going to happen. Stay calm. If you are distressed about your child's impending hospitalization, your child will sense your distress, and he will be worried, too.

- Be sure to explain why he is going into the hospital.
- Tell him honestly and simply what he can expect, even when it comes to the unpleasant parts such as needle sticks, tests, surgery, and other procedures.
- Visit your community library to borrow age-appropriate books and videotapes to help your child prepare for his hospital experience. If none are available, ask the hospital admissions office or nursing department.
- Tell your child exactly when you will be with him, and when you will be away from him. If you will be rooming-in, assure him that you will be there the whole time. If you will be going home at night, prepare him for your absence.
- Before arriving at the hospital, ask your child how he feels, and if there is anything he is afraid of. If there is, you might be able to soothe his fears.

For young children, the prospect of being away from their parents is usually the most frightening part of a hospitalization. Today, most children's hospitals allow a parent to stay with a child 24 hours a day. Some also have a rooming-in policy; in these hospitals, a parent is given a place to sleep in the child's room or in a nearby location. If rooming-in is not available and you will be far from home, ask about nearby hotels and motels and whether they offer discounts to families of hospitalized children. Ronald McDonald Houses are available in some cities. These houses make it possible for families to stay together at no cost or low cost during extended hospitalizations.

Finally, prepare yourself and the rest of your family for the hospitalization. The more organized your home life is prior to your departure, the more easily they will adjust to your absence.

- Make appropriate arrangements with your work.
- Make arrangements with your child's school for his absence. Arrange to take school books and assignments with you, and for homework assignments to be sent to the hospital so your child will not fall behind.
- Make arrangements for care of other children and pets during your absence.
- Hold a family meeting to discuss each family member's responsibilities during the hospitalization. Determine who will be responsible for cooking, cleaning, grocery shopping, laundry, and other tasks.

- Cook and freeze food in advance if possible, so the family can eat while you are away from home, and so food can be fixed easily when you and your child first return.
- Ask family members and friends to visit your child in the hospital as appropriate.

During the hospitalization. The hospital environment can be stressful. You may not always know what's going to happen or what is wrong with your child. One thing you can do is find out as much as possible about daily routines and other aspects of the hospital environment. By asking questions in advance—and also as new situations arise—you may be able to handle the hospital experience better, and you'll certainly be better equipped to support your child.

Here are some other things you can do to help your child feel comfortable in the hospital:

- Tell the hospital staff by what name your child likes to be called, and ask them to use it.
- Bring familiar things from home to the hospital if they are allowed. A favorite blanket, pajamas, toys, stuffed animals, or family photos from home are comforting to a young child. A radio with headphones, as well as favorite tapes and books, can be soothing for a child of any age.
- If your child is admitted for elective rehabilitation, bring comfortable street clothes such as sweat pants, T-shirts, and sneakers. Most children's hospitals do not require children to be in pajamas all day, and your child will be more comfortable doing therapy in "workout" clothes. Bring a bathing suit if pool therapy is scheduled.
- Keep your child's routines as normal as possible. Bedtime, nap time, television time, bath time, and so on ought to be as close as possible to what they would be at home.
- Maintain good communication with the hospital staff. Be sure to share information about your child's past experiences with medications, allergies, surgeries, and therapy; informing the hospital staff will help make certain your child receives the finest care possible. If something bothers you about the care your child is receiving, tell a nurse or doctor, rather than keeping the complaint to yourself.

  By the same token, if you feel that your child is receiving considerate, high-quality care, tell the staff. Your feedback helps the staff learn about caring for children like yours in the hospital. Your comments can help them to provide better care for other children in the future.
- Find out what time the doctors make rounds and have your questions ready when they arrive. If the doctors make rounds in the morning, be dressed and ready for their arrival.

- Learn the hospital routine and adapt to it. Find out when meals are served, when nap or quiet time is, and when televisions and radios should be turned off at night. Comply with hospital policies concerning over-the-counter medications, having food in rooms, smoking, and visiting hours.
- Ask people to identify themselves—and their role, function, or position—to you. Be sure you know who each person is and what role each person plays in your child's care. If your child is old enough, these care providers will almost certainly introduce themselves to your child. If this doesn't happen, you should step in and introduce the person to your child. Your child will have contact with many types of people in the hospital, and not all of them will wear uniforms. It's a good idea for him to be able to recognize as many of the people who are taking care of him as possible.

Some children's hospitals have family participation programs. Family participation units encourage parents to participate in their child's care as a way of decreasing the child's anxiety during the hospitalization. Parents are often asked to be responsible for bathing, feeding, and dressing their children, helping to keep track of fluid intake and output, and supervising tooth brushing. Parents may also be asked to make their child's bed, keep their child's room neat and clean, and help to observe safety precautions such as keeping bed rails up, supervising play, and keeping dangerous objects out of reach. Having a parent rather than a stranger do these household duties makes the child feel more comfortable.

Many medical centers with pediatric rheumatology programs are teaching hospitals. This means that the hospital is affiliated with a medical school and is dedicated to providing education and training to physicians and other health professionals. If your child is hospitalized in a teaching hospital, you and your child will probably come in contact with fellows, residents, interns, medical students, nursing students, and therapy students.

In teaching hospitals, it's likely that your child will be part of the teaching rounds, when medical students and others visit patients with a physician on the staff to learn about different diseases as well as patient care. The physician and the students will stand around the bed and ask questions and probably examine your child. This experience is valuable for the students. You should know, however, that you have the right to refuse to have your child participate in teaching rounds.

Planning for discharge. Discharge planning usually begins the day your child is admitted to the hospital. Prepare for your child's homecoming by taking these steps *before* your child comes home:

- Become familiar with your child's medications and their dosage levels and schedules. Obtain prescriptions as needed.
- Obtain needed equipment, supplies, or monitoring devices and know how to use them.
- Become familiar with any special care procedures such as wound dressing or cast care.
- Become familiar with any home therapy program you will be expected to perform with your child. Find out whether your child has any activity restrictions.
- Understand any special dietary restrictions.
- Know when your child can return to school.
- Find out who to call with questions after discharge.
- Obtain appointment times for follow-up visits with doctors, therapists, and other health professionals.
- Obtain any referrals needed to physical or occupational therapy, nursing agencies, equipment vendors, or other community providers.

Surgery

Most children with rheumatic diseases will never need surgery. For a few children with arthritis, however, surgery may be advised. Surgery may be recommended if he must use a wheelchair to get around or if he is in a great deal of pain, is limited in his functional abilities, or has a correctable deformity.

Some insurance plans *require* that the patient get a second opinion before undergoing surgery. Sometimes the insurance company will even provide a list of surgeons whom you might visit to get this second opinion. But getting a second opinion before undergoing surgery may be a good idea in any case. You can ask your surgeon to provide the names of surgeons who are qualified to provide a second opinion. Getting a second opinion is standard medical practice, and surgeons are used to being asked this, so no good surgeon will be offended by the question. You may also ask your child's pediatrician or pediatric rheumatologist for the names of qualified surgeons.

Preparing for surgery. If surgery is recommended for your child, you can follow all of the steps outlined in this chapter for children who are hospitalized. In addition, you will want to ask your child's surgeon the following questions:

- What are the risks and benefits of the surgical procedure? What are the potential complications?

- Are there alternatives to surgery? If so, how do they compare to the recommended surgery in terms of benefits and length of treatment?
- Have you performed this particular procedure on children with the same diagnosis as my child? If so, how often? What were the results? Can I talk to another parent whose child has had this procedure performed by you?
- Can the surgery be delayed until a more convenient time, such as school vacation? Can it be delayed another year or two?
- Does my child need to participate in any special physical therapy to "get in shape" prior to surgery?
- Will my child require general anesthesia? (If so, be sure to tell the anesthesiologist if your child has limited mobility of his neck or any respiratory problems such as asthma.)
- Can my child donate his own blood in advance to avoid receiving blood bank products?
- How long will the operation last? How soon can I see my child after surgery?
- How much pain will my child have during and after the surgery? What kind of pain medication will be available?
- Will my child's medication be changed before and after the surgery? (There may be an increased risk of bleeding if some medications, such as NSAIDs, are not stopped before major surgery.)
- What is the total cost of the procedure likely to be? How much of this cost will be covered by my insurance plan? If necessary, can a payment plan to the hospital and the surgeon be worked out?

You will also want to find out what is likely to happen after surgery. Ask the surgeon these questions:

- What is the usual postoperative course?
- When will my child begin receiving physical therapy? When will he begin walking and going up and down stairs?
- How much therapy will be required after the surgery? What will it entail?
- How long will the benefits of the surgery last?
- What effect will this surgical procedure have on my child's growth?
- What can you expect my child's level of function to be at the time of his discharge from the hospital? What will his functional status be 2 weeks, 6 months, and 1 year following the surgery?

Types of surgical procedures. Surgery that may be recommended for children with arthritis includes the following:

- *Soft tissue release* (surgical stretching of tendons or ligaments) may be used to improve the position of a joint that has been pulled out of line by a contracture.
- *Arthroscopic surgery* is joint surgery in which a small microscope and surgical instruments are inserted through a small incision. Many corrective procedures can be performed during arthroscopic surgery.
- *Synovectomy* is the removal of the inflamed joint lining.
- *Bunionectomy* is the removal of painful deformities of the ball of the foot.
- *Arthrodesis* is a fusion of the bones in the joint; it is performed to stabilize a joint.
- *Total joint replacement* surgery involves replacing the entire joint with an artificial prosthesis.

Total joint replacement. The modern era of joint replacement surgery began in the early 1960s with the development of a plastic and metal artificial hip joint. Since then, advances in technology have improved the design of artificial joints and allowed for the reconstruction of many different body sites, most successfully hips and knees. Orthopedic surgeons have also been working to perfect artificial shoulders, elbows, wrists, finger joints, and ankles.

Once it became clear that total joint replacement was reasonably safe and effective in adults, the technology was applied to children, beginning in the 1970s, especially hip and knee replacements. Less commonly, other joints, such as shoulders and knuckles, have been replaced in children. For a child who has intense or constant pain or who has lost function because of joint deformity, a joint replacement may be the best therapy.

As many children with arthritis and their families know, pain can interfere with school, sleep, and normal daily activities. When pain has not responded to medication and other conservative measures, surgery may be indicated. When pain is associated with significant damage to the joint and adjacent bone, the child may be a candidate for a total joint replacement. Pain relief is often dramatic following this type of surgery. Some children with JRA, however, do not have a significant degree of pain, but rather gradually lose motion and function in a joint.

An example of deteriorating function would be the child with systemic or polyarticular JRA who has increasing difficulty in getting around. He may end up spending more and more time in a wheelchair and eventually lose the strength and range of motion needed to walk. Even if the child is not having significant pain, total joint replacement may be indicated if there is significant joint damage and other conservative measures have not resulted in restored function.

Joint replacement surgery has now been performed in children as young as 10, although most children having this surgery are older than that. Ideally a child will have completed most of his growth before having joint replacement surgery. Children with severe polyarticular JRA are often small, both in weight and in height, and complete most of their growth by the time they are 13 or 14. This actually works to the advantage of the patient and the surgeon, since the metal and plastic components will last longer in a person who is relatively light in weight.

Though there are a number of different types of artificial joints available, the choice is largely dependent on the surgeon and the patient. Some older JRA patients may do well with an off-the-shelf prosthesis, but many younger children undergoing this procedure will require custom-made implants. Some orthopedic centers will design and construct the implant in advance based on careful X-ray and computed tomographic (CT) scan measurements; others use a computer-assisted design during the operation itself. Because of the unique technical problems involved, this surgery should be performed by an orthopedic surgeon who has had a great deal of experience performing joint surgery on children.

The complication rate for children following joint surgery is fairly low: infections, hematomas (collections of blood), nerve injury, and joint dislocation are all possible but uncommon events. The major long-term complication is loosening of the joint implant, but most experienced surgeons nowadays predict that the artificial joint will survive for 15 to 20 years, depending on the size and activity of the patient. A second operation to revise the artificial joint may replace the loosened implant with a new artificial joint or may fuse the joint in a functional position.

Children and young adults who undergo joint replacement surgery need to be motivated and need to understand that there is an extensive rehabilitation process required following surgery. Patients remain in the hospital for 7 to 14 days following total hip or knee replacement, then continue their therapy on an outpatient basis. Despite the immediate discomfort following surgery, most children who undergo joint replacement surgery report much less pain, greater mobility, and improved function. It remains to be seen, however, how long the joint implants will last and who the best candidates for this type of surgery are.

Unproven Remedies

There is nothing that children and their parents and doctors want more than an immediate cure for the child, with total relief from all symptoms. That, unfortunately, is exactly what pediatric rheumatologists cannot offer. One of the most difficult truths for parents to learn about the childhood rheumatic diseases is that there is no cure. Treating a childhood rheumatic disease takes patience and diligence. The pediatric rheumatologist will work with the parent to identify the safest, most effective regime of medicines and physical therapy. This will take time, and improvement will occur only gradually.

In contrast, many of the arthritis "cures" and home remedies that are offered by individuals and health food suppliers promise complete relief from arthritis symptoms with none of the dangerous side effects associated with some medical therapies. These unproven remedies are popular: arthritis sufferers each year in the United States spend nearly one billion dollars on them.

As proof of their claims to "cures," the sellers of these products, who usually have no medical or scientific credentials, offer testimonials of former "arthritis sufferers" who claim to have recovered after taking their products. These claims often cannot be substantiated. There may be no evidence that the individuals had rheumatic diseases to begin with, or that they achieved full and lasting remissions. We all need to view these claims with a healthy skepticism.

It's a very different story with medications used in traditional treatment regimes, which have been approved by the U.S. Food and Drug Administration (FDA). The FDA, which must approve all medications before they are released into the marketplace, has specific guidelines for the conduct of scientific studies to demonstrate a drug's safety and efficacy. These studies, or trials, require that large samples of patients be given the medication at the same time that other large samples of patients are given a *placebo* (a substitute for the actual medication with no active medicine in it). In these trials, neither the doctor nor the patients know who is receiving active medication and who is receiving placebo.

Because of the episodic nature of many rheumatic diseases, it may be difficult to tell when medications or other treatments are effective. For example, if a child's arthritis quiets down while he is taking a certain medication, the improvement may be related to that medication, or it may be a result of the natural course of the child's illness. Similarly, in the drug trials, some patients in both groups will improve because they enter a period of decreased disease activity. Overall, however, if more patients in the drug group do better than those in the placebo group, the drug is considered to be effective in treating arthritis.

Side effects are also evaluated in these trials. Unwanted symptoms that occur more frequently in the drug group are attributed to the drug's activity. The drug in question is considered safe to use if the potential side effects are less serious than the consequences of uncontrolled arthritis.

Scientists who publish the results of drug trials in medical journals must provide information about the number of patients in the study and their medical histories, the manner in which the study was conducted, and how the results were analyzed.

From this information, other physicians and scientists can carefully scrutinize the results for accuracy and replicate the experiments to determine whether the results are reliable. Unproven remedies are not subjected to this type of rigorous scientific investigation. It is impossible for scientists to interpret the claims of effectiveness made by those who promote these remedies.

Many home remedies that claim to treat arthritis and are available to consumers are considered "foods" (not "drugs") by the FDA and are therefore not subjected to stringent testing for purity, safety, and efficacy. These remedies may have a mixture of ingredients, some of which may have significant side effects. Rarely have these unproven remedies been tested in children to learn what doses are appropriate, or even if they are effective.

Parents considering the use of an unproven remedy should first consider its potential to cause serious harm, particularly in growing children. Some unconventional treatments, like copper bracelets, are not harmful but should not be used *in place of* traditional medical therapy. Others, such as vitamins, do not cause a problem when used in reasonable doses. Some preparations sold as arthritis cures, however, may cause illness or unwanted side effects.

Because long-term follow-up is rarely done with patients taking unconventional remedies, harmful long-term effects are completely unknown. It is tempting to believe that all home remedies and "natural therapies," such as those from plants, are completely harmless. But we have to remember that "natural" substances, such as poisonous mushrooms, can be dangerous, and that plants often are the basis for drugs with potent side effects, such as digitalis, used for heart disease, and salicylates, the plant forerunners of aspirin.

Of course, all treatments are unproven until they have been studied scientifically, and we are hopeful that new treatments or even a cure for rheumatic illnesses will be discovered. We also want to protect our patients from harmful unproven remedies, and our patients' parents from unnecessary (and often prohibitive) expense. If you believe that an unproven remedy may help your child and you are considering using it, please discuss this with your child's rheumatologist before taking another step. Here are some of the unproven remedies for the childhood rheumatic diseases:

Vitamins
Diet therapy
Copper bracelets
Chicken collagen
Vinegar
Gin-soaked raisins
Mushroom tea
Honey
Healing baths
Bee venom
Bee sting therapy
Laser treatments
Allergy diets

Before starting an unproven remedy for your child, follow these steps:

- Ask for a complete listing of all ingredients before you buy anything. Review this list with your doctor to be certain there are no dangerous ingredients.
- Ask if the remedy has been used in children and, if so, what the safety profile is. What is the dosage for children as compared to adults?
- Ask for a listing of reported side effects. Be suspicious if the individual selling you the treatment claims there are none. This usually means they have never asked those who take the remedy if they have encountered problems.
- Ask if there is long-term follow-up of individuals who have taken this treatment.
- Ask about costs. Many unproven remedies are very expensive, and they are rarely covered by insurance.

QUESTIONS AND ANSWERS ABOUT UNPROVEN REMEDIES

Does fish oil help children with rheumatic diseases?

Fish oil has gained attention as a treatment for a variety of inflammatory conditions, including arthritis. There is a low incidence of inflammatory disease among populations whose diets contain large amounts of fish (such as the Japanese or Inuit), suggesting that taking fish oil has a possible therapeutic benefit. Some studies have shown that fish oil supplements decrease inflammation. In adults with arthritis, patients receiving fish oil had fewer swollen and tender joints, less morning stiffness, and decreases in various laboratory measures of inflammation. Patients who received a placebo (in this case, olive oil) also did better, however.

Before running out and stocking up on fish oil, keep in mind these precautions. First, all fish oils are not alike. The beneficial effect appears to derive from a specific component of fish oil known as eicosapentaenoic acid. Different fish oil preparations have different amounts of this component. Therefore, you should ask your doctor to help decide on the correct dose for your child depending on the preparation available. Second, fish oil may have side effects, including suppression of the immune system. The effects of fish oil supplements in growing children have not been investigated. Finally, although the oil comes in a tablet preparation, many people find that it tastes unpleasant. Because of its potent effects, fish oil should be considered a drug and should be given to a child only with a physician's guidance.

My local health food store is selling evening primrose oil as a "cure" for arthritis. Is there any truth to this claim?

An ingredient in evening primrose oil called gammalinoleic acid (GLA) has recently been studied as a treatment for arthritis. In adults with arthritis, those taking GLA had modest improvements in the number of swollen and tender joints and morning stiffness as compared to those taking a placebo. The investigators in this study concluded that GLA may be beneficial as an additional treatment for arthritis, to be used in conjunction with conventional medications.

Although it is unlikely that GLA is a "cure," it certainly may offer some benefit, and side effects are minimal. GLA is found in both evening primrose oil and borage seed oil. The dose needed depends on the preparation, as different amounts of active GLA are found in different preparations.

The effects of GLA on children with arthritis have yet to be studied, and dosing for children has not yet been worked out, so it's probably best not to give evening primrose oil to young children.

Should I put my child on a special diet to help her arthritis?

Many parents wonder whether giving their child extra vitamins, taking away certain foods, or using a special diet will cure or help arthritis. There are books available that claim that certain diets will cure arthritis, or that arthritis is due to an "allergy" and removal of the offending food will cure the disease. To date, there is no evidence that any of these claims are true. For children, some of these diets may be hazardous.

Eliminating nutrients that are necessary for growth may have negative long-term effects on a child's physical development. Children with rheumatic disease require a high-calorie diet to keep up with increased needs imposed by inflammation and growth. To avoid undernutrition, the best approach to feeding your child is to provide a well-balanced, nutritious diet.

Chapter 6

•

Monitoring Your Child's Progress

A parent is in a good position to observe day-to-day changes in his or her child's condition and to monitor how the child responds to different therapies. Because parents can watch these changes on a daily basis, and also because parents care so much about their children, they are important participants in monitoring their children's health. The purpose of this chapter is to provide parents with a framework for maintaining their own personal record of all aspects of their child's health, including symptoms, treatments, and response to therapy.

If you are a parent or a grandparent or the primary caregiver of a child with rheumatic disease, this record will be useful for you, for your child, and for your child's health care providers. For example, over the course of your child's illness, she will be seen and treated by many health care providers; having a record of these visits helps when the time comes to make decisions about future treatment. Although much of this information will be in your child's physician's chart, it's possible that you will have the only *complete* record of your child's medical care. The rheumatology clinic may have some of it, the pediatrician may have some of it, the pediatric rheumatologist or the surgeon may have some of it. But you will have all of it, and all of it will be easily available to you whenever you need it.

It's helpful, too, to have a written record on those numerous occasions when you will be asked to summarize your child's medical history. This will happen, for example, when your child:

- Enrolls in preschool, kindergarten, school, or college.
- Wants to participate in school sports.
- Visits a new doctor, such as a new pediatrician or pediatric rheumatologist.
- Needs to obtain a second opinion regarding treatment of the rheumatic disease.
- Is being prepared for a surgical procedure or hospitalization.
- Is about to begin taking a new drug or having other new therapy.
- Has a significant medical event, such as an allergic reaction or a gastrointestinal problem, that requires specialized medical care.

• Is applying for an entitlement program, such as Supplemental Security Income (SSI), Medicaid, and some health insurance programs.

You probably received a small health record or health journal for your child when she was born. Over the years, you may have recorded her height and weight at each well-child visit, and kept track of vaccinations, illnesses, and other information. When your child has a rheumatic disease, it can be helpful to expand on this concept by keeping records about the illness and your child's response to treatments.

This health care record for your child will help you to organize current information about your child's illness and treatment plan, and it will provide a permanent record of the course of the illness and your child's response to past treatments. The personal health record should help you to understand your child's illness, coordinate her care, and talk intelligently with health care providers. The health care record will help you report accurate information about your child to physicians, therapists, and other care providers.

The suggestions in this chapter come from parents who have had good success in keeping such a record. We include some blank forms that may help you to keep track of various aspects of the treatment plan. You can photocopy the forms as needed, using whichever ones you find helpful, or create new forms as you need them. You may wish to make extra copies of some of these blank forms and keep them in your health record, for convenience's sake.

You should use whatever information in this chapter helps you to create your health care record, and disregard the rest. We don't want this record keeping to add to your burden. We hope that it makes things easier for you.

Many parents have found that keeping the health record in a three-ring binder makes sense, because materials can be added in a logical sequence. Dividing the notebook into sections labeled, for example, "Directory," "Medical History," "Office Visits," "Schedule of Treatments," and "Other" may help you find what you're looking for. If you want to number the pages, it works best to start over again with page 1 for each section, because you will be adding new pages to each section. It's a good idea to keep each section of your health care record in chronological order.

Suppose, for example, that your child is scheduled for a visit to the rheumatology clinic. You will insert a clean copy of the "Clinic or Office Visit Summary" into the notebook, following the records of the earlier visits, and insert a new page number. If you take the notebook with you to the clinic, you can fill in the form with the information from the visit. Each time your child visits a health care provider, you will complete a new "Clinic or Office Visit Summary" and place it in the health record.

If you take the health care notebook with you on each visit to a health care provider, you can also use the information recorded there to help you describe your child's interim history (what's happened since the last visit). And if the physician or the therapist or someone else you see during your visit gives you a written handout (such as a description of an exercise program or a medication fact sheet), you can insert it directly into the health record.

The record you maintain will be individualized to your own child's needs. Don't feel that you have to fill in every blank or write down every laboratory value. Record only the information that is important to you, and organize the notebook in a way that works for you. If you would like help in setting up the health care record, you might ask the nurse in the specialty care clinic to get you started.

Directory of Health Care Providers

We've all had the experience of searching through piles of papers, combing through desk drawers, and lamenting our poor memory when we need to come up with an important name or telephone number. To avoid having this happen to you, you may find it convenient to make the first section of your health care record a directory of your child's health care providers, from the pediatric rheumatologist and team members at the specialty care center, to community health care providers and the relevant staff at your child's school. Having information about health insurance companies and public health agencies close at hand can also be a time saver.

The forms provided in this section may be copied and inserted into this section of the notebook. Begin by recording the name, address, and phone number for each of your child's current health care providers; when appropriate, include your child's account number or medical record number. It may take some time to enter all the information into the directory, but you'll save time in the long run by not having to search for information when you need to contact someone about your child's services.

The directory will be a convenient reference for you whenever you need to contact providers, make appointments, or share information among providers. Say, for example, that the physical therapist in the specialty care center notices an increase in your child's knee flexion contracture, and would like to review management strategies with the local physical therapist. If you have your health care record with you, you'll find the community therapist's name, address, and phone number right at your fingertips, and you will be able to help these two therapists communicate with each other.

Remember to keep the information in your directory current. Update it when substitutions or additions are made on your child's health care team, or when one of the health care providers has a change of telephone number or address. Information that changes frequently can be entered in pencil to make it easier to enter new information as needed.

Form 1. Specialty Care Center Information

Hospital name	
Clinic name	

Hours of operation *Office hours* *Clinic days and times*	Address
Phone numbers *During office hours* *After office hours (evenings and weekends)*	Emergency phone number (if different)

Other information (if different) *To make an appointment* *To obtain test results* *To obtain prescription refills*	*Phone*	*Contact person*

Form 2. The Health Care Team at the Specialty Care Center

Name	Position	Phone
	Pediatric rheumatologist	
	Pediatric rheumatology fellow	
	Nurse	
	Physical therapist	
	Occupational therapist	
	Social worker	
	Nurse's aide	
	Secretary	
	Secretary	

Form 3. Community-Based Health Providers

Name	Service Provided	Phone	Address
	Pediatrician		
	Physical Therapist		
	Occupational Therapist		
	Eye Doctor		
	School Nurse		
	Pharmacist		

Form 4. Health Insurance

Primary Health Insurance

Insurance company name	Policy number	Group number
Address	Phone	Contact person (name/title)
Name of policyholder		
Group policyholder (i.e., employer)(omit if nongroup policy)	Group benefits manager, name and phone number/extension	

Secondary Health Insurance

Insurance company name	Policy number	Group number
Address	Phone	Contact person (name/title)
Name of policyholder		
Group policyholder (i.e., employer)(omit if nongroup policy)	Group benefits manager, name and phone number/extension	

Form 5. Public Health Agencies

Primary Agency

Agency name	Child's ID number
Address	Phone

Contact person (name/title)

Other Agency

Agency name	Child's ID number
Address	Phone

Contact person (name/title)

Other Agency

Agency name	Child's ID number
Address	Phone

Contact person (name/title)

Form 6. School

School Information
Name of school

Address	Phone
Teacher	School nurse
Physical education teacher	Principal

Other teachers or service providers *Name*	*Subject taught or service provided*

School District Information
Name of school district
Address

Superintendent (name and phone)	Special education director (name and phone)

The Medical History

The second section of the health record can be used to create a summary of your child's medical history for conditions other than her rheumatic disease, as well as an ongoing record of her routine medical care. Information on immunizations, medical conditions, medications, hospitalizations, and surgeries, as well as a family history, can be recorded there.

A family history of rheumatic disease can provide diagnostic clues for the physician, while a history of other chronic illnesses in parents, grandparents, aunts, uncles, and cousins alerts the physician to the possibility that the child may develop certain hereditary diseases, such as diabetes. If your child or someone in the family has a chronic medical condition, that should be noted in the health care record, even if the condition seems to be unrelated to a rheumatic illness and even if it seems like a nuisance disorder (like mild psoriasis, for example). The medical history form can be photocopied and used to keep track of these medical illnesses and routine medical care.

Form 7. Medical History

Date of birth _____   Birth weight _____

Complications_____

Immunizations					
Type	Date	Date	Date	Date	Date
DTP (diphtheria, tetanus, pertussis)					
MMR (measles, mumps, rubella)					
HIB (*Haemophilus influenzae* type b)					
Polio					
Tuberculin tine test (TB)					
Hepatitis B					
Influenza					
Chicken pox					

Child's Medical Conditions Other Than Rheumatic Illness			
Condition	Date	Condition	Date
Allergy		Hernia	
Asthma		Inflammatory bowel disease	
Chicken pox		Kidney disease	
Congenital anomaly		Measles	
Convulsions		Mumps	
Diabetes		Poliomyelitis	
Developmental delay		Rheumatic fever	
Ear infections		Scarlet fever	
Fractures		Strep throat	
German measles		Tuberculosis	
Hearing impairment		Other	
Heart disease		Other	

Form 7. Medical History (continued)

Child's Medications Other Than for Rheumatic Illness	

Child's Hospitalizations

Description	Date	Physician	Hospital

Child's Surgeries

Description	Date	Physician	Hospital

Family History of Rheumatic Illness

Name of Illness	Relative's Relationship to the Child	Name of Illness	Relative's Relationship to the Child
Adult rheumatoid arthritis		SLE	
Ankylosing spondylitis		Osteoarthritis	
Dermatomyositis		Other	
Inflammatory bowel disease (colitis)		Other	
Juvenile rheumatoid arthritis		Other	

Recording Office Visits

In this section of the health care record, you can record information about your child's doctor visits. This section can help you prepare for clinic visits and keep track of observations and recommendations made by your child's physician and other health care providers. You can summarize the information you receive at each visit to a health care provider, whether it be the pediatrician, eye doctor, rheumatologist, or community-based providers.

It's a good idea to prepare for the visit in advance, before you leave home. Write down any questions you would like to ask during the visit as well as any concerns you have about symptoms or medicines or other treatments. Also record any changes you have noticed in your child's condition, including improvement. If you have concerns about your child's overall well-being, make a note of those, too. Record the duration of morning stiffness.

During the visit, write down the doctor's observations and answers to your questions. Take notes about any problems that are identified and write down the suggestions the doctor makes for addressing these problems. If specific goals are identified, write them down and note how long the doctor expects it to take your child to achieve them. List any X rays, lab tests, or other procedures that are done, and briefly note the results when you learn them.

Finally, document treatment recommendations, such as new medications or changes in dose, and physical and occupational therapy programs. If the doctor makes referrals to other specialists, such as dermatologists and ophthalmologists, or to community-based health care providers, write this information down, even if the doctor makes the arrangements for your child to see the other care provider.

The form for a clinic or office visit summary can be used to help you organize this information. Use a separate form for each visit, and keep all completed forms in your health care record. As suggested earlier, you may wish to make extra copies of these blank forms and keep them in your health record.

Form 8. Clinic or Office Visit Summary

Doctor's/provider's name _____ Date of visit _____

Complete before visit
Duration of morning stiffness
Questions, concerns, and observations

Summary of visit
Health care provider's observations (current symptoms, changes in disease activity, response to therapy)

Lab tests, X rays, other procedures, and results

Treatment recommendations

Schedule of Treatments

This section of your health care record is designed to help you keep track of medications, splints, therapies, and other treatments, and how well they work. It will also help you keep track of when and where follow-up visits are needed. This section may be the best place to keep any written instructions you receive regarding your child's care, such as physical and occupational therapy home exercise programs. We've included three different forms here—a follow-up schedule, a prescription record, and a record of additional treatment—to help you organize information related to your child's treatment and follow-up schedule.

The Follow-up Schedule

This form is designed to help you keep track of appointments or procedures that must be repeated at regular intervals, such as monthly lab tests and periodic eye exams. Record both the date of the current procedure and the recommended frequency for that procedure, and it will be easy to remember when the next appointment should be scheduled. You can also record test results and other observations here. Keep a blank form in your health record and make copies as needed. A completed form might look something like the sample reproduced below.

Form 9. Sample Completed Follow-up Schedule

Procedure, Test, etc.	Recommended Frequency	Date	Location	Results, Observations, etc.
Blood tests	Monthly	4-12-96	Ayer Community Hospital	Results OK
Eye exam	Every 3 months	5-1-96	Dr. Smith, Concord	No iritis

Form 9. Follow-up Schedule

Procedure, Test, etc.	Recommended Frequency	Date	Location	Results, Observations, etc.

The Prescription Record

The prescription record form provides a valuable summary of your child's prescription medicine use and is useful in a number of ways. When you call your child's doctor to get a prescription refilled, for example, you can refer to this form for the name of the medication and the dose, and you'll be able to tell the doctor how long your child has been taking the medication as well as what other medications your child is taking. Be sure to have an estimate of your child's weight on hand, because the dosage prescribed for your child will change as your child grows. Also be sure to have your pharmacy phone number handy when making the call, in case the doctor wishes to call the prescription in directly (there's a place for the pharmacy name and number in the directory section of the health care record).

This form will also be useful to you when you call the pharmacy to order prescription refills. Be sure to have the prescription number (Rx #) available when you call. The Rx # can be found on the prescription label and is usually needed by the pharmacist for refills.

When you record the name of a medicine in your health record, write down its strength, as well (for example: Naprosyn, 250 mg). In the *dose* column, record both the number of tablets (or spoonfuls of liquid medicine) taken at one time, and the number of doses taken each day. In the *observations* column, record any side effects or other important observations about how the medication affects your child. A completed form might resemble the sample reproduced below.

Form 10. Sample Completed Prescription Record

Date Started	Medicine Name (Strength)	Dose (Amount and Frequency)	Rx Number	Date Stopped	Observations
2-19-93	Naprosyn, 250 mg	1 tablet, 2 times/day	423378	5-17-93	Didn't help
5-17-93	Tolectin, 200 mg	1 tablet, 3 times/day	622391		

Form 10. Prescription Record

Pharmacy name _____   Pharmacy phone number _____

Child's approximate weight _____

Date Started	Medicine Name (Strength)	Dose (Amount and Frequency)	Rx Number	Date Stopped	Observations

The Additional Treatment Record

The additional treatment record form can be used to summarize treatments other than medications. Other treatments might include resting splints, shoe lifts, joint injections, diagnostic procedures, physical or occupational therapy, and assistive devices. Make a record here of hospitalizations, visits to the emergency room, and consultations with other health care providers, such as orthopedic surgeons and gastroenterologists. Use the *observations* column to note any unexpected results, to comment on effectiveness, or to describe why the treatment was stopped. An example of a completed form is presented below.

Form 11. Sample Completed Additional Treatment Record

Date Started	Treatment (Splint, Shoe Lift, etc.)	Description	Date Stopped	Observations
5-19-96	Wrist splints	Right wrist, night and naps		Wrist stiff for 10 minutes in morning
5-17-96	Therapy--putty	Green--hard		Moves fingers better

Form 11. Additional Treatment Record

Date Started	Treatment (Splint, Shoe Lift, etc.)	Description	Date Stopped	Observations

Growth Chart

Pediatricians and pediatric rheumatologists use a growth chart to record and monitor a child's growth in height and weight over time. You can keep your own record of your child's growth by plotting his or her height and weight according to his or her age on one of the following charts. It is not particularly important which line of the growth chart your child is on (that is, the 5th, 30th, or 60th percentile). What is important is that your child maintains a steady rate of growth without dramatic jumps from one percentile to another.

If you are concerned about your child's growth, review her growth chart with the pediatrician or pediatric rheumatologist. If your child is not growing properly, you and the doctor may want to make changes in her diet or medications to improve her rate of growth.

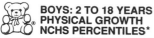

BOYS: 2 TO 18 YEARS
PHYSICAL GROWTH
NCHS PERCENTILES*

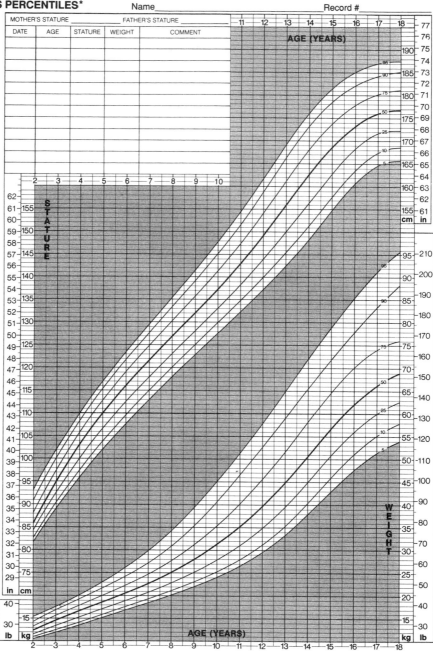

*Adapted from: Hamill PVV, Drizd TA, Johnson CL, Reed RB, Roche AF, Moore WM: Physical growth: National Center for Health Statistics percentiles. AM J CLIN NUTR 32:607-629, 1979. Data from the National Center for Health Statistics (NCHS), Hyattsville, Maryland.

© 1982 Ross Products Division, Abbott Laboratories

GIRLS: 2 TO 18 YEARS
PHYSICAL GROWTH
NCHS PERCENTILES*

Name_____ Record #_____

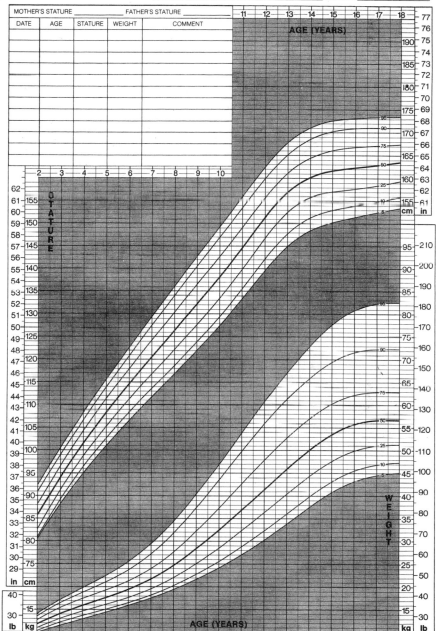

**BOYS: BIRTH TO 36 MONTHS
PHYSICAL GROWTH
NCHS PERCENTILES***

NAME_____   RECORD #_____

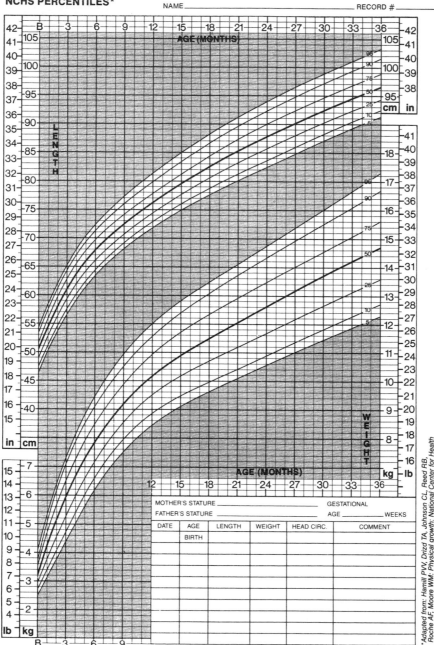

GIRLS: BIRTH TO 36 MONTHS
PHYSICAL GROWTH
NCHS PERCENTILES*

NAME_____ RECORD #_____

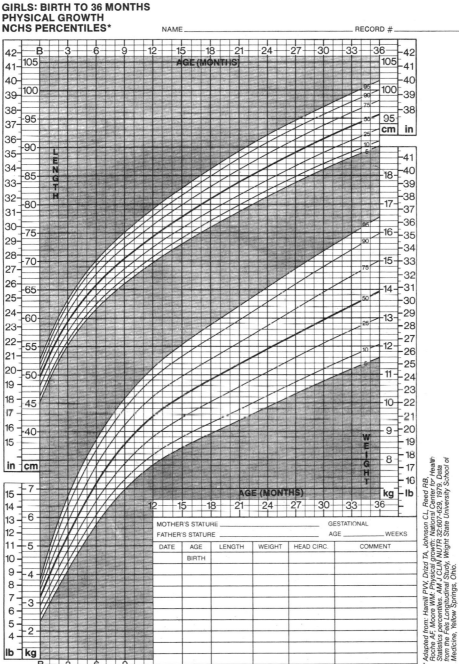

MOTHER'S STATURE _____ GESTATIONAL
FATHER'S STATURE _____ AGE _____ WEEKS

DATE	AGE	LENGTH	WEIGHT	HEAD CIRC.	COMMENT
	BIRTH				

* Adapted from: Hamill PVV, Drizd TA, Johnson CL, Reed RB, Roche AF, Moore WM: Physical growth: National Center for Health Statistics percentiles. AM J CLIN NUTR 32:607-629, 1979. Data from the Fels Longitudinal Study, Wright State University School of Medicine, Yellow Springs, Ohio.

© 1982 Ross Laboratories

Miscellaneous

This final section of the health record can be used to organize the written information you receive from health care providers and other sources that doesn't fit anywhere else. Information you may want to keep in this section includes:

- Diagnosis fact sheets given to you by your physician describing your child's illness.
- Medication fact sheets describing your child's medication and possible side effects.
- Information about physical and occupational therapy.
- Diet recommendations.
- Techniques to reduce pain or relieve morning stiffness.
- Information designed to help your child in school.

Chapter 7

•

Creating a Positive School Environment

Children spend a great deal of time in school, where they not only learn and absorb information but also develop the confidence and skills they will need to succeed as adults. Anything that interferes with a child's education, including a chronic illness, naturally poses a concern for parents.

The childhood rheumatic diseases don't impair a child's intellectual ability, but they can make it more difficult for children to function at their best in the structured environment of school. Fortunately, the problems that rheumatic illnesses cause for children in school can be overcome. Even children who have rather severe rheumatic illness attend school regularly and participate in a wide variety of activities with their classmates.

There are a number of steps you can take to help your child do well in school. The first, of course, is to understand just how the illness affects your child's ability to meet the routine demands of the school day. Parents and school personnel should work together to develop solutions that will allow the child to participate fully in school activities and achieve to the best of his ability. Often, this can be accomplished by making minor adjustments in routine school practices.

It's important to emphasize one point, and that is that *all children in the United States are entitled to a free, appropriate public education.* Federal and state laws require all public schools to provide whatever support and services are needed to help children with disabilities and chronic illnesses benefit from public education. The Education of the Handicapped Amendments of 1986 (P.L. 99-457, Part H) deal with educational services for children from birth to 3 years of age. Educational services for children aged 3 to 21 are covered by the Individuals with Disabilities Education Act of 1990 (IDEA).

This chapter describes the kinds of problems your child may encounter in school because of his rheumatic illness and offers suggestions for overcoming these difficulties. The federal and state laws governing public education are also described. The information in this chapter can help you to understand the basic provisions of the laws and to obtain services under these laws, if necessary. The process of obtaining services can be complicated and difficult, so you may wish to obtain more detailed information about this process from other resources, such as those listed in Appendix 2.

Good communication among students, parents, school personnel, and health care providers is essential to create a rewarding school environment. In this chapter we also suggest ways to make this communication more effective.

At the end of this chapter there are two checklists: one for your child to complete to identify problems he is having in school, and one that parents can use when developing a plan of school services and provisions. A variety of sample letters are included. These letters can be used as templates for your own letters to school staff. A telephone log for recording contacts with teachers and other school personnel is also included.

Reducing the Impact of Rheumatic Illness in School

You have probably heard it said that, as parents, you are your child's best advocates. This is certainly true. No one understands your child's needs and cares for him the way you do. Unlike health care providers and school personnel, you observe your child's activity in every area of his life. The dictionary defines an *advocate* as a person who acts on behalf of another individual to ensure that person's rights and proper treatment. By advocating for your child's needs in school, you can help to create a positive educational experience for him.

Before requesting assistance for your child, you need to identify his specific needs. You should, of course, ask him about any problems he is having in school. Some children, particularly younger ones, may have difficulty expressing their problems clearly, and you may need to ask very specific questions. A child may say that his teacher is mean or unfair. This can mean any number of things. Maybe the teacher *is* mean or unfair. Or maybe the child was disciplined for arriving late to class by a teacher who did not understand that he needs extra time to move from place to place within the school building. Older children may deny that they have any problems in school; they dislike being identified as "different" and may be unwilling to volunteer any information about school at all.

If your child is reluctant to go to school or is not achieving up to his potential, find out what the problems are. A checklist is provided at the end of this chapter that you and your child can use to help identify problems that occur in school. Talk with your child's teachers about problems they may have noticed. Visit the school and observe his classroom and other activity areas, such as the cafeteria, playground, library, and gym. Do this as unobtrusively as you can, on days when other parents are visiting the school if possible, to avoid embarrassing your child in front of his classmates.

Do not be discouraged by the number of *potential* school problems listed in this chapter. Most children who have rheumatic illnesses have only a few of these difficulties in school, and some have none at all. By keeping school personnel informed about your child's illness and needs, you can prevent a lot of problems from occurring in the first place, and quickly resolve those that do. With careful planning and good communication, most problems are easily resolved. There is every reason to expect that your child will have a rewarding and enjoyable school experience.

Two resources that are available from the Affiliated Children's Arthritis Centers of New England (see Appendix 2) may help school personnel to understand the special needs of children with rheumatic disease. The first, *Just One of the Kids*, is a videotape for teachers and school personnel that can be shown at a meeting with school staff to help explain what JRA is and how it affects school functioning. The other, *School Nurse Standards of Care for Children with Juvenile Rheumatoid Arthritis*, is a document that provides guidelines for the school nurse, who will play a large role in managing your child's health care needs in school.

Dealing with Variations in Symptoms and Need for Assistance

Children who have chronic rheumatic illnesses experience considerable variation in their symptoms from day to day, and even at different times during the same day. Because their symptoms fluctuate, their need for assistance in school will also change frequently. It is important to explain the variable nature of the disease to teachers and other school personnel. Otherwise, your child may be accused of faking his symptoms to avoid school activities he does not enjoy. Teachers should also realize that your child will not always need help with activities that are only difficult when symptoms are present. To encourage independence and build skills, children should only be given help when it is needed. There should be a simple mechanism in place to enable your child to get help when he needs it, without drawing undue attention to himself.

Establishing a Balance between Help and Independence

Many children who have rheumatic illnesses will need some help from teachers and classmates in school. Parents and teachers have the important responsibility of preparing children for full participation in an independent life as adults. As children develop, they are given increasing amounts of freedom and responsibility for taking care of themselves and making their own decisions. The same level of independence should be encouraged in dealing with problems caused by chronic illness or disability. At home, you provide clothing with fasteners your child can handle himself, rather than dressing him for school each morning. Similarly, teachers should provide tools and support that minimize the need for direct assistance, while making it possible for the student to keep up with his classmates. Doing things for the student should be avoided. Whenever possible, the environment should be changed to permit the student to do things for himself.

Assistance in school should be given for the purpose of increasing the student's ability to function independently, not for the convenience of teachers or to comply with the school's daily routines. For example, it may be easier or less expensive to excuse children with hand involvement from lengthy written assignments, but it is better to require the same amount of work and provide the tools needed (perhaps a computer) to get the work done. Instead of cutting out project pieces for a student, the art teacher should provide large-handled scissors that cut with less effort. Even when direct assistance is required, it should be viewed as improving independent function in another area. Helping a child get on or off the school bus makes it possible for him to attend school with his peers. As children get older, they should be given increasing responsibility for identifying areas of difficulty in school and developing their own solutions.

Creative Problem Solving

Later in this section, solutions are suggested for a variety of problems children might encounter in school, but you know better than anyone else how your own child responds to difficulties. Be creative in developing solutions that will work best for your child. Just because something has not been done before does not mean that it cannot work. One young child who had difficulty walking rode his tricycle around the school. He got to class on time, had access to all areas of the building, and got terrific exercise! Furthermore, his young classmates did not see him as being disabled, as they might have done if he had used a wheelchair. Children can be wonderfully creative. Ask your child to help think of ways to solve the problems he encounters.

School Policy and Exceptions to the Rule

Schools develop policies to establish the structure and discipline necessary to keep schools safe and promote a constructive learning environment. In school, there are regulations governing most aspects of student behavior, including areas such as acceptable dress, attendance, tardiness, and hallway, locker, and rest room use. All students are expected to abide by the regulations, and disciplinary action is taken against those who fail to do so. Because school policies are written to apply to the entire school population, they may fail to account for the special needs of a student who has a chronic illness or disability. For example, a regulation forbidding students to carry backpacks between classes should be relaxed for a student with arthritis for whom carrying heavy books in the arms is difficult or inadvisable. School policies do not carry the force of federal or state legislation and cannot be used to deny a child any rights to which he is entitled under federal or state law. The following example illustrates this point:

Lisa is a ninth-grade student who has JRA. She missed school on Friday because she had a clinic visit at the pediatric rheumatology center located 2 hours from her home. When Lisa arrived at the Homecoming Dance later that evening, she was not permitted to attend. School policy prohibits students from attending after-school activities on days when they are absent from school. Lisa's absence was legitimate, and she was well enough to attend the dance. By denying her admission, the school was guilty of discrimination against Lisa because of her disability. Lisa had been told, in effect, that she could not participate in a school activity because she had received necessary treatment for her medical condition. This strict application of school policy violated federal antidiscrimination statutes.

To avoid conflicts with school regulations, parents and students need to be intimately familiar with the policies in effect in their own schools and school districts. The school policy is usually published in a student handbook and distributed to students at the beginning of the school year. Contact your child's principal if you have not received a copy. Also ask about any unpublished rules and regulations. Review the policy with your child to identify potential problems. Meet with the principal to discuss exceptions to school policy for your child before a difficult situation arises. Any approved modification of school policy should be put in writing and kept in your child's student file.

Developmental Issues in School

A child's education does not begin when he turns 5 and enters kindergarten, nor does it end with graduation from high school. The early childhood years are spent developing important skills and independence that prepare a child for formal learning in school by the time he is 5 or 6. During high school, teenagers identify interests and sharpen skills in preparation for college or vocational training that will lead to successful and rewarding careers. Parents of a young child or teenager with a chronic rheumatic illness who are aware of the impact such an illness can have on school readiness, career choices, and career training are better able to help the child make the most of educational opportunities. At each stage of a child's life, parents need to pay attention not just to the issues relevant at that age level, but also to preparing the child for the next stage of development.

Infants and toddlers. Infants and toddlers who have JRA or other rheumatic illnesses can experience developmental delays that leave them unprepared to enter kindergarten with other children their age. Pain and stiffness in the hands make it more difficult for toddlers to learn to dress themselves and manipulate small objects like crayons and scissors. Involvement of the legs and feet interferes with walking. It is not uncommon for children with significant illness to remain dependent on their parents, both emotionally and for assistance with difficult tasks.

Early detection of developmental delays gives parents, health care providers, and educators the opportunity to intervene with services that can help the child catch up and avoid future delays. The type of intervention necessary depends on the child's particular needs. In many cases, all that is required is careful observation and encouragement toward independence. Other young children benefit from community recreation programs, play groups, or preschool. Physical, occupational, or speech therapy may also be required. A parent who is concerned about developmental delays or school readiness needs to discuss those concerns with the child's pediatrician or pediatric rheumatologist, or with a social worker.

Teenagers and young adults. The high school years are a period of transition between childhood and adult life. Teenagers are faced with difficult decisions regarding their future life of independence from parents. Teenagers who have rheumatic conditions need to consider the impact of their illness when making decisions about college, vocational training, and careers, but they should not limit their choices because of *unfounded* or *incorrect* beliefs about disabilities. Knowledgeable and sensitive guidance counselors can help high school students choose and prepare for appropriate careers. They can also help students select colleges that are equipped to meet the special needs of students with chronic illnesses or disabilities.

High school students and their parents should be familiar with federal and state laws regarding educational services and civil rights for teenagers and young adults. The Individuals with Disabilities Education Act of 1990 (IDEA) requires high schools to provide transition planning services for children 16 years of age or older. Civil rights laws, including the Rehabilitation Act of 1973 (P.L. 93-112) and the Americans with Disabilities Act (ADA), prohibit employers and adult education programs from discriminating against an individual on the basis of disability. (More information on these laws is provided later in this chapter.)

Specific Problems and Suggestions

Absences. Pediatric rheumatologists consider regular school attendance to be of such significance that they frequently use the number of days missed from school as a measure of treatment effectiveness. Children who have acute illnesses, like ear infections or strep throat, stay home to recuperate and to avoid passing the infection to classmates. Children who have chronic rheumatic illnesses, however, do not get better after a few days at home, and their illnesses are not contagious. Frequent or prolonged absences limit academic achievement and isolate children socially. They also prevent children from developing effective coping strategies. Children who attend school regularly learn to succeed despite their chronic health problems, whereas children who are kept at home learn to expect less of themselves.

This does not mean that children should just "tough it out" and go to school when they are not feeling well. You should work with school personnel and your child's health care providers to create a school environment that accommodates your child's needs. Of course, some absences cannot be avoided. The following suggestions may help your child avoid falling behind when he does miss school:

- Many children live a considerable distance from their specialty care center and must miss school on days when they have clinic visits. Because these absences are planned, your child can ask his teachers to give him that day's work in advance, so he can keep up with his classmates.
- At the beginning of a flare, a child may need a day or two to adjust to the change in his condition, and on exceptionally bad days he might not feel well enough to attend school. Call your child's teachers early in the day to ask for reading and other assignments that can be done at home. Consider sending your child to school for a part of the day, perhaps in the afternoon when stiffness has worn off, or in the morning if fatigue and endurance are problems later in the day.
- Occasionally, hospitalization may be necessary. You should work with your child's teachers to develop a plan to continue his education during any prolonged absence. Many school districts require an absence of 2 weeks or longer before they will provide tutoring. You may be able to arrange for home or hospital tutoring to begin earlier, at the school's expense, if your child has an Individualized Education Plan (IEP). (IEPs are discussed in greater detail in the next section.)
- Teachers should give students a reasonable amount of additional time to complete assignments missed because of illness.

Getting to and from school. Getting to and from school can be a problem for children who have difficulty walking. Some children have trouble getting on and off school buses, and some experience considerable pain from the jostling that occurs in crowded bus seats. You cannot be required to drive your child to and from school if he cannot walk or ride the school bus: your school must provide appropriate transportation. Even children who live within walking distance from school are entitled to transportation services if a medical condition makes walking difficult. Get a letter from your child's doctor that explains why alternative transportation is needed and what type of transportation is appropriate. Contact your school principal or other administrator to arrange appropriate transportation. Here are some suggestions for resolving transportation problems:

- When a child cannot ride a regular school bus, schools use cars or specially equipped vans to provide door-to-door service. Some schools contract with taxi companies to provide transportation for children who are able to ride in a car.
- If your child is able to ride the regular school bus but the bus stop is too far from home for him to walk, the bus can be rerouted to stop closer to your home or even at your home.
- If crowding is a problem, ask for a reserved seat near the front of the bus that your child can share with at most one other child (crowded buses frequently have three children in each seat). Safety regulations prohibit children from standing while the bus is in motion.
- Arrange to have the bus driver, an aide, or other responsible adult help your child on and off the bus.
- Arrange a visit to the bus company before the first day of school so your child can practice getting on and off the bus.

Getting around in school. In large schools, or in schools with more than one floor, children who have rheumatic illnesses often have difficulty getting to classes on time and using facilities like the library and cafeteria. Your child should have access to all areas of the school that are used by his classmates. Newer schools, and those that have recently undergone extensive remodeling, are required to be completely accessible to students with disabilities. School districts are not usually required to bring older buildings up to this level of accessibility if that would require expensive remodeling projects, such as the installation of elevators. A number of relatively simple modifications can make it easier for children to move between classes and access special areas of the school, however. They include the following:

- Children who need extra time should be given it. Perhaps all your child needs is an additional 5 minutes to move from one class to the next and to use his locker.
- Another student can walk with your child between classes to help with books and doors if necessary.
- Children who have difficulty using stairs should be given an elevator pass or key. If your child is very young or could not use the elevator safely on his own, he should be escorted by a teacher or aide. Older children should be allowed to use the elevator independently.
- Classes can be relocated to make it unnecessary for the child to walk long distances between classes and to specialty rooms, such as the library and cafeteria.
- Although wheelchair use is discouraged for children who have arthritis, children who otherwise cannot attend school should have use of a wheelchair during school.
- If your child has any difficulty at all moving about the school, school administrators should develop an emergency evacuation plan that will ensure that he gets out of the building safely in the event of fire or other emergency. The plan should be tested during routine fire drills. The plan should charge one or two responsible adults with the responsibility for seeing that the child has safely left the building.
- Short flights of stairs can be equipped with a ramp.
- All staircases should be equipped with sturdy hand railings.
- If the school building that your child would normally attend cannot be made accessible for him, the school district is required to provide an equivalent education at another school, and to transport him there, at no cost to the parents. This option should only be used when no other solution is available for keeping your child in his regular school.

Written assignments and homework. Rheumatic involvement of the hands and wrists can make it difficult for a child to hold a pencil properly or write for very long without tiring. This makes it hard to complete written assignments, and it can also affect a child's ability to do well on timed tests. For the same reason, children with hand involvement of rheumatic disease may not be able to complete projects that require coloring, painting, or cutting.

Being able to communicate clearly in writing is one of the most important skills children develop in school, but children who have difficulty with handwriting may not get enough writing practice to become proficient communicators. Although it can be helpful to eliminate some of the copying work children do in school, it is not a good idea *routinely* to shorten writing exercises or substitute oral assignments. All children need to learn how to take essay tests and write book reports and term papers. The following suggestions may be helpful for children who have trouble with writing:

- Children who need it should be given extra time to complete tests and in-school assignments.
- Built-up pens and pencils and inexpensive pencil grips can make writing easier for some children. Your child's occupational therapist can make specific recommendations and help locate the necessary equipment.
- Children who find it very difficult to write should have access to a computer and be trained in keyboard skills. When a child writes using a computer, he can develop his work from an outline and make corrections and revisions just as he would if he were writing on paper. Presenting reports orally does not develop the same skills. Even children in the earliest grades can begin to learn how to use a computer.

  Computer use offers the secondary benefit of exercise to keep the fingers from becoming stiff. In fact, the only drawback to using a computer is the expense. Many schools have computers available for students to use on a limited basis. Any child who has an illness that makes handwriting difficult should be given additional opportunities to use the school computers. Having an IEP is the best way (and sometimes the only way) to guarantee that a child has adequate access to a computer in school.
- A tape recorder can be used if a child has difficulty taking notes in class, but it will take the child or a helper extra time after school to make notes from the tapes. Alternatively, teachers or other students can provide copies of their own notes.
- Teachers can help students keep up with their classmates by taking some of the busy-work out of assignments. Teachers of young children can pre-cut small pieces or partially assemble difficult projects. (Larger, adult-type scissors are easier to use than most children's scissors, but their use by young children should be carefully supervised.) To help older students, teachers can copy worksheets and shorten practice assignments for subject areas in which the student excels.
- Oral reports and tests should be used infrequently in place of written reports and exams. They are most appropriately substituted when the student's writing difficulty is temporary.

You may wish to purchase a computer for your child's home use. Check newspapers and computer stores for bargains—used equipment may be available at considerable cost savings. Private organizations, including some Arthritis Foundation chapters, may have limited funds available to assist with the purchase of a computer. Unfortunately, computer purchases are not usually reimbursable by insurance companies. A number of computer programs are available that are designed to teach children how to type, including *Mario Teaches Typing* (Interplay Productions, Irvine, California) and *Mavis Beacon Teaches Typing* (The Software Toolworks, Novata, California).

Physical education class. Physical education classes help children develop strength and coordination, learn new sports, and learn to work as part of a team. They also provide valuable opportunities for social interaction. Children who have rheumatic illnesses should participate in regular physical education classes whenever possible, perhaps taking adaptive physical education in addition to regular gym classes. If a child is unable to participate in regular gym classes, he or she can be offered adaptive physical education classes.

Stiff, painful joints, fatigue, and limited endurance sometimes make it difficult for children to participate in gym classes of any kind. The following suggestions may make things easier:

- Children should be given extra time, if needed, for changing into gym clothes.
- Children should be allowed to set their own pace for strenuous activities.
- Physical education teachers can modify activities, or choose alternative activities, so that *all* members of the class can participate.
- If the school has a pool, extra swimming classes may be substituted for other types of activities.
- Adaptive physical education can help children gain the skills and confidence that will make them more comfortable in regular gym class.
- When participation in gym class is not practical, the child may be able to use the time to do a home therapy program and earn physical education credit for doing it.
- Children should be encouraged to participate in school and community sports programs. In addition to playing on the team, children may serve as team managers, scorekeepers, coaches, and referees. A child does not have to be a star player to enjoy the excitement and camaraderie of team sports.

Carrying books and the cafeteria tray. Children whose hands, arms, or shoulders are affected sometimes find it difficult to carry books and other heavy or bulky objects. You may be able to ease your child's burden by following these suggestions:

- Ask the school to provide a second set of books for your child to keep at home. In school, it may be easier for your child to keep his books in the classrooms where they are used rather than in his locker.
- If your child does not have shoulder involvement, suggest that he carry his books in a backpack. A backpack worn over both shoulders distributes the weight of heavy objects best. Avoid bags that are carried over one shoulder.
- Arrange to have a classmate help by carrying your child's lunch tray or other items, if necessary.

Dressing and using the bathroom. Personal hygiene problems can cause severe embarrassment if they are not handled with discretion and concern for the child's feelings. If your child has difficulty dressing or using the bathroom, make certain that school personnel are aware of his particular needs in advance. Review the school's plans for helping your child in these situations, to be sure that your child will not be unnecessarily embarrassed. In addition, you can:

- Provide clothing that is easy to put on and take off, like elastic-waist pants. Some children find zippers easier to manage than buttons. Velcro closures can be a big help, particularly on boots and shoes.
- In the winter, allow your child to keep a pair of shoes in his locker to wear after removing his boots. That way he won't have to carry an extra pair of shoes back and forth to school each day.
- Ask to have a chair placed near your child's locker so that he can sit to remove his boots. He can also use the chair to hold books and other items while he's using his locker.
- School bathrooms should have at least one stall that is handicapped accessible, with grab bars and a raised seat. For small children, the standard toilet seat is the proper height.
- If your child needs help using the bathroom, make arrangements for him to use the one in the nurse's office or faculty room so that he will have more privacy.

Field trips and other activities. Field trips and extracurricular activities are both fun and educational. Your child has a right to go on field trips with his class. Your child should also be able to participate in all regular school activities, such as assemblies, recess, and art and music programs. Many schools offer a variety of optional extracurricular activities. Help your child pick appropriate, optional activities that interest him. To avoid having your child miss out, try the following:

- Ask for early notification of field trips, preferably while the trips are being planned. This will help you identify any potential problems for your child and give school personnel time to develop solutions. Special transportation can be arranged to accommodate your child's needs. Walking and stair climbing can be minimized. An aide can accompany your child to help with other problems.
- Volunteer to chaperone for a field trip, but do not go on every field trip with your child. The school cannot require that you accompany your child on field trips.
- Visit your child's school to make sure that special activity areas, like the auditorium and playground, are accessible. If you discover that they are not, work with the school to overcome any barriers that exist.

Teasing and other social problems. The effects of rheumatic illnesses cannot always be seen, and they can vary from one day to the next. This can lead to teasing by children who may feel that the child with a rheumatic illness is given special attention. Your own child may feel uncomfortable talking about his illness with classmates. Special attention or assistive devices can cause embarrassment. He will probably go out of his way to fit in and be just like his classmates. The following suggestions can help make your child and his classmates more comfortable:

- Teach your child how to explain his illness. Provide simple answers to common questions. Holding practice sessions, where you play the role of a classmate, can help build your child's confidence.
- Some children write term papers or create projects that explain or incorporate information about their rheumatic condition. If this idea appeals to your child, you might want to cue a teacher to provide the appropriate assignment.
- Provide the teacher with copies of the *Learn About JRA* workbooks offered by the Affiliated Children's Arthritis Centers of New England (see Appendix 2). The series teaches elementary schoolchildren basic facts about arthritis and encourages them to be sensitive about people's individual differences. Separate workbooks are provided for kindergarten through grade 2, grades 3 to 5, and grades 6 to 8. Teachers' guides are also available.
- Suggest that the school invite a representative from the local Arthritis Foundation chapter to the school to present a *Kids on the Block* puppet show about childhood arthritis. Many chapters have trained volunteers who can do this, and there is usually no charge for this program. Lesson plans and a coloring book entitled *Yard Sale* for third and fourth graders are available from the American Juvenile Arthritis Organization (see Appendix 2).

• If your child is upset about teasing and has been unable to solve the problem himself, ask his teacher to intervene in an appropriate way. It is not usually productive to contact the other child's parents. This can escalate a problem, and your own child may feel like a snitch. If the problem is serious, however, you may need to involve the school's administrators to resolve the problem.

Medications at school. Most schools have policies that prohibit children from taking medicine at school unless there is a written note from the child's doctor on file. Even then, in most cases the medicine must be kept in the nurse's office and administered by the nurse or another member of the school staff. If your child must take medicine in school, you cannot be required to come to the school each day to give it to him. You *are* required to supply the school with any medications your child needs. Following these precautions can help to ensure that your child's medicine is administered properly:

• Some medications are available in "long-lasting" or "time-released" forms. Ask your child's doctor if there is another form of the medication that can be given in fewer doses to avoid the need for the medication to be taken during school hours.

• Ask the school nurse for extra copies of the school's medication permission form. Keep the extras in your personal health record and take them with you to clinic visits. If the doctor changes your child's medications or dosages, he or she can complete the new medication form at the same time. You will be able to keep your child's school medications up to date and will avoid the extra effort required to obtain signed medication forms after returning home.

• Make sure that the school has identified a back-up person to administer your child's medications on days when the school nurse is absent.

• Provide the school nurse with information on medication side effects and indications of an overdose. Make sure that the school nurse knows what to do in case of an adverse drug reaction.

• Provide the school nurse with juice or other foods that your child uses at home to make it easier for him to take his medications.

Physical or occupational therapy during school. Children who have IEPs can receive physical and occupational therapy in school if they have a documented, educational need for these services. More information about obtaining services under an IEP is provided in the next section. Following these procedures may help to ensure the delivery of appropriate physical and occupational therapy services:

- Ask the therapists at your child's pediatric rheumatology center to provide specific exercises for your child's school therapy program.
- Provide your school-based therapists with copies of *Physical Therapy Practice Guidelines for Children with Chronic Arthritis* and *Occupational Therapy Practice Guidelines for Children with Chronic Arthritis*, developed by the Affiliated Children's Arthritis Centers of New England (see Appendix 2).
- Encourage communication between your rheumatology center and school-based therapists. Provide addresses and phone numbers. Ask your child's therapists to share evaluations with the therapists at the school or the clinic.
- Make sure that the school provides an appropriate location for the delivery of therapy services as well as providing all necessary equipment. The location should provide privacy.
- Schedule school therapy sessions to avoid taking children out of important classes.

Pain and stiffness. Rheumatic illness can make it hard for a child to perform all of the activities required during the school day. Try these techniques for accommodating pain and stiffness:

- If your child has significant morning stiffness, wake him up early enough to take a warm bath and do stretching exercises before going to school.
- If your child develops stiffness after sitting for a long time at his desk, ask the teacher to provide opportunities for him to get up and move around the classroom. The child can distribute papers or run errands to relieve stiffness. It may help to locate his desk at the end of a row, near the back of the classroom, so he can stand and stretch as needed without disturbing classmates.
- Your child's desk and chair should fit him properly so that he can sit comfortably.
- If your child has stiffness in his neck, a book rest can be used to hold reading materials at a comfortable angle on the desk.
- If painful joints or poor balance make your child uncomfortable in crowds, ask that he be allowed to go to his locker and change classes a few minutes early, when the halls are less crowded. A locker located at the end of the row will give him more room to maneuver.
- If your child tires easily, arrange for a short rest period during the day.
- Arrange for your child to have help opening milk cartons and other packaged lunch foods if it is needed.

Resources for Training and Information

To help their children who have chronic rheumatic illnesses obtain an appropriate education, parents need to be educated about programs, services, and the laws related to educational and civil rights. At first all of this may seem overwhelming, and there's no question that there *is* a lot to learn. But there are a variety of excellent resources available to help parents develop the knowledge and skills needed to advocate effectively for their children's educational needs.

The Statewide Parent Information Network (SPIN), funded by a grant from the U.S. Office of Special Education, provides a variety of services to help parents advocate for their children's educational needs. SPIN programs include basic and advanced workshops on special education laws, IEP clinics where parents receive individual technical assistance with their children's IEPs, and information and referral services by phone. SPIN projects also provide extensive training to prepare interested parents for roles as Parent Consultants and volunteer educational advocates. The SPIN project in your state may be able to help you locate a volunteer advocate if you are having difficulty dealing with the school system. The SPIN project is coordinated by the Federation for Children with Special Needs in Boston, Massachusetts, with Parent Training and Information (PTI) Centers in most states.

The American Juvenile Arthritis Organization (AJAO) offers a *Partners in Education* workshop as part of its Partnership Training Program. The workshop focuses on the abilities of children with rheumatic illnesses, and provides information on educational rights and entitlements as well as training in communication skills. *Partners in Education* training is available to parents through most Arthritis Foundation chapters at no charge, or for a minimal fee (10 to 15 dollars) to cover the cost of the workshop materials. It may also be offered at the annual national conferences of the AJAO. Contact your local Arthritis Foundation chapter for additional information.

There are also a number of excellent books, pamphlets, and manuals on educational rights, special education laws, and effective communication and advocacy techniques. Listed in Appendix 2 are references and the addresses of the organizations named above as well as other agencies that provide educational services or information.

Federal and State Laws Governing Education and Civil Rights

A number of federal laws protect the educational rights of children who have chronic illnesses and disabilities. These laws overlap in many areas, and they do not all apply to every child who has a rheumatic illness. The following guidelines can help you determine which laws are applicable to your child's situation. Parents should rely on the Individuals with Disabilities Education Act of 1990 (IDEA) to obtain a free, appropriate public education for children who require special education and related services. The Education of the Handicapped Amendments of 1986 (P.L. 99-457, Part H) can be used to obtain assessment, case management, and, in some states, intervention services for children from birth to 3 years of age who have developed or are at risk of having developmental delays. Both Section 504 of the Rehabilitation Act of 1973 and the Americans with Disabilities Act provide various protections against discrimination on the basis of disability. In most cases, parents should seek protection against discrimination in public education through the provisions of Section 504 of the Rehabilitation Act. Additional information on each of these laws is provided in this section. Before parents make decisions or take any action, however, we strongly advise them to obtain more detailed information from the resources listed in Appendix 2.

State laws regulating regular and special education vary so much from one state to another that it is not possible to provide detailed descriptions here. Suffice it to say that, no matter where you live, there are important provisions of state laws that you should be aware of when planning for your child's education. Obtain information about these provisions from your state's Department of Education.

Individuals with Disabilities Education Act of 1990

The Individuals with Disabilities Education Act of 1990 (IDEA, P.L. 94-142) guarantees a free, appropriate public education for all children with disabilities. IDEA is an amended version of the Education of All Handicapped Children Act (P.L. 94-142), which was passed by congress in 1975. Before the passage of the earlier law, it was not uncommon for children with disabilities to receive inadequate educational services or, in some cases, no educational services at all. IDEA ensures that children with disabilities have access to educational services that meet their individual needs in such a way as to provide educational opportunity equal to that offered to children without disabilities.

IDEA eligibility requirements. Children between the ages of 3 and 21 who have disabilities that affect their ability to benefit from regular public education programs are entitled to services under IDEA. IDEA defines eligible children as those who are:

> Mentally retarded, hard of hearing, deaf, speech impaired, visually handicapped, seriously emotionally disturbed, orthopedically impaired, other health impaired, deaf-blind, multi-handicapped, or as having specific learning disabilities, who because of those impairments need special education and related services.

It is important to note that disability alone does not qualify a child for services under IDEA. The disability must be related to an educational need. Children who have chronic rheumatic illnesses can qualify for IDEA under the orthopedic impairment or other health impairment categories.

Provisions of IDEA. IDEA entitles children with special needs to the following:

- *Free, appropriate public education.* States are required to provide a free, appropriate public education for children with special educational needs. To be "appropriate," educational services must meet the student's individual needs. These services must be "free"—that is, provided without charge to the student or his family.

- *Identification of children with special educational needs.* School districts are responsible for identifying, locating, and evaluating children with special educational needs. School districts conduct annual screening programs to identify the needs of children who are just beginning school. Teachers, parents, and others may refer any child suspected of having special educational needs for further evaluation.

- *Comprehensive evaluation.* Children identified through routine screening and those referred for evaluation are entitled to a comprehensive evaluation that may include cognitive and psychological assessments; medical assessment; evaluation by physical, occupational, or speech therapists; and other assessments necessary to identify a child's individual needs. These assessments are conducted by school personnel or professionals selected and compensated by the school. When parents disagree with the assessments, they are entitled to an independent evaluation by professionals of their own choice at school expense. A school may initiate a due process hearing to show that the original evaluations are appropriate. If the hearing officer finds in favor of the school, parents are still entitled to obtain independent evaluations, but at their own expense.

- *Individualized Education Plan (IEP).* Children are entitled to an educational plan that meets their specific individual needs. All services and program modifications required to address the student's individual needs must be listed in the IEP. The IEP must also indicate who is responsible for providing services; when, where, and how often the services are to be provided; specific educational goals and objectives; and methods for evaluating student progress. All services identified in the IEP must be provided. The child's needs, not the availability of services or funding, determine the elements of the IEP.

- *Timeliness.* The school has 10 days to respond to a referral, and 30 days to complete evaluations after permission for the evaluations has been obtained from the parents. The IEP must be written within 30 calendar days after the child is found to need special education and related services. The IEP must be implemented with no undue delay after it is approved by the child's parents.

- *Parent participation.* Parents must give approval before an evaluation for special needs can be conducted, and parents must approve the IEP before services can be provided. Parental consent for evaluation and service delivery is voluntary and may be revoked at any time. Parents must be given the opportunity to meet with the planning team and participate in the IEP planning process.

- *Annual review.* A child's IEP must be reviewed at least once a year and must be updated to reflect the child's current educational needs. Parents may request a review at any time.

- *Equal opportunity.* Children with special educational needs are entitled to services that provide educational opportunity equal to that available to students without special educational needs. This provision applies to school-sponsored extra-curricular and social activities, resources, and transportation as well as to academic programs.

- *Least restrictive environment.* Children are entitled to receive educational services in the least restrictive environment possible. To the maximum extent possible, children must be educated with peers who have no special educational needs.

- *Related services.* Schools must provide related services that are necessary to meet a child's special educational needs and that are specified in the IEP. Related services include services such as appropriate transportation and physical, occupational, and speech therapy.

- *Assistive devices.* Schools are required to provide assistive devices that are necessary to meet a child's special educational needs and that are listed in the IEP. This provision does not apply to personal items such as eyeglasses, hearing aids, splints, or crutches.

- *Student records.* Parents have a right to review and copy records, and they can request that erroneous or misleading information be removed or amended. Student records are confidential. Parental consent must be given before information contained in student records is shared with individuals outside the school system or with school personnel who have no legitimate interest in the student.

- *Transition planning.* The IEP of students aged 16 years or older must include a statement of needed transition services, including the names of the agencies responsible for providing the services. IDEA does not provide an entitlement to services needed to accomplish an appropriate transition from public education, but it does require identification of the types of services necessary and agencies capable of providing those services.

- *Due process.* Students and their parents are entitled to have settled in a court of law any disputes regarding the appropriateness of the IEP or failure to implement the IEP. Parents' rights to access and amend student records, keep records confidential, obtain independent evaluations, and revoke consent are similarly protected. Other options for managing complaints include mediation and Department of Education hearings.

Obtaining services. The first step in obtaining services under IDEA is to set up a referral for evaluation of the child's need for special education services. If the child has not been referred for an evaluation by a teacher or other member of the school staff, the parent should make the referral. The referral should be made in writing and be addressed to the Director of Special Education in the child's school district. The letter should indicate the types of evaluations needed, and request that copies of all evaluation reports be sent to the parents.

You may wish to request a pre-evaluation conference to talk with school personnel about which evaluations are necessary, who will be doing them, and how and when they will be conducted. You must give written consent before the evaluations can be done. If you disagree with any evaluation, you are entitled to an independent evaluation at the school's expense.

Once the evaluations are complete, an IEP planning committee or team will meet to determine the need for special education and to develop the IEP. Members of the team include you, a school administrator, your child's teacher, the child himself if he is of an appropriate age, and any or all of the individuals who conducted the evaluations. You may also bring a member of your child's health care team, a friend or relative for support, an advocate, or anyone else you choose to the IEP planning meeting. The result of the meeting may be a finding of no need for special education services or the development of an IEP that identifies the special education and related services that will be provided.

After the IEP is completed you will be given a copy of the IEP and a consent form. The IEP cannot be implemented until you give written consent. You may reject all or part of an IEP. Provisions that you accept must be implemented without unnecessary delay. The IEP planning team may reconvene to consider any disputed issues. If you cannot reach agreement with the IEP planning team, a number of complaint management options are available. These are discussed in the next section.

The IEP must be reviewed at least annually and updated as necessary to meet the student's changing needs for special education and related services. Changes to the IEP or discontinuation of services are subject to the same parental review and consent as the initial IEP process. You are entitled to receive periodic progress reports that can help alert you to any need for a change in services.

Sample letters for requesting evaluations, records, IEP planning team meetings, and mediation or due process hearings are provided at the end of this chapter.

The complaint management system. IDEA provides both parents and school districts the option of instituting due process hearings to resolve disputes regarding eligibility for special education and related services or the provisions included in the IEP. In addition, the U.S. Education Department General Administrative Regulation (34 C.F.R. 76) requires each state education agency to adopt written procedures for "receiving and resolving" complaints of noncompliance with any of the federal education statutes, including IDEA. Many states have also established mediation and arbitration procedures that can be utilized to resolve complaints if both parties (the parents and the school district) consent. Finally, parents may also file complaints under Section 504 of the Rehabilitation Act of 1973, which prohibits discrimination on the basis of disability. Here are the options available to you for complaint resolution:

- *Complaints filed with the state education agency.* Parents may file a complaint with the state education agency when the school district violates, or is about to violate, any requirement of IDEA. The complaint must be made in writing and must detail the nature of the violation. The state education agency has 60 days to investigate and resolve the complaint. If parents are dissatisfied with the state education agency's resolution, they may request review by the U.S. Secretary of Education. If they continue to be dissatisfied, parents may initiate a due process hearing.
- *Mediation.* Mediation is an informal proceeding in which a trained mediator will try to help the parents and the school reach agreement. The mediator cannot impose a decision on either party. If mediation fails to achieve an agreement, the parents or the school may initiate a due process hearing.
- *Arbitration.* When a parent and school district agree to arbitration, both parties waive their right to a due process hearing. An arbitrator will be assigned to consider both parties' arguments and make a decision. The decision of the arbitrator is binding and final.
- *Due process hearing.* Both a parent and the school district have the right to initiate a due process hearing. A due process hearing must be requested in a written letter to the school district. If the school district initiates the due process hearing, parents must be informed in writing. The state education agency may conduct the hearing, which can then be appealed to a state or federal court. In

some states, the local school district may conduct the initial hearing, which can then be appealed to the state education agency, and then to state or federal courts.

Unless it is appealed, the hearing officer's decision is considered to be final and is binding on both the parents and the school district. Written notice of the hearing officer's decision must be mailed to both parties within 45 days after receipt of the request for a hearing. Parents may be entitled to reimbursement for lawyers' fees if the decision is in their favor.

Education of the Handicapped Amendments of 1986

Public Law 99-457 (Part H) is federal legislation that addresses the early intervention needs of infants and toddlers with disabilities. Part H services are intended to minimize the impact of early childhood problems on a child's development and his ability to benefit from public education when he reaches school age. P.L. 99-457 (Part H) encourages the development and implementation of a "statewide, comprehensive, coordinated, multidisciplinary, interagency program of early intervention services for handicapped infants and toddlers and their families."

Each state will develop its own plan for providing early intervention services. State plans must be approved by the U.S. Department of Education before they can be implemented. Currently, many states offer assessment and care coordination for children who qualify for services under P.L. 99-457 (Part H).

Eligibility requirements. P.L. 99-457 (Part H) applies to children from birth to 3 years of age. Children and their families are eligible for services if the child is "experiencing developmental delays" or if the child has a "diagnosed physical or mental condition that has a high probability of resulting in a developmental delay." An infant or toddler who has a rheumatic illness that limits his ability to walk or perform other activities typical of children his age would qualify under this provision. In some states, children who are at risk of developmental delay because of early life experiences, such as extreme poverty or disruptions in family life, are also eligible for Part H services.

Planning early intervention services. After an initial screening to determine eligibility, an Individualized Family Service Plan (IFSP) is developed for each child found to have, or to be at risk for, developmental delays. The IFSP is developed with input from families and agency staff. Families and staff share information that will assist parents in making an informed decision about the early intervention services they desire. It is important to note that parents, not agencies, make the final decisions about the services they wish to incorporate in the IFSP. Services will vary from state to state but can include a variety of early childhood enrichment programs (for example, Head Start, preschool, play groups), therapeutic services (physical, occupational, or speech therapy), and counseling services. A case manager from the early intervention program is assigned to help the family locate and gain access to services.

Obtaining services. Contact the Department of Education or Department of Public Health for more information about specific services and entitlements under your state's plan for implementation of P.L. 99-457 (Part H). You may be entitled to planning services that result in the development of the IFSP, but you may not be specifically entitled to the services named in the plan. In some cases, you will be placed on a waiting list for services that are available for only a limited number of children. The social worker in your pediatric rheumatology center and local Parent Training and Information Centers can provide additional information on application procedures and services.

Section 504 of the Rehabilitation Act of 1973

Section 504 of the Rehabilitation Act of 1973 (P.L. 93-112) protects a child's right to a free, appropriate public education by prohibiting discrimination against students who have disabilities. Section 504 of the Rehabilitation Act of 1973 provides that "no otherwise qualified handicapped individual ... shall, solely by reason of her handicap, be excluded from the participation in, be denied the benefits of, or be subjected to discrimination under any program or activity receiving federal financial assistance."

When this law was first passed in 1973, it applied only to discrimination in employment practices. The Rehabilitation Act Amendments of 1974 (P.L. 93-516) extended protection against discrimination to all areas of civil rights, including elementary and secondary education; postsecondary education, vocational training, and employment; and health, welfare, and other social service programs. The Rehabilitation Act and its amendments apply only to programs receiving federal financial assistance.

This section deals primarily with the application of Section 504 protections for students in elementary and secondary schools. Postsecondary education and vocational training are covered to a lesser degree. More information about the Rehabilitation Act of 1973 is available from the U.S. Department of Education, Office for Civil Rights.

Definition of disability. To qualify for protection from discrimination under Section 504, children must satisfy the definition of "handicapped individual" provided in the law. Section 504 defines a handicapped individual as any individual who:

- Has a physical or mental impairment that substantially limits one or more major life activities.
- Has a record of such an impairment.
- Is regarded as having such an impairment.

Children with JRA or other rheumatic illnesses who have significant difficulty walking, caring for themselves, or participating in school satisfy this definition.

Schools and other institutions covered by the law. All public elementary and secondary schools that receive federal financial assistance are required to provide a free, appropriate public education to all children living in their school districts. In addition to regular education programs, public schools must provide special education programs and related aids and services to meet the individual needs of children with disabilities. Nearly all public school systems accept federal funding.

Private elementary and secondary schools that receive federal assistance are required to admit students with disabilities who are able to participate in the school's regular programs with minor modifications. These schools are not required to develop special education programs to meet the needs of individual students. Private schools that operate without federal financial assistance are not covered by Section 504.

Postsecondary and vocational education programs that receive federal financial assistance are prohibited from discriminating against individuals with disabilities who meet the academic and technical admission requirements for their programs. These programs cannot discriminate in the areas of recruitment practices, admissions, housing, course selection, recreation, transportation, and others. Students with disabilities must be given an equal opportunity to participate in and benefit from programs offered in these settings.

Section 504 applies to preschools and day care facilities that receive federal financial assistance. Preschools and day care facilities must take into account the special needs of children with disabilities in determining what assistance and services are offered to participants in their programs.

Definition and requirements of "free, appropriate public education." A "free, appropriate public education" must provide educational opportunities to students with disabilities which are equal to those offered to other students. Public elementary and secondary schools are required to make regular education programs accessible to students with disabilities, and to provide special education, support services, and related services (such as physical and occupational therapy) that are necessary to meet the student's individual needs. These services must be provided at no cost to the students' families. Specific requirements of a "free, appropriate public education" include:

- Public elementary and secondary schools must provide a "free, appropriate public education" for all school-aged children in their school districts regardless of the extent of the disability.
- The needs of a student with a disability must be met to the same extent as the needs of students with no disabilities.
- A student's individual needs may be met through a combination of regular education services, special education services, related services (such as transportation and physical and occupational therapy), and assistive equipment.
- Students who have disabilities must be educated with students without disabilities to the maximum extent that is appropriate.
- Students who have disabilities must be given equal opportunity to participate in extracurricular activities such as recreational sports, clubs, and field trips.
- Schools must establish nondiscriminatory methods for evaluating the performance of students with disabilities.
- Schools must conduct periodic re-evaluations to ensure that a student's individual needs continue to be met.
- Schools must conduct annual screening evaluations to identify children whose individual needs are not being met.
- If a school cannot meet the individual needs of a student, placement in another public or private school is permitted. The student's home school district is responsible for all costs associated with services received in another setting, including tuition, room and board, and transportation.
- The school cannot charge a fee for any services required to provide an appropriate public education for a student who has a disability, except for those fees that are also charged to students with no disabilities. For example, a student who has a disability would have to pay the same fee to cover field trip costs as all other students. If the school incurs additional transportation costs for the student with a disability, it cannot pass those costs on to the student or his family.
- Schools are only required to make structural modifications to existing facilities (such as the installation of an elevator) when there are no other means of making programs equally accessible. Nonstructural modifications that have the effect of segregating individuals with disabilities are not acceptable. For example, a school would be allowed to relocate first-grade classes and activities to an architecturally accessible area of the school to accommodate the individual needs of a first grader with disabilities. The school would not be allowed to

create a separate lunchroom for students with disabilities who are not able to reach the cafeteria.

Requirements for postsecondary education programs. Postsecondary education programs include two- and four-year colleges, trade schools, and other adult education programs. Section 504 prohibits federally assisted postsecondary education programs from discriminating against individuals who have disabilities. Unlike public primary and secondary education programs, postsecondary programs have no obligation to identify students who have disabilities. In fact, Section 504 prohibits preadmission inquiries into an applicant's disability status. Postsecondary students with disabilities who require services or accommodations bear the responsibility for making their needs known. Specific requirements for postsecondary programs include the following:

- Students who meet the academic and technical requirements for admission cannot be denied admission because of disability.
- Students who have disabilities must have an equal opportunity to participate in and benefit from all programs and activities.
- All programs and activities must be offered in the most integrated setting possible.
- Students who have disabilities must be given an equal opportunity to participate in housing programs. Housing must be accessible, and it must be comparable in convenience and cost to that which is available to students without disabilities.
- Students who have disabilities must be given an equal opportunity to benefit from financial assistance programs.
- Students who have disabilities must be given an equal opportunity to participate in job placement programs. Guidance offered by career counseling services must be based strictly on students' abilities and interests, without regard to disability.

Procedures for filing a complaint of discrimination. If you believe that a school covered by Section 504 has discriminated against your child because of his disability, you should file a complaint with your regional Office for Civil Rights of the Department of Education. Your complaint should include the following information:

- The name of the child discriminated against
- A description of the discriminatory act and the date that it occurred
- The name of the school you believe to be guilty of discrimination
- Names, addresses, and phone numbers (yours and the school's)

- Other information that you believe to be relevant to your complaint
- Your signature

Complaints must be made in writing. You can contact the regional Office for Civil Rights by phone for help in preparing the complaint. Unless you obtain an extension, complaints must be filed within 180 days of the discriminatory act.

Americans with Disabilities Act of 1990

The Americans with Disabilities Act (ADA, P.L. 101-336) provides protection against discrimination on the basis of disability in a number of areas where Section 504 of the Rehabilitation Act does not apply. (Section 504 protections apply only to schools and other agencies that receive federal financial assistance.) ADA, however, provides few additional protections in the area of education. In most cases, IDEA and Section 504 of the Rehabilitation Act should be used to obtain educational services for children who have chronic illnesses or disabilities. ADA is described only briefly in this section. Additional information about ADA is available from the U.S. Department of Justice.

ADA is divided into five sections referred to as "Titles." Each Title addresses a different area of responsibility for compliance with ADA regulations, as described below:

- *Title I: Employment.* Employers with fifteen or more employees cannot discriminate against individuals on the basis of disability in hiring and promotion practices. Covered employers must provide "reasonable accommodations" for employees who have disabilities.
- *Title II: State and Local Governments.* Departments and agencies of state and local governments cannot discriminate against individuals on the basis of disability in any programs or services they provide, regardless of whether they receive federal financial assistance. Facilities, services, and communications must be accessible, as defined by Section 504 of the Rehabilitation Act.
- *Title III: Public Accommodations.* Places where private entities conduct business or offer services to the public are considered places of public accommodation. These include retail stores, restaurants, hotels, theaters, doctors' offices, day care facilities, private schools, and many others. Public accommodations cannot discriminate against individuals on the basis of disability. Public accommodations must provide necessary aids and services to individuals with disabilities, unless this would result in an "undue burden." Physical barriers to accessibility must be removed, if removal is "readily achievable." New construction must be accessible. Religious organizations are not covered by Title III. Private clubs

are only covered to the extent that their facilities are made available to the public.

- *Title IV: Telecommunications.* Companies that provide telephone service to the general public must provide services to individuals who have hearing impairments.
- *Title V: Transportation.* New public buses, train cars, and stations must be accessible. Where existing bus or train services are not accessible, public transportation systems must provide comparable special transportation services for individuals with disabilities, unless this would result in an "undue burden" on the public system. Air travel is covered by the Air Carrier Access Act, not by ADA.

Individuals are covered by ADA if they satisfy the definition of disability established by Section 504 of the Rehabilitation Act. In addition, individuals who have a known association or relationship with a person who satisfies the Section 504 definition are covered by Titles I and III. This provision protects the families and other associates of individuals with disabilities from discrimination. For example, an employer cannot refuse to hire someone whose child has a disability because of a concern that the potential employee would frequently be absent from work to care for the child.

ADA generally requires only "reasonable accommodation" to the needs of individuals with disabilities. Accommodations that are very costly or those that would require changes in the essential nature of a service are not required. Similarly, accommodations that would place an "undue burden" on an agency or business and those that are not "readily achievable" are not required. These terms are specifically defined in the language of ADA.

State Education Regulations

Regular and special education services are also regulated by state laws. States that accept federal funding for public education—and most do—cannot enforce regulations that provide a level of service less than that required by federal legislation. Some state laws provide more educational services and protections for children with disabilities than federal laws require. In these states, the higher standard established by the state applies. For example, IDEA requires public schools to provide services that are necessary for a child to "benefit" from his educational program. Massachusetts state law requires schools to provide services that "assure maximum possible development" for children with special needs. In Massachusetts, public schools are held to the higher state standard when developing IEPs for students with special educational needs.

Each state has different laws. You should obtain a copy of your own state's regular and special education regulations from the state department of education. The state laws define the specific procedures parents must follow to obtain educational services for children who have chronic illnesses or disabilities. They also include definitions of terms you will need to know, the types of services available, eligibility requirements, and procedures for filing complaints. The address for the Department of Education in your state can be found in the blue "Government" section of your telephone book (look under "Education").

Strategies for Effective Communication

Parents are often intimidated at the prospect of meeting with teachers and principals, particularly if an earlier meeting has gone poorly. It may help parents to know that teachers and principals frequently have similar concerns about meetings with parents. It is normal to feel apprehensive in any unfamiliar setting, and even more so when matters as important as your child's educational plan are being discussed. Remember, you are as much an expert on your child's needs as school personnel are about educational theory and practices. Your insights and suggestions are just as important as the teacher's. Good teachers and administrators will welcome your input.

Unfortunately, meetings between parents and school personnel do not always go as well as we would wish. Conflicts arise when there is disagreement over the amount and type of services a child needs. Parents who are skilled in negotiation and communication techniques are better able to avoid conflicts in the first place, and can help to re-establish a spirit of cooperation when conflicts do arise. These skills are based on courtesy and common sense, and can be learned without much difficulty. *Getting to Yes,* by Roger Fisher and William Ury, is an excellent short book that teaches easy-to-use techniques for resolving all types of disagreements. Here are some specific strategies for more effective communication:

Do not respond out of anger. We frequently say and do things when we are angry that we regret later. Certainly, an angry response will put others on the defensive and make future cooperation more difficult. Anger is a legitimate emotion, however, and you should let others know when you are unhappy with their proposals. The best way to deal with anger is to take time out to regain your composure and reconsider your strategy. If you are in a meeting, ask for a short break to give everyone a chance to calm down, or suggest that the meeting be rescheduled for a later date. Use the time to collect your facts and develop a rational response to any objections that have been raised against your recommendations.

Be prepared. Before calling or meeting with school officials, collect all information that is relevant to the topic under discussion. Prepare a list of the specific issues you wish to address and write down any questions you have. Make sure that you are familiar with school regulations and state and federal laws regarding educational rights and discrimination. If you are properly prepared, you will save yourself and school personnel valuable time and will ensure that important issues are not forgotten.

Avoid confrontational language and finger pointing. A negotiation is not a disciplinary proceeding. Your goals are to obtain the services your child needs and to change the attitudes and practices that interfere with his education. Placing blame on teachers and administrators is counter-productive. Instead of saying "You are not giving my child the help he needs," say, "My child is having difficulty in school and needs more help with (identify specific needs)."

Respect the professional expertise of teachers and other school personnel.   Remember that your child's teachers and other school personnel have completed formal training in educational theory and practices. They may also have many years of professional experience. Their opinions and suggestions should be given careful consideration. This does not mean that you should always accept their recommendations or that they are always right. You are the expert on your own child. You should be treated with the same level of respect, and your recommendations should be given equal consideration.

Be open to compromise.   There often is more than one solution to a problem. If you are willing to compromise, you can often get services started sooner and maintain good will with school personnel. Remember, though, that a compromise requires give and take on both sides. It is not a compromise if you are the only one giving up something. Furthermore, you should not accept a compromise that fails to meet your child's needs. There can be honest disagreement over necessary services.

One possible compromise is an agreement to implement services recommended by the school for a short trial period followed by an evaluation to determine whether they were effective. Your compromise agreement should specify the length of the trial period and clearly define expected results and evaluation techniques. The agreement should also include an alternative plan for providing services if the trial is not successful.

Do not delay. Problems tend to get bigger if they are not dealt with right away, and your child will spend a longer time struggling without assistance if you delay. Failure to take prompt action when a problem arises can give school personnel the impression that you do not believe the problem is serious or warrants their attention. Furthermore, special education regulations establish strict timetables for developing an IEP and implementing services. Always return phone calls and answer letters promptly.

Follow proper channels. Always try to solve a problem by working with the person most directly involved. Contact your child's teacher about problems that occur in the classroom. If the problem is related to building accessibility, transportation, school policy, or routine school practices, work with the principal. Do not involve a staff person's supervisor unless you cannot reach a satisfactory agreement otherwise. Unnecessarily "going over someone's head" threatens that person professionally and can make future interactions more difficult for both of you. You should involve a supervisor when the person you are dealing with is uncooperative or does not have the authority to approve necessary services or program modifications. The usual chain of command is teacher, principal, special education director (if your child receives special education services), superintendent of schools, school board, state department of education, federal agencies.

Get all agreements in writing. Get a written description of all services your child will receive and any modifications in his school plan or exceptions to school policy. If your child receives services under the Individuals with Disabilities Education Act (IDEA), you will receive a formal Individualized Education Plan (IEP). Services that are provided under less formal agreements should also be documented in writing. It is a good idea to write letters to request services or other accommodations, or to schedule meetings, instead of relying on the phone. When you do communicate by phone, follow up with a short note to the person you spoke with, summarizing the content of your conversation, any agreements reached, and any further action that is to be taken. Keep a copy of such letters for your records.

Keep complete and accurate records. In addition to keeping documentation of your child's current educational services, you should save records of previous services, evaluations, and all letters related to school services written by you, school representatives, and members of your child's health care team. Use the telephone log at the end of this chapter to record the dates and important details of phone conversations with school personnel.

Emphasize the educational, rather than the medical, need for services. Remember that schools are not required to provide services to address strictly medical needs, although some services that are necessary to meet educational needs may have a medical component. For example, schools are required to administer medications to children who need them during the school day. If the medications were not available in school, the children would have to stay home and they would not receive an appropriate education. Therefore, the child has an educational need to have his medications available in school.

Physical and occupational therapy are other examples of services that have both educational and medical components. Pain, stiffness, decreased strength, and limited range of motion affect a child's ability to keep up with classwork and participate in other school activities. Physical and occupational therapy can relieve symptoms that interfere with a child's ability to function optimally in school. Therapists can also teach children alternative techniques for dealing with difficult situations, and they can advise teachers regarding appropriate program modifications. Without necessary, school-based physical and occupational therapy services, some children are unable to receive an appropriate education.

When requesting services that include a medical component, be sure to emphasize the educational need.

Stay focused. Keep your attention focused on the specific issues the meeting was called to address. If new issues arise, deal with them after completing your scheduled business. Never agree to negotiate over a newly raised issue if you are not prepared with the necessary information and documentation. Request a meeting at a later date to discuss those issues.

Obtain the services of an advocate or other support person. If you are unable to reach an agreement regarding school services on your own, try to find an advocate to assist you. Advocates are trained in educational rights and have experience working with school personnel to obtain services. Volunteer, lay advocates are usually other parents of children who have chronic illnesses or disabilities. Their services are provided free of charge. Professional advocates usually have more training than lay advocates, but they also charge a fee for their services. The availability of advocacy services varies, depending on where you live. Contact parent support agencies in your area, including Parent Training and Information Centers, for the names of advocates who may be available to help you.

In addition to advocates, family members, trusted friends, or health care providers can also provide support and assistance at school meetings. It can be helpful to have someone with you to take notes, so that you can concentrate on what is being discussed. Your support person can also make sure that you do not forget to discuss important issues. Health care providers can explain the nature of your child's illness and suggest appropriate services and program modifications. As a matter of courtesy, inform the school in advance that you will be bringing other people with you to a meeting.

QUESTIONS AND ANSWERS ABOUT SCHOOL ISSUES

We recently moved from Vermont to Massachusetts. Does the new school district have to implement the IEP that was in effect at my son's school in Vermont?

Yes. Massachusetts special education law specifically requires the new school district to immediately implement the IEP that was in effect for your son at his school in Vermont. This regulation applies whether you moved to your new community from another district within Massachusetts or from another state. The previous IEP will remain in effect until the new school completes an evaluation and a new IEP is written and accepted by the parent.

The regulations pertaining to implementation of federal and state special education laws differ from state to state. Individuals living in other states should contact their state's department of education and local parent advocacy groups for information specific to the state's regulations.

My 8-year-old daughter has arthritis. Should I be doing anything about her school needs during the summer break?

Most people try not to think about school in the summertime. Vacation is here, the weather is warm, and education is the furthest thing from our minds. It is, however, very important to think about school during the summer months when your child has a rheumatic disease. September is an important transition time. Regardless of your child's grade or level of disability, it is important to develop plans for her school program during the summer so that they will be in place on the first day of school. Perhaps your child is entering a new school or going off to college for the first time. Planning early will make the transition easier and may help eliminate potentially difficult situations for your child. Time spent educating the school staff in advance can make a world of difference.

When should I consider purchasing a computer for my child, who has hand arthritis? Are there special features I should look for in a computer?

Many children with hand arthritis can benefit from a computer. Most children with arthritis can type efficiently even if their hand function is limited. Having a computer allows them to complete all of the necessary work at school. With an appropriate computer, your child will be able to keep up academically with the increased writing demands of high school and college. It may also promote free time writing skills for children who like to keep a diary, write stories or poems for fun, or catalog baseball cards. The only drawback to getting a computer is the expense. You may be able to get financial assistance from the school or from other local charitable organizations, such as your local Arthritis Foundation chapter office, Kiwanis, Shriners, or others.

Children with hand arthritis should begin learning to touch-type and use a mouse to point and click at as early an age as possible; many children begin at age 4. A computer can be purchased at any age a parent feels appropriate. Many parents purchase a computer when the child enters high school because the writing demands increase at that time. A computer is practically a prerequisite for college. A child who is planning to attend college should have a computer and be proficient in its use in his senior year of high school.

There are several considerations when purchasing a computer. Because computer technology is changing rapidly, you should do extensive research prior to purchase. Make an educated purchase by considering your child's present and future needs. An inexpensive fixed-based unit may seem all that is needed now, but a more expensive laptop may be needed in the future for note-taking in high school or college. Portable computers often have a memory and work capacity equivalent to fixed-base units. Portable units are a must if your child will be using the computer to take notes in school or needs to bring work between home and school or the library.

If you are purchasing a laptop computer, be sure to get one with a full-sized keyboard. Some laptops have a compressed keyboard with smaller-sized keys that are difficult for a person with arthritis to use. Also consider weight when purchasing a laptop. Unit weight varies widely, from 4 to 10 pounds; the heavier models can be difficult for children with arthritis to move, lift, and carry. Finally, consider the position of the track-ball on the laptop, and whether it is protuberant or recessed; your child may have difficulty manipulating some models.

Another consideration is the operating system. The choices include MS-DOS and Windows (IBM compatibles) or Macintosh. Both Windows and Macintosh have user-friendly point-and-click menu systems that even young children can learn easily. You should consider things like compatibility with existing school and home computer systems, ease of use, and current and future needs.

Most important of all, plan to make several trips to the computer store to research and try the available models. Be sure to have your child "test drive" the various computers, as one may be far easier to use than another.

Checklist for Students with JRA

Every student has different problems, and to help an individual student, the school needs to know what his specific problems are. To make it easier for the student to identify problems, we've included a list of the most common school-related problems affecting children and adolescents with JRA. After reading through this list, the student can check off the problems that apply to him. The list should then be returned to the student's doctor or any of the rheumatology team members.

Checklist for Students with JRA

Student's name:_____ Date:_____

School:_____ City:_____ Grade:_____

_____ 1. Getting to school is difficult for me.
_____ 2. I have to wait for the bus or my ride outside, sometimes in the cold.
_____ 3. I get stiff when I have to sit too long.
_____ 4. I'm stiff in the morning, even after I take a warm bath.
_____ 5. I'm stiff in the morning, but I don't have time to take a warm bath before school.
_____ 6. My hands hurt when I write.
_____ 7. I can't write fast enough during tests or when taking notes.
_____ 8. Writing on the chalkboard is difficult for me.
_____ 9. I have trouble raising my hand to ask or answer questions.
_____10. I sometimes forget to take my splints to school.
_____11. I don't have the equipment at school that I need, such as splints, a tilt board, a wheelchair.
_____12. It's hard for me to take off my coat, boots, or shoes.
_____13. It's hard for me to turn door handles or open my locker.
_____14. It's hard for me to carry my books or lunch tray.
_____15. I have trouble eating at school.
_____16. I have trouble using the bathroom at school.
_____17. I don't have enough time to change classes.
_____18. My classes, the bathroom, or the cafeteria are too far away for me.
_____19. Staircases are a problem for me.
_____20. I have trouble with fire drills or earthquake drills.
_____21. I have trouble changing my clothes in Physical Education (PE) class.
_____22. I have trouble taking a shower in PE class.
_____23. I don't have time to exercise at school.
_____24. I'm too tired after school to exercise at home.
_____25. PE is too much for me.
_____26. My school day is long, and I'm very tired when I get home.
_____27. I need a rest in the middle of my school day.
_____28. I have trouble standing in long lines, like the cafeteria.
_____29. I have trouble doing all of my homework on time.
_____30. I can't keep up with the other students in my school work.
_____31. I'm absent from school a lot (one week or more is "a lot").
_____32. My school makes me keep my medicine with the school staff.
_____33. I sometimes forget to take my medicine at school.
_____34. I feel different when I have to go to the office for my medicine.
_____35. Some of the other students make fun of my arthritis.
_____36. I don't know how to talk to my classmates about my arthritis.
_____37. My teacher doesn't understand my arthritis.
_____38. My teacher babies me.
_____39. My teacher forgets that I have arthritis.
_____40. Other_____

Checklist of Items for Consideration in Developing
Individualized Education Plans (IEP) for Students with
Physical Disabilities or Special Health Needs

The following checklist contains items often identified by parents and professionals as important components of appropriate educcational plans. Not all items will be important to all students; some students may have needs that are not reflected here.

TRANSPORTATION
    [ ] Regular bus
    [ ] Van
    [ ] Wheelchair car
    [ ] Special equipment
    [ ] Seat belt
    [ ] Car seat
    [ ] Other _____

[ ] Special assistance
    [ ] To and from home to vehicle
    [ ] To and from school to vehicle
    [ ] Aide
    [ ] Positioning
    [ ] Other _____

    NOTES:_____

ACCESSIBILITY
    [ ] Use of elevators
    [ ] Bathrooms
    [ ] Classrooms
    [ ] Gym
    [ ] Cafeteria
    [ ] Library

[ ] Vocational areas
[ ] Auditorium (stage)
[ ] Administrative offices
[ ] Locker location
[ ] Other _____

    NOTES:_____

THERAPIES
    [ ] Occupational therapy
    [ ] Physical therapy
    [ ] Speech therapy

[ ] Other_____
[ ] Other _____
[ ] Other _____

    NOTES:_____

SELF-HELP SKILLS
    [ ] Eating
    [ ] Dressing
    [ ] Toileting
    [ ] Student needs
        [ ] Assistance
        [ ] Training

[ ] Grooming
    [ ] Bathing/washing
    [ ] Tooth brushing
    [ ] Other _____

    NOTES:_____

POSITIONING
- [ ] Wheelchair
- [ ] Car
- [ ] Classroom
- [ ] Gym
- [ ] Lunch
- [ ] Other _____

- [ ] Aids
    - [ ] Prone board
    - [ ] Back supports
    - [ ] Other _____
    - [ ] When _____

NOTES:_____

STAMINA
- [ ] Scheduling concerns
- [ ] Length of day
- [ ] Effect on testing, especially timed
- [ ] Breaks/rest periods
    - [ ] As needed
    - [ ] Regularly scheduled

- [ ] Identifiable signs of fatigue
- [ ] Whose responsibility
- [ ] Whose authority
- [ ] Role of student

NOTES:_____

FIRE SAFETY
- [ ] Plan
- [ ] Who is responsible
- [ ] Backup person

NOTES:_____

FIELD TRIPS
- [ ] Early notification
- [ ] Transportation

- [ ] Aide
- [ ] Other_____

NOTES:_____

EXTRACURRICULAR ACTIVITIES/PROGRAMS (This is a section 504 issue)
- [ ] Special learning opportunities
    - [ ] Drivers education
    - [ ] Work experience
    - [ ] Job placement programs
    - [ ] Other _____
- [ ] Extended day programs
- [ ] Clubs

- [ ] Sports programs
- [ ] Social events
- [ ] Transportation
- [ ] Aide
- [ ] Accessibility

NOTES:_____

HOME/HOSPITAL TUTORING
- [ ] Needed now
- [ ] Possible needed later
- [ ] Outline plan (even if tentative)

NOTES:_____

CURRICULUM

[ ] Materials to be modified
    [ ] Taped
    [ ] Written in large print
    [ ] Computer software
    [ ] Other _____
[ ] Timelines set
[ ] Responsibilities assigned

[ ] Methods to be adapted
    [ ] Timelines for completing
        tasks/assignments/tests
    [ ] Written *and* spoken
    [ ] Use of computer

NOTES:_____

CLASSWORK

[ ] Backup tutoring
    [ ] Regularly scheduled
    [ ] As needed

[ ] Make-up assistance
    [ ] Regularly scheduled
    [ ] As needed

NOTES:_____

PHYSICAL EDUCATION

[ ] Regular program
[ ] Modified regular program
[ ] Adaptive physical education program
[ ] Other _____

[ ] Special equipment
[ ] Special staff
[ ] Other _____
[ ] Other _____

NOTES:_____

ENRICHMENT CLASSES/ACTIVITIES

[ ] Art
[ ] Music
[ ] Computer
[ ] Other _____

[ ] Modifications needed
    [ ] Special equipment
    [ ] Special staff
    [ ] Other _____

NOTES:_____

EQUIPMENT NEEDED

[ ] Typewriter
[ ] Computer
[ ] Special grip pencils

[ ] Communication devices
[ ] Extra set of books for home
[ ] Other _____

NOTES:_____

SPECIAL HEALTH NEEDS AT SCHOOL

[ ] Regular basis
[ ] As needed
[ ] Use of bathroom as needed
[ ] Other _____

[ ] Specify
    [ ] Who
    [ ] What
    [ ] Backup person

NOTES:_____

MEDICATIONS
- [ ] Who administers
  - [ ] Student
  - [ ] Nurse
  - [ ] Teacher
  - [ ] Backup person
- [ ] Side effects implications for
  - [ ] Regular school schedule
  - [ ] Test schedule
  - [ ] Special events/activities

- [ ] Storage
- [ ] Recordkeeping, logs
- [ ] Instructions on self-administering for student

NOTES:_____

_____

SPECIAL SUPPLIES OR EQUIPMENT
- [ ] Storage
- [ ] Whose responsibility
  Other considerations: _____

- [ ] At school only
- [ ] Shared between home and school

NOTES:_____

_____

BACKUP MEDICAL SUPPORT
List specific health-related emergencies that may occur: _____
_____
_____
Whom to contact:_____
Where to go:_____
What to do in an emergency:_____
_____
_____

NOTES:_____

_____

MOBILITY
- [ ] Need for assistance
- [ ] Regular method/person
- [ ] Backup person
- [ ] Use of elevator
- [ ] Other _____

- [ ] Proximity considerations for developing schedule
- [ ] Classrooms
- [ ] Lunchrooms
- [ ] Gym
- [ ] Other _____

NOTES:_____

_____

Sample Letters

Sample Letter Requesting an Evaluation

(Remember to keep a copy of the letter you actually sign and send for your records.)

Your street address

City, State, Zip

Date

Name

Administrator of Special Education

_____ Public Schools

Street address

City, State, Zip

Dear Mr. or Ms. (name of local special education director shown above):

I am requesting a TEAM evaluation for my child, (child's name and date of birth), who is presently at (name of your child's school and grade/program).

I understand that the evaluation is to be provided at no charge to me, and I would like the assessment to include testing in the following areas:

(List here any area in which you feel your child should be tested.)

I would appreciate meeting with the TEAM Chairperson before the testing begins so that I might share information about (your child's name) with (her/him), and discuss the evaluation procedures. I would like a copy of the written report from each evaluator so that I can review them before the TEAM Meeting.

I understand that I have to give my permission for these tests to be done. Please send me the proper forms to sign.

I will call you in three days to set up an appointment with the TEAM Chairperson. Thank you for your prompt consideration in this matter.

Sincerely,

(Sign your name here)

(Print your name here)

Developed by the Federation for Children with Special Needs. Reprinted with permission.

Sample Letter Requesting an Independent Evaluation

(Remember to keep a copy of the letter you actually sign and send for your records.)

> Your street address
>
> City, State, Zip
>
> Date

Name

Administrator of Special Education

_____ Public Schools

Street address

City, State, Zip

Dear Mr. or Ms. (name of local special education director shown above):

I am requesting an independent evaluation for my child, (child's name, date of birth, name of your child's school and grade/program). I understand that the independent evaluation is to be provided at no charge to me, and must be equivalent to those originally done by the school. I would like the assessment to include testing in the following areas:

(List here any area in which you feel your child should be tested.)

I plan to have the independent evaluation done by (name of evaluator) in (organization, town).

Please contact (name of evaluator) to arrange payment for these services. Thank you for your prompt consideration in this matter.

Sincerely,

(Sign your name here)

(Print your name here)

Developed by the Federation for Children with Special Needs. Reprinted with permission.

Sample Letter Requesting Records
(Remember to keep a copy of the letter you actually sign and send for your records.)

<u>Your street address</u>

<u>City, State, Zip</u>

<u>Date</u>

<u>Name</u>

Administrator of Special Education

_____ Public Schools

<u>Street address</u>

<u>City, State, Zip</u>

Dear Mr. or Ms. (<u>name of local special education director shown above</u>):

This letter is a request to review all my child's records that are collected, maintained, or used by the school.

Please bring my child's file, (<u>child's name, date of birth, name of your child's school and grade/program</u>), to one location where I may inspect the file and get copies, if necessary.

Your cooperation in this matter is appreciated. I look forward to hearing from you within the next two days.

Sincerely,

(<u>Sign your name here</u>)

(<u>Print your name here</u>)

Developed by the Federation for Children with Special Needs. Reprinted with permission.

Sample Letter Requesting a TEAM Meeting

(Remember to keep a copy of the letter you actually sign and send for your records.)

Your street address

City, State, Zip

Date

Name

TEAM Chairperson

_____ Public Schools

Street address

City, State, Zip

Dear Mr. or Ms. (name of TEAM chairperson shown above):

I am requesting a TEAM meeting concerning my child, (child's name and date of birth), who is presently at (name of your child's school and grade/program). The purpose of this meeting will be:

(List the issue[s] you want to discuss here.)

I am available (date[s] and time[s]). Your cooperation in this matter is appreciated, and I look forward to hearing from you within the next five days.

Sincerely,

(Sign your name here)

(Print your name here)

Developed by the Federation for Children with Special Needs. Reprinted with permission.

Sample Letter Requesting Mediation or a Hearing
(Remember to keep a copy of the letter you actually sign and send for your records.)

Your street address
City, State, Zip
Date

Bureau of Special Education Appeals
(Your state's name) Department of Education
Street address
City, State, Zip

To Whom It May Concern:

I am requesting a formal hearing to resolve a dispute with (name of your town) school system.

The dispute involves special education services for my child (name of your child). (If you wish, you may include a general statement about the issue being disputed.)

I understand that you will set a date for this hearing within five days, and that the hearing will be held within _____ days (use the time frame that is required by the laws in your state).

I look forward to hearing from you regarding the hearing date and the hearing officer as soon as possible.

Thank you for your help in this matter.

Sincerely,

(Sign your name here)

(Print your name here)

Developed by the Federation for Children with Special Needs. Reprinted with permission.

Telephone Log for School-Related Issues

The School Information form in the directory section of your personal health record provides spaces to record names, addresses, and phone numbers of school personnel you may need to contact. It's a good idea to complete that form and keep it handy when you call the school to discuss your child's need for assistance or program modifications. For documentation purposes, you may also wish to record all of your contacts in the log reproduced on the following page, and keep this record in your health record for reference. (You may wish to make additional copies of this log for future use.)

Form 12. Telephone Log for Contacts with School Personnel

Date	Name, Title, and Phone Number/Extension of Person Spoken With	What Was Discussed	Action to Be Taken and Who Is Responsible

Chapter 8

*

Financing Health Care

Few of us can manage to pay the high costs of medical care without having some form of health insurance coverage. This is especially true when a member of the family develops a chronic illness. Because there is tremendous variation among health insurance plans, ranging from private insurance to publicly funded programs, choosing the right plan, or even determining the extent of your existing coverage, can be difficult. Public sources of funding for medical care involve many different state and federal agencies, and each has complicated eligibility guidelines and application procedures. To get the most benefit from your health insurance or public health care plan, you must understand the plan's coverage and limits, and know how to file a claim or appeal an unfavorable decision.

This chapter provides information about private and public sources of funding for health care. The first few sections define terms and clauses that are frequently included in health insurance policies. The most common types of privately available health insurance plans are compared. The section on public financing describes the most traditional programs available to children and identifies the responsible state and federal agencies. Eligibility for public sector programs is discussed, along with information on covered services. Another section of this chapter provides suggestions for resolving disputes with your insurance company or health care agency. A worksheet is included to help you compare the costs and benefits of different insurance policies. You will also find a log sheet that you can use to keep track of your communications with insurance companies or funding agencies about disputed claims.

This chapter cannot answer all of your questions about health care financing, but it's a good starting point. If you have specific questions about your own coverage, you should be in touch with representatives of your health insurance company or state health agency. A social worker on the staff at your child's rheumatology center or elsewhere may be able to help determine which programs suit your needs. There are excellent books and pamphlets (many of them listed in the Bibliography at the end of this book) that provide additional information.

Regulations and legislation governing health care financing are changing rapidly. It is critical for you to get up-to-date information that is relevant to your specific situation.

Health Insurance: Terms and Common Practices

Whether you are choosing a new plan or trying to get the most out of an existing one, it is important to know what benefits the policy provides and what those benefits will cost you. You must read the policy carefully. Be sure that you are reading a complete copy of the policy (available from the insurance company or your employer), not just the benefit summary that is frequently given to customers.

When a family member has a pre-existing chronic illness, insurance companies may refuse coverage altogether, charge extremely high premiums, or exclude coverage for services related to the chronic condition. It can be difficult to obtain adequate health insurance if your child has a rheumatic illness, and even those families who have insurance may find that it fails to cover a significant portion of their health care costs. Many standard policies put severe limits on the benefits available for some of the health care services that are necessary for the proper treatment of rheumatic illnesses, particularly physical and occupational therapy.

A number of terms used by the health insurance industry are defined below, along with some standard health insurance practices that significantly affect people with chronic illnesses.

Covered Services and Exclusions

A health insurance policy is a contract between you and the insurance company: the company will pay a specific set of benefits in return for your payment of a fixed premium (premiums are paid periodically, usually monthly, quarterly, or semi-annually). Read your policy carefully to determine exactly what benefits are offered. Your insurance company will pay only for services it has agreed to cover; these are listed in the policy document as covered services or benefits. The insurer will not pay for any other health care services, whether or not those services are medically necessary.

In addition to covered services, your policy will also list services that are specifically excluded. Typically excluded are such services as experimental therapies, routine eye care, medications, and expensive treatments like organ transplants. The list of covered services and exclusions varies dramatically depending on the policy.

Riders or endorsements may be attached to your policy to provide additional coverage or further restrict benefits. Prescription drug and durable medical equipment riders are common. These extend the coverage provided by the basic policy to include payment for most prescription medications and certain types of durable medical equipment.

Copayments and Deductibles

Health insurance is designed to *limit*, not eliminate, your out-of-pocket expenses for health care. It does not cover all of the costs, even for covered services. *Copayments and deductibles* are the amounts you must pay for services that are covered by your health insurance plan. Copayments are usually required for each health care service you obtain. Managed care plans, like health maintenance organizations (HMOs), usually charge a small, fixed copayment of $5 or $10. Traditional health insurance plans generally require a copayment that is a fixed percentage (typically 20 percent) of the fee for services. The copayment rate may vary depending on the type of service.

A deductible is the amount of out-of-pocket expenses you must incur before your insurance company pays for covered services. Until you have paid an amount equal to your deductible, you are responsible for paying 100 percent of the cost of covered services. After you have met the deductible, the insurance company pays its share of the costs for a specific medical procedure or treatment, and your copayment covers the rest.

Family plans usually have individual and family deductibles. Each family member's health care costs are considered separately. Coverage for an individual begins after his own deductible has been met or the family deductible has been reached. The family deductible is usually equal to three times the individual deductible. In this case, a family with four or more members would exhaust its deductible after three family members incurred covered expenses in excess of the individual deductible. Copayments and payments for services not covered by the plan cannot be used to offset the deductible. The following example demonstrates the effect of deductibles:

> A family of four has an insurance plan that requires payment of a $200 individual deductible with a family deductible of $600 and a copayment of 20 percent. One member of the family incurs $3,000 in health care expenses, of which $500 are for services not covered by the plan. A second family member is billed for $150 of covered services.
>
> The insurance company would pay 80 percent of the covered services exceeding the deductible for the first family member, or $1,840. This figure is reached by

subtracting $500 from $3,000 ($2,500), then subtracting $200 (the individual deductible) from $2,500 ($2,300), and taking 80 percent of that figure ($1,840 that the insurance company would pay). The family would be responsible for paying $500 in noncovered services, the $200 deductible, and $460 for the copayment (20 percent of $2,300), for a total of $1,160. The family would also be responsible for the entire $150 bill for the second family member, which would be applied to his individual deductible. Although the family's out-of-pocket expenses were $1,310, the family deductible was reduced by only $350.

Copayments and deductibles are sometimes referred to as the cost-sharing provisions of a health insurance policy.

Reasonable and Customary Charges

Insurance companies base their payments on the reasonable and customary charge for the service provided. The reasonable and customary charge is supposed to be the fee that is typically charged for a specific procedure by health care providers in your area of the country. Insurance companies determine the reasonable and customary charges themselves and update them periodically. With health care costs rising annually, it is not uncommon for the reasonable and customary charges set by your insurance company to lag behind the actual fees charged by health care providers.

Your insurance company will pay its share of the lesser of the actual fee charged and the reasonable and customary fee. If you are billed $60 for a service and the reasonable and customary charge is only $50, the insurance company will pay its share (say, 80 percent) of the $50 fee. You will be responsible for your usual copayment (based on a $50 fee) as well as the $10 excess charge, *unless* your health care provider has an agreement with the insurer that he or she will accept payment of the reasonable and customary fee as payment in full for the service. In that case, you are responsible for paying only the usual copayment.

Benefit Limits

Most health insurance plans limit benefits for covered services by restricting the number of service instances it will cover or by setting a maximum dollar amount it will pay for particular types of services. For example, a plan may cover up to fifteen visits per year for mental health care or a maximum of $2,000 for the purchase or rental of durable medical equipment. Different limits may apply to each type of service covered by your plan. To monitor your health insurance coverage, you must know not only which services are covered but also how much coverage you have for each type of service you expect to use.

Limits on physical and occupational therapy. Coverage for physical and occupational therapy varies widely among health insurance plans. Many limit coverage of physical and occupational therapy to between 60 and 90 *consecutive* days of coverage per diagnosis, per year, regardless of the frequency of services during this period. The coverage period begins with the date of the first therapy session and ends 60 to 90 days later. If additional therapy is required after the coverage period ends, it is generally not covered, even if services were provided for less than the full coverage period initially. For example, if your child receives physical therapy for one month in February, she may not be eligible for an additional month of services in July. Although she needed therapy for a total of only 60 days, your coverage period for therapy ended 60 to 90 days after the first session in February. Other insurance plans limit the total number of physical and occupational therapy visits covered per year.

If your insurer denies coverage for physical or occupational therapy, you can appeal the decision—and it is usually a good idea to do so. Therapy benefits are designed to meet therapy needs resulting from accident or injury, and therefore the rules governing them are often disadvantageous to people who have chronic conditions. When applying for coverage or appealing a decision, it's best to explain the exact nature of the services to the insurer, as illustrated in the following examples:

- Some insurance plans will not cover occupational therapy for improvement of daily living skills (like dressing or feeding) but will cover therapy to strengthen the muscles and increase joint range of motion in the hands and arms. Make the purpose of the therapy clear to the insurer.
- Many children who have JRA are evaluated by physical and occupational therapists during periodic visits to the pediatric rheumatology clinic and do most of their own therapy at home. Because of a 60- or 90-consecutive-day limit on physical and occupational therapy benefits, the insurance company may deny coverage for these services after the first or second clinic visit each year. Insurance may cover these services, however, when it is clear that they are done for evaluation or diagnostic purposes, and not as ongoing rehabilitative therapy.
- Coverage for physical and occupational therapy is usually limited to one period of therapy *per diagnosis* per year. The diagnosis used for the therapy referral should be more specific than JRA. Your child may be covered for a period of physical therapy to address a specific problem such as a knee contracture. In the same year, he might then be covered for therapy to address a different problem, such as limited range of motion in the shoulder.
- Some insurers will grant an extension of benefits, usually for another limited period of time, if you can provide evidence of continued improvement with therapy.

- Occasionally, insurers will cover physical and occupational therapy if you can prove that more expensive corrective procedures, such as surgery, will be necessary if the therapy is not done. It may help to have the pediatric rheumatologist write a letter to the insurance company supporting the need for continuing therapy for your child.

Lifetime Maximums

Many health insurance plans place a limit on lifetime benefits payable under the plan. Once the lifetime benefit has been reached, the insurance is terminated and no further reimbursements will be made. This situation is often referred to as "maxing out." Some plans place lifetime benefit limits on various types of services, such as mental health or physical therapy, while others limit the lifetime benefit for all services combined.

Your policy should clearly indicate whether lifetime maximums are in effect. If so, you need to make sure that you are sent periodic reports indicating the amount of coverage remaining. If your insurance company does not provide this information automatically, you should request updated reports at least annually, and more frequently as you near the limits of coverage. Do not wait until your benefits have expired to explore other health insurance options. In rare instances, insurance companies may offer an extension of the lifetime maximums if you file a written appeal.

Stop-Loss Clause or Out-of-Pocket Maximum

Some health insurance policies include a stop-loss clause that limits your annual out-of-pocket expenses. When your out-of-pocket costs for covered services exceed the specified limit, the insurance company pays 100 percent of the remaining costs for services covered under the plan. Copayments and deductibles are no longer required.

Prolonged Illness or Catastrophic Illness Clause

Similar to a stop-loss clause, a prolonged illness clause extends your benefits for services related to a long-term illness. A prolonged illness clause may extend the policy limits or increase the rate of coverage for covered services. These extended benefits apply only to services provided for the treatment of the specified prolonged illness. The usual policy limits apply to all other health care services required by any family member. You will continue to pay deductibles and copayments for these other services. The application for prolonged illness benefits requires a statement from your physician detailing the nature of the illness and the need for continued services. Not all plans offer a prolonged illness provision. Check with your insurer for availability and application procedures.

Pre-existing Conditions and Waiting Periods

A pre-existing condition is any condition that is present prior to enrollment in a health plan. Some insurers limit the look-back period to a number of months or years. Conditions not treated during this period of time before enrollment are not considered pre-existing conditions for purposes of evaluating insurability. Other insurers consider a condition as pre-existing if it has been diagnosed or is known about at any time before enrollment.

Insurance company policies regarding pre-existing conditions vary. In some cases, the insurer may refuse to enroll an individual or family because of the pre-existing condition. In other cases, a higher premium is charged for the same policy, or a policy is offered with reduced benefits. Insurance companies frequently impose a waiting period for benefits related to a pre-existing condition. During the waiting period, treatment for the pre-existing condition is not covered. Some plans begin covering pre-existing conditions after the waiting period has expired, but others will do so only if there was no treatment for the pre-existing condition during the waiting period. This provision effectively eliminates all coverage for the rheumatic illness for children who require ongoing treatment.

Every time you change your health insurance policy you may be subject to exclusion or increased premiums due to a pre-existing condition. Before making decisions that will affect your current health insurance coverage, such as changing jobs or moving, be sure to examine the health insurance options that will be available to you. If your child is nearing the age at which he can no longer be covered under your family policy (usually age 21 or 23, or after graduation from college), it is important to begin planning for continued coverage before her present health insurance lapses.

Open Enrollment Periods

Open enrollment periods offer consumers the opportunity to purchase health insurance without regard to pre-existing conditions. During the open enrollment period, all eligible applicants for health insurance are accepted into the plan. Eligibility requirements vary. For employer-based plans, the applicant must be a current employee working full time or working a predetermined minimum number of hours per week. HMOs usually require applicants to live within their service areas. A spouse and dependent biological, adopted, and step-children are eligible for enrollment in a family plan if they live with the applicant and the children are under the age limits set by the plan. Applicants who are confined to a hospital at the time of application, or who have exceeded another plan's lifetime benefit maximum, are usually not eligible for enrollment in the plan. The existence of a known medical condition, such as JRA, does not affect eligibility during the open enrollment period.

Many employers provide annual open enrollment periods, during which you may obtain coverage for the first time or choose a different health insurance plan. Open enrollment may also be offered when you start a new job, or after a short period of time (3 to 6 months) of working in a new job. You also may be able to add dependents to a family plan without consideration of pre-existing conditions if you do so within a fixed time period after the change in family status occurs (for example, within 30 days after the birth of a baby or completion of adoption proceedings).

Coordination of Benefits

When an individual is covered by more than one insurance policy, benefits are coordinated to prevent duplicate coverage. This is likely to occur if both you and your spouse receive health insurance benefits from your employers. The policy offered by your own employer, on which you are the named insured, is your primary policy. If you are also covered by your spouse's plan, that plan provides you with secondary coverage. Whenever there is coverage by more than one health insurer, you must submit health care bills to the primary insurer first. Only those expenses not covered by the primary plan will be considered for coverage under the secondary insurance.

The rules for determining which policy has the primary responsibility for the health care costs of dependents vary; the insurance policy documents should define coverage of dependents. Often, the determination of primary and secondary coverage for dependents is based on the birth dates of the policy owners. In this case, if your birthdate is earlier in the year than your spouse's, your policy will provide your children's primary coverage. Your spouse's plan will be considered your children's secondary plan. Ask your insurers about the specific formula they use to determine which policy provides primary coverage for each of your dependents.

Maintaining duplicate health insurance policies can be expensive. Your employer may offer alternative benefits or cash payments for employees who elect not to be covered by their company's health insurance plan. Some employers will make payments to a Health Care Reimbursement Account (HCRA) in your name if you choose not to enroll in an employee health insurance plan because you are covered by another plan. Funds deposited in an HCRA are not taxable and can be used to pay for medical expenses that are not covered by health insurance, including copayments and deductibles. (HCRAs are described in more detail later in this chapter.) Check with your employer's benefits manager about substituting another benefit for health insurance if you are already covered by a health insurance plan.

Continuation of Coverage (Conversion)

Losing health insurance coverage is a special problem for individuals who may be denied coverage in other plans because of pre-existing conditions. You can lose coverage if you move, change jobs, retire, are laid off, go on strike, exceed your lifetime maximum, or reach the age limit for dependent children. When wage earners are disabled or die, their dependents risk losing the coverage previously provided through the wage earner's employer.

Many health insurance policies contain provisions for continuing your coverage. The details will be spelled out in the policy's continuation of coverage or conversion clause. If you are covered under a group plan, you may be able to convert to nongroup coverage by paying higher premiums when your group eligibility ends. If you have been covered as a dependent, you may be able to purchase an individual policy when your dependent status changes.

Generally the insurer is under no obligation to offer the same benefits in a policy begun under a conversion clause as were included in the original policy; in addition, the premium may be substantially higher in a policy begun under a conversion clause. Provisions for continuation of coverage differ among policies. In all cases, you must request conversion of your policy and begin paying the new premiums within a specified time period after termination of your original policy benefits, usually 30 days, or you will lose the right to continuation.

State and federal legislation may protect you from loss of health insurance in some cases. A federal law known as COBRA (P.L. 99-272) guarantees the right of an employee and his or her family to continue group coverage under an employer-based group plan for 18 to 36 months after a change in job or dependent status, divorce, or the employee's death. You will be responsible for paying the full insurance premium, but you will have the advantage of paying the lower group rate. COBRA regulations apply to employers with twenty or more employees. State regulations regarding continuation of coverage vary. Contact your state's commissioner of insurance for more information (look under *insurance* in the state government listings in the blue pages of the Yellow Pages).

Private Health Insurance Plans

There are four major types of private health insurance plan: traditional (indemnity) plans, health maintenance organizations (HMOs), preferred provider plans (PPOs), and hybrid plans that combine the benefits of traditional coverage and HMO coverage. The plans are distinguished by the manner in which providers are reimbursed for services and the degree of freedom allowed in the choice of health care providers and facilities. The four types of plan are described in this section. Keep in mind that within each type of plan, there are significant differences in benefits and costs among different insurers and in different geographic regions.

Each of these four types of health insurance plan can be offered as group or nongroup (individual) policies. Group coverage rates are based on the *average* risk for all members of the group, whereas individual coverage rates are based on a rating of the health insurance risk of the individual seeking coverage. In group insurance, the risk of a small number of members having high health care costs is shared by all group members, and this results in lower individual premiums. It is always cheaper to purchase health insurance through a group plan; the larger the group, the smaller the premium will be.

Most group plans are offered through large employers, but unions and associations of small businesses may also offer group coverage to their members. Before you purchase a nongroup health insurance policy, look for ways to join a group. Check with the officers of the associations or organizations that you belong to, or that you are eligible to join, to find out whether the organization offers group health insurance for members. You can also talk with other individuals in situations similar to yours, to find out what health insurance strategies have worked for them.

Traditional (Indemnity) Plans

Traditional health insurance plans (such as Blue Cross/Blue Shield) offer greater freedom in the selection of health care providers but usually cost more than HMOs and PPOs. In addition to higher annual premiums, traditional plans require the insured to pay the first portion of health care costs (the deductible) and a percentage of the remaining costs up to an annual out-of-pocket limit. The copayment amount is usually 20 percent, with the health insurance plan paying 80 percent of covered health care costs after the deductible is met. Most of these plans cap annual out-of-pocket expenses by paying 100 percent of covered medical costs in excess of the annual out-of-pocket maximum specified in the policy.

Deductibles and out-of-pocket maximums vary. Typical deductibles range from $250 to $500 per individual and $600 to $1,500 per family. Annual out-of-pocket maximums are also different in different plans. Some traditional plans place a limit on the total benefits they will provide an individual for a lifetime. Once the insurance company has paid benefits equaling the lifetime maximum, no further coverage is available under the policy.

Although traditional health insurance plans give you considerable freedom in your choice of health care providers, you are not completely free to choose health services. Only covered health care expenses for medically necessary treatment will be paid by the insurance company. Most plans exclude or limit coverage for physical, occupational, and speech therapy, mental health services, eye exams, experimental therapies, and durable medical equipment. Many traditional plans require pre-approval for surgery and hospitalization. If you fail to obtain preapproval when required, the expenses you incur will not be covered. Only covered expenses can be used to meet your deductible and annual out-of-pocket maximum. The lists of covered services, limits on services, and exclusions can be found in your policy contract.

Some plans offer prolonged illness coverage or extended benefits for people with chronic illnesses. These options generally pay 100 percent of the cost of medically necessary, covered treatments for the chronic condition. Some limits on services may be relaxed, as well, and lifetime maximum benefits may be extended. A letter from the physician is usually needed to activate prolonged illness coverage or extended benefits. The period of extended coverage is generally limited to a few years.

If you have a traditional health insurance plan, it is important to keep careful records. You will usually have to pay for services at the time of treatment and then submit your bills to the insurance company for reimbursement. Some providers will bill the insurance company directly for hospitalizations or expensive procedures, but you will still be liable for deductibles and copayments. Furthermore, the insurance company will determine what are reasonable and customary charges for the services you receive. The reasonable and customary charge is often less than you were billed. Although you often are liable to the provider for the entire amount, the insurance company bases its reimbursement on the reasonable and customary charge. (Some providers, as noted earlier, will accept payment of reasonable and customary charges as payment in full.)

Health Maintenance Organizations

Belonging to an HMO can significantly decrease your health care costs if you are able to obtain all necessary medical services from HMO physicians at participating facilities. Premiums are usually lower for HMOs than for traditional health insurance plans, and there are no deductibles for most services. Copayments for doctor visits range from $2 to $10, with higher copayments (typically $25) for emergency room treatment. Most HMOs provide 100 percent coverage for the cost of hospitalization, surgery, X rays, and laboratory tests. Like traditional health insurance plans,

HMOs limit benefits for physical, occupational, and speech therapy, mental health services, eye exams, experimental therapies, and durable medical equipment. There is often a deductible that applies to the purchase or rental of durable medical equipment.

HMOs control health care costs by contracting with physicians and health care facilities for reduced rates, and by limiting access to medical specialists by HMO members (patients). HMO members must choose a primary physician who will manage all of their health care. Each family member may choose his or her own primary care physician from among those affiliated with the HMO. The HMO will pay for all covered services that are ordered by the primary physician and obtained in HMO-approved facilities.

The primary physician determines whether additional services are needed and, if so, refers the patient to HMO-affiliated specialists for care. If the primary physician determines that the patient needs covered medical services that cannot be obtained within the HMO, he or she may refer the patient to a non-HMO specialist for treatment. If the HMO approves the out-of-plan referral, the patient's health care expenses will be paid by the HMO at the same rate as in-plan services.

The patient is responsible for paying the entire cost of out-of-plan treatment obtained without a referral. (If you forget to get a referral, contact your HMO immediately; they will occasionally issue a referral retroactively for a service they would normally have covered.) All HMOs make provisions for emergency care needed while you are out of their service area. Usually, you must notify the HMO within 48 hours of receiving emergency care from non-HMO providers.

The major disadvantage of HMOs is that they severely limit your choice of health care providers. Large HMOs contract with many primary care physicians, making it likely that you will be able to obtain satisfactory primary care services. However, you will have very little, if any, choice of specialty care providers. This restriction may be even more severe for children with highly specialized medical needs. Most HMOs have a limited variety of pediatric specialists on staff or under contract. To keep costs down, HMOs frequently deny out-of-plan referrals for pediatric specialty care and, instead, refer children to adult specialists who are in the plan.

As noted earlier in this book, children who have JRA or other rheumatic diseases should be cared for by pediatric rheumatologists, who are trained to deal with the unique physical, emotional, and social issues of childhood rheumatic illness. The adult rheumatologist associated with an HMO probably has no specialized training in pediatric rheumatic illness and little experience treating children. (Some adult rheumatologists have treated a large number of children over many years and are competent to care for children with rheumatic illnesses. But these rheumatologists are usually affiliated with large medical centers, not with HMOs. An out-of-plan referral will usually be needed to obtain their services, as well.)

HMOs may also make it more difficult to coordinate specialty care. If you are given a referral to a pediatric rheumatologist, you may still be required to have X rays and laboratory and other tests done at the HMO's facilities. This can double the number of health care visits you have to make, increasing the amount of time you lose from work and your child loses from school. Test and X-ray results must be communicated to your pediatric rheumatologist in a timely fashion so that he or she has the information needed to treat your child appropriately. Worse than the inconvenience, this lack of service coordination can result in additional, unpleasant experiences for a child who is fearful of health care providers. To avoid unnecessary out-of-pocket expenses, it is important to tell health care providers at the pediatric rheumatology clinic which tests and procedures you can have done at the clinic and which must be done at the HMO's facility. The HMO's customer service representatives can provide this information.

One final advantage of HMOs is the reduction in paperwork. There are no claim forms to fill out. Health care providers are paid directly by the HMO. The only paperwork you need to be concerned with is the written referral from your primary care physician for all specialty care and out-of-plan services.

Preferred Provider Organizations

In PPO plans, the insurance company contracts with physicians and health care facilities for reduced rates. When you obtain care for covered services from participating providers, you pay less. You are also free to obtain services from nonparticipating providers, but will pay more of the costs.

These plans take many different forms. Some of them pay 100 percent for covered services provided by participating providers and 80 percent after the deductible has been met for services obtained from nonparticipating providers. Other PPO plans provide 80 percent coverage with a deductible for in-plan services and 70 percent coverage with a higher deductible for out-of-plan services.

Annual premiums for PPO plans are usually higher than HMO premiums and lower than premiums for traditional health insurance. PPOs give you greater freedom in choosing providers than HMOs, but you will pay more for covered services obtained from nonparticipating providers. Reimbursement procedures vary. Participating providers may or may not bill the insurance plan directly. You will have to pay nonparticipating providers at the time of service and submit your bills to the plan for reimbursement.

Hybrid Plans

A few employers now offer plans that combine the advantages of HMOs and traditional health insurance. Under such a plan, you enroll in an HMO and receive the standard benefits of that HMO for all services ordered by your primary physician. But you also have the freedom to choose health care providers who are not part of the HMO, and receive reimbursement as you would under a traditional health insurance plan. When you obtain services outside the HMO without an approved referral, your traditional plan benefits are in effect. You pay a deductible and a percentage of costs, and the plan reimburses you for a fixed percentage of the remaining reasonable and customary charges.

The annual cost of premiums for hybrid plans is usually between the cost of an HMO and the cost of traditional health insurance. Deductibles, copayments, and annual out-of-pocket maximums are usually higher than for traditional plans alone. The amount of paperwork will also be moderate. You will need to obtain referrals from your primary physician for specialty services to be covered under your HMO. In-plan providers will bill the HMO for their services. For non-HMO medical treatment, you will have to pay the provider at the time of service and submit your bills for reimbursement.

One disadvantage of hybrid plans is that there is little incentive for the HMO to provide referrals for specialty services not available in-plan. It's likely that you will have to rely on the benefits of the traditional plan for the specialty care you need that is not available from the HMO's own providers.

Hybrid plans seem to offer the best of both worlds, and they can be a good choice if your child has a chronic illness requiring specialty care. If you are happy with the HMO's primary care physicians, if you receive most of your family's health care within the HMO, and if you require limited services from outside specialists, a hybrid plan can give you the choices you need while keeping costs down. However, if you rely on non-HMO providers for most of your care, a traditional health insurance plan will probably be cheaper.

Table 3 compares the different health insurance plans discussed above.

Choosing the Right Health Insurance for Your Family

If you have the option of choosing your health insurance plan, you'll want to take the time to examine each plan carefully and review your expected medical expenses before making a decision. It's a very good idea to review your medical bills from the previous year to determine the amount and types of medical services you are likely to use. It can also be helpful to talk with other people who are already insured by the plans you are considering. Keep in mind, however, that people's health insurance

TABLE 3. SUMMARY OF DIFFERENCES AMONG HEALTH INSURANCE PLANS

Features	Type of Plan			
	Traditional	HMO	PPO	Hybrid
Premium	Highest	Lowest	Moderate	Moderate
Deductible	Applies to all services; some preventive services may be exempted	None, except on specified services	Varies; larger for services of non-participating providers	Like HMO for in-plan services; like traditional plan for non-HMO providers, but higher
Copayment	Percentage of fee charged for services	Small, fixed-dollar amount per service (possibly higher for equipment and mental health services)	Varies, but higher for services of non-participating providers	Like HMO for in-plan services; like traditional plan for non-HMO providers, but higher
Benefit limits	Yes	Yes	Yes	Yes
Lifetime maximum benefit	Common	Less common	Varies	Common on non-HMO services
Annual out-of-pocket premium	Common	Not applicable	Varies	Applies only to services of non-HMO providers
Choice of providers	Yes	Restricted to HMO participating providers	Yes, but higher cost for using non-participating providers	Yes, but higher cost for using non-HMO providers
Preapproval for covered services	Required for some services, like surgery	Referral required for all services not provided by primary physician	Required for some services, like surgery	Under HMO coverage, referral required for all services not provided by primary physician, like traditional plan for non-HMO coverage
Method of payment for covered services	Submit bills to insurance company for reimbursement after paying provider at time of services	Provider bills HMO directly	Varies; usually similar to traditional plans	Like HMO for in-plan services; like traditional plan for non-HMO providers

needs are different. The best plan for one family may not be the best plan for you. If the policies that are offered include any provisions that you do not understand, particularly provisions about referral policies and limits on covered services, you can call the insurance companies and ask for clarification.

If the cost of medical care is your family's greatest concern, an HMO may be your best choice, but only if it covers the services you need. If you place a higher value on your freedom to choose health care providers, you will probably be more satisfied with a traditional plan. PPOs and hybrid plans may offer a reasonable compromise when costs and choice of providers are equally important.

Other policy provisions can also influence your choice of health plans. A generous conversion option may be the most important factor if you have a child who is nearing the age when she will no longer be eligible as a dependent on your plan. Pre-existing condition clauses and lifetime benefit caps will also influence your decision.

Use the "Health Insurance Policy Comparison Worksheet" to help you decide which plan will be best for your family. Complete the worksheet for each plan available to you, then carefully consider the pros and cons of each plan.

Public Health Care Financing

Medicaid is the major source of public funding to provide for the medical needs of children with disabilities or chronic illnesses. Funding for some medical or medically related services may also be available through state-run programs for Children with Special Health Care Needs, called Title V Programs or Maternal and Child Health (MCH) Block Grant Programs. Some states also offer high-risk pools or Medicaid buy-in programs for families who cannot qualify for Medicaid or Title V services and cannot purchase sufficient private insurance. Medicare is a federally funded program for people over 65 and those with severe, chronic kidney disease. Medicare coverage is not usually available to children with chronic health conditions.

This section of the chapter contains information about eligibility, benefits, and application procedures for each of the public sector programs. These programs have strict eligibility requirements and complex application procedures, so you may want to contact the appropriate state agency for further information and assistance with the application. (Look in the state government listings in the blue section of the Yellow Pages under "Health and Mental Hygiene." Under that heading there generally is a subsection with a heading such as "Medical Care Operations" or "Medical Care Policy Administration," with listings for "eligibility.") Social workers and hospital billing departments may also help you with these tasks.

Form 13. Health Insurance Policy Comparison Worksheet

Plan 1 _____

Plan 2 _____

Plan 3 _____

	Plan 1	Plan 2	Plan 3
Basic Provisions			
Choice of providers			
Service area restrictions			
Pre-existing condition restrictions			
Waiting period			
Prolonged illness clause			
Age limit for dependent children			
Conversion option			
Your Costs			
Annual premium			
Deductible: individual/family			
Annual out-of-pocket maximum			
Lifetime maximum on benefits			
Benefits Indicate copayment rate, separate deductibles, any limits on number or duration of services, and whether a referral or preapproval is required.			

Physician services
  Office visits
  Routine exams
  Surgical charges			

Form 13. Health Insurance Policy Comparison Worksheet (continued)

Benefits (continued)	Plan 1	Plan 2	Plan 3
Immunizations			
Prescription drugs			
Lab tests and X rays			
Outpatient surgery			

Inpatient hospital care
  Room and board
  Physician services
  Other hospital services
  Drugs and supplies			

Emergency care			

Psychiatric care
  Outpatient visits
  Inpatient care			

Physical therapy			
Occupational therapy			
Speech therapy			
Eye care			
Durable medical equipment			
Other benefits			

Medicaid

Medicaid is jointly funded and administered by the federal and state governments. The federal agency responsible for Medicaid is the Health Care Financing Administration (HCFA) of the U.S. Department of Health and Human Services. At the state level, the Medicaid agency is usually the state's public health or human services agency. Each state develops its own Medicaid plan and makes decisions about covered services and eligibility. The state plan must be approved by HCFA. Medicaid recipients are generally free to choose their own health care providers for Medicaid services.

When you have been approved for Medicaid coverage, you will be given a Medicaid card that must be presented to the health care provider every time you obtain covered services. The provider will submit the bill to the Medicaid agency, which will reimburse the provider directly. If you use your card to obtain services that are not covered, Medicaid will refuse the claim and you will be responsible for any costs incurred. If you are not sure whether a particular service is covered by Medicaid, you should obtain prior approval for the service from your Medicaid agency. You may also appeal the decision of the Medicaid agency if it refuses payment for a service that is medically necessary.

Medicaid eligibility. Medicaid eligibility is determined in a variety of ways. Families who are receiving Aid to Families with Dependent Children (AFDC) are automatically eligible for Medicaid. In most states, individuals are also automatically eligible for Medicaid if they receive Supplemental Security Income (SSI) through the Social Security Administration. To qualify for SSI, children must satisfy the federal standard for disability and meet the financial means test. A list of specific diagnoses is used to determine whether an SSI applicant is qualified to receive Medicaid coverage on the basis of disability. Children may also qualify when their particular diagnosis is not listed, if the disability is severe and significantly interferes with daily functioning.

A 1990 Supreme Court ruling called the Zebley ruling expands the definition of disability for children applying for SSI. For children under 18, the family's assets and income are considered in determining a child's financial eligibility for SSI. If the child is hospitalized for a period of 30 days or longer, the family's resources are not considered in determining financial eligibility during the period of hospitalization. When the child leaves the hospital, eligibility is re-evaluated and the family's resources are again taken into account.

In some states, Medicaid eligibility is granted to families who are determined to be "medically needy." The definition of medically needy is separately determined by each state that offers this eligibility category. Frequently, families become eligible under these guidelines after their out-of-pocket medical expenses are sufficient to bring their income and resources down to the standard Medicaid levels. Under medically needy provisions, families may not be entitled to the full range of Medicaid services. Medicaid eligibility is re-evaluated periodically, usually every 6 to 12 months. Any change in family income, family size, or dependent status can affect eligibility.

Medicaid benefits. Federal guidelines mandate a minimum set of services that must be covered by Medicaid programs. (States may provide additional, optional services, depending on the availability of health care funds.) The following services must be covered in all states:

- Inpatient hospital services
- Outpatient hospital services
- Rural health clinic services
- Lab and X-ray services
- Skilled nursing facility services and home health services for individuals 21 years of age or older
- Physician services
- Family planning services
- Nurse-midwife services
- Early and periodic screening, diagnosis, and treatment (EPSDT) for individuals under 21 years of age

Optional services offered by a specific state may include any combination of the following:

- Services of other licensed health care providers, including optometrist's services; dental services; physical therapy; occupational therapy; speech, hearing, and language disorder therapy; and rehabilitative services
- Drugs and devices, including prescription drugs, prosthetic devices, and eyeglasses
- Outpatient services, including screening services, preventive services, diagnostic services, clinic services, and emergency hospital services
- Intermediate care facilities (ICFs), including ICf services, ICf for the mentally retarded, and inpatient psychiatric services for individuals under age 21
- Skilled nursing facilities for individuals under age 21
- Personal care services and private duty nursing

Obtain the complete list of services covered in your state from your Medicaid agency. States may place limits on coverage for both mandatory and optional services. For example, there may be limits on the number of times you can have access to a particular service each year, or on the number of inpatient hospital days covered during a specific period of time.

Early and periodic screening, diagnosis, and treatment program (EPSDT). EPSDT is a part of the Medicaid program that is available to all Medicaid-eligible children who are younger than 21. EPSDT provides screening for actual and potential health problems. For any problem identified during the screening process, the state must provide all medically necessary diagnostic and treatment services that are covered in the state. Under the EPSDT program, the state has the option of providing additional, medically necessary services that are not normally covered by Medicaid, or of extending the usual limits on covered services. This important provision may be used to supplement traditional Medicaid services for chronically ill, Medicaid-eligible children, but the child must participate in EPSDT screenings and receive preapproval for any additional services. Many families and health care providers are not aware of EPSDT services. Be sure you ask for further information from your Medicaid agency.

Medicaid buy-in programs. Some states permit families to purchase Medicaid-like coverage for individuals who meet the Medicaid disability guidelines but whose financial resources exceed Medicaid limits. Premiums are usually based on a sliding fee scale. The greater the family's resources, the higher the premium for this coverage. These programs can be used to purchase insurance for individuals who are uninsurable in the private sector because of existing medical conditions. Medicaid buy-in programs can also be purchased as supplemental coverage for people whose private insurance is not sufficient to meet the high costs of care for chronic illness. These programs provide Medicaid benefits only to the individual who meets the definition of disability, and not to other members of the family.

Medicaid waivers. States have the option to offer Medicaid waivers, which expand the range of covered services or relax eligibility criteria. Waivers are generally granted to provide home health care for children whose Medicaid eligibility would otherwise depend on continued hospitalization. If care can be provided in the home that is equal in quality to that provided in the hospital, and if home care is less expensive, then a Medicaid waiver may be granted to cover the costs of in-home medical care. A waiver must be applied for, and waivers are seldom granted for children who do not require life-sustaining equipment or daily nursing care.

Title V (MCH Block Grant) Programs

Title V programs used to be called Crippled Children's Services but are now more frequently known as programs for Children with Special Health Care Needs (CSHCN), although different states have different names for these services. (Your pediatrician or other health care provider can tell you the name of the program in your state.) CSHCN programs are jointly administered by state health agencies and the Bureau of Maternal and Child Health (MCH) of the U.S. Department of Health and Human Services. The federal government provides funding for CSHCN programs through block grants. In some states the funds are augmented with state moneys.

You will receive a Title V card to present to health care providers. As with Medicaid, providers bill the state CSHCN program for reimbursement. You are not free to choose your own providers. You must obtain services from designated Title V providers and clinics.

Title V eligibility. Title V eligibility, which is based on both medical and financial need, varies dramatically from state to state. Many states limit services to children who have specific diagnoses, but Title V *income* limits are often more generous than Medicaid's. Contact your state's CSHCN program to receive a list of covered conditions and financial eligibility requirements.

Title V services. Because the federal government does not mandate which services must be covered by state Title V programs, there is tremendous variability among the states. Many states used to operate clinics to treat children with specific diagnoses, and some still do. In other cases, the Title V agency contracts with individual providers and facilities for the delivery of covered services. States are free to determine which types of services will be covered based on available funding, need, and health care priorities. Most state Title V agencies provide diagnostic services, care coordination, and limited treatment services. Request a list of covered services from the Title V agency in your state.

Supplemental Security Income

The Social Security Administration provides Supplemental Security Income (SSI) for individuals who meet disability and financial need criteria. SSI provides a monthly income based on the applicant's financial resources. The family's income and financial assets are considered in determining the size of the monthly stipend for a child. In most states, SSI recipients are automatically eligible for Medicaid. (Information on SSI eligibility criteria is provided in the section on Medicaid above.)

Other Funding Sources

High-Risk Pools

A high-risk pool offers health insurance to individuals or families who are unable to purchase standard policies because of expensive health conditions. High-risk pools are not available in every state. They are usually created by state laws that require insurers operating in that state to form an association to provide coverage for high-risk individuals.

High-risk policies are usually similar to traditional health plans. The insurance provides reimbursement for covered services listed in the policy. The insured person pays deductibles, copayments, and the full cost of noncovered services. Benefit limits and lifetime maximums may be in effect. Insurance coverage purchased from a high-risk pool is often very expensive. Premiums, deductibles, and copayments can be very costly, and the list of covered services may be quite limited. If you are unable to obtain health insurance from any other source, however, the cost of joining the high-risk pool may be less than going without any insurance at all.

Contact your state's insurance commissioner for more information about the high-risk pool. Find out what this insurance costs, who is eligible, and how to apply. Ask whether the state mandates a minimum set of covered services or benefits. If so, ask that a copy of the list of mandated covered services and benefits be sent to you.

Free or Reduced-Cost Care

Some health care providers, usually hospitals, offer free or reduced-cost care to individuals with limited family income and no other source of payment for health services. Eligibility for free or reduced-cost care is based on family size, family income and other assets, other health insurance, and the amount of unpaid medical bills. In some states, certain types of institutions are required to provide a specified amount of free care. Hospital emergency rooms are usually required to provide lifesaving emergency care regardless of the patient's ability to pay, but they are not under any obligation to provide free medical care for an illness or an injury sustained in an accident that is not immediately life-threatening.

If you are having difficulty paying for a provider's services, ask to speak with someone in the patient services or billing department, and find out whether you qualify for free or reduced-cost care. Even if you are not eligible, the billing department will usually work with you to develop an interest-free repayment plan to help you pay off large bills in small monthly installments.

Private Organizations

Private community groups and volunteer health organizations provide limited funds for the purchase of medical equipment or services not covered by insurance. None of the programs that disperse these funds are designed to provide ongoing support; instead, they make it possible for families to purchase specific items or services, such as wheelchairs or special shoes. Funding for these programs often is provided by individual donors, some of whom specify the conditions under which the funds are dispersed. The funds may allow only one grant per individual, or one grant per year, for example.

The Arthritis Foundation chapters in a number of states have limited funds available for people who have rheumatic illnesses. Many Arthritis Foundation chapters offer scholarships for children to attend summer arthritis camps. Some Shriner's hospitals, such as the Shriner's Hospital in Springfield, Massachusetts, offer free care to children who have JRA or other rheumatic diseases.

Health Care Reimbursement Accounts (HCRAs)

Internal Revenue Service (IRS) regulations allow individuals to establish personal accounts for the purpose of covering medical expenses not reimbursed by health insurance. These accounts, called Health Care Reimbursement Accounts (HCRAs), are set up and managed by employers.

To develop an account, the employee makes regular contributions through automatic payroll deductions. The employee is reimbursed from his or her account when receipts for medical bills are submitted to the employer (generally through the payroll or human resources office). The amount of the employee's salary that is subject to withholding for federal taxes, Social Security, and sometimes state and local taxes is reduced by the amount contributed to an HCRA.

The IRS also permits individuals who file itemized income tax returns to deduct health care expenses, but only medical costs that exceed an individual's adjusted gross income by 7.5 percent can be deducted. There are two advantages to establishing an HCRA. First, when you use an HCRA, you pay for health care with pretax dollars. Your taxable income is reduced by the entire amount of your HCRA contributions, regardless of your adjusted gross income.

The second advantage of HCRAs is that they make it easier to budget for health care expenses. A small weekly deduction of $25 will result in an HCRA worth $1,300 annually. Furthermore, the total amount of your annual contributions is available to you from your first day of participation in the program. If you have contributed $100 to your HCRA by the end of January and have reimbursable out-of-pocket expenses of $500 during that period, you will be reimbursed for the full $500 when you submit your receipts in February. Subsequent contributions to your account repay the amount reimbursed.

There are certain disadvantages of using HCRAs, as well. First, any unused funds remaining in your HCRA at the end of the year are forfeited. It is important to estimate your expenses carefully before setting your contribution rate, since if you cannot submit bills or insurance records showing out-of-pocket expenses totaling the amount of your account, you will lose the portion of your account that exceeds your expenses. You should also be careful to submit requests for reimbursement without delay. You usually have until March to submit reimbursement requests for expenses incurred in the preceding year.

Another disadvantage is that, because HCRA contributions reduce the amount of your salary subject to Social Security tax, you may receive a slightly lower Social Security benefit when you retire or if you become disabled. The tax advantages of an HCRA usually are greater than any reduction of Social Security benefits, however.

If you can estimate your out-of-pocket medical expenses fairly accurately, you will save money by establishing an HCRA. You can enroll in an HCRA when you begin a new job or during annual open-enrollment periods. You cannot change your contribution except during open enrollment, and contributions must be made through payroll deduction. You can stop payroll deductions at any time, but you will only be able to submit reimbursement requests for expenses incurred while you were enrolled in the program. You may be able to make changes to your HCRA without waiting for open enrollment when there are certain changes in your family status, such as the birth or death of a dependent or change in job status. There is a limit to the amount you can contribute to your HCRA.

Most out-of-pocket medical and dental expenses can be reimbursed through an HCRA. Generally, the same health care expenses that IRS regulations allow to be taken as deductions on itemized income tax returns are eligible for HCRA reimbursement. HCRA-reimbursable expenses include deductibles and copayments, eyeglasses and contact lenses, orthodontics, dentists' and doctors' fees, and hospital charges. One reimbursable expense that is often overlooked is automobile mileage, parking, and tolls for travel to health care. Your HCRA cannot reimburse for health insurance premiums or for medical costs that are reimbursed by other sources. Expenses for cosmetic surgery, health club dues, meals and lodging while away from home for medical treatment, and custodial care are not reimbursable from your HCRA.

Your employee benefits or personnel manager can provide complete information on HCRA application procedures and reimbursable expenses.

Resolving Disputed Claims

The best way to avoid problems with your health care claims is to understand your coverage thoroughly. Your policy is a contract between you and the insurance company for specific benefits. The insurance company must provide the coverage spelled out in the policy that you purchase through periodic premium payments. You are responsible for following the specified procedures for getting care (for example, using approved providers, obtaining required pre-approvals and referrals, giving prompt notification of emergency care received). Federal and state laws govern the practices of insurance companies. Contact your state's commissioner of insurance for information on health insurance regulations (look under "Insurance" in the state government listings in the blue pages of the Yellow Pages).

Public health agencies must follow very strict guidelines in evaluating eligibility and determining specific coverages. These agencies provide information about the health care programs they offer. If you are eligible for a public health program, you are entitled to receive the benefits provided by the program. You are responsible for following the agency's regulations and submitting required documentation. You can ask to have any unfavorable decision reconsidered if you are denied eligibility or if you are denied coverage for a specific medical service. The agency must explain the reasons for its decision and give you an opportunity to appeal.

If you believe that you have been denied coverage unfairly, contact the insurance company or appropriate public health agency immediately. Some disputes are resolved very easily with a single phone call. Insurance companies and public agencies do make mistakes, and they will correct any errors made in handling your claim. You may be asked to provide further documentation to clarify the nature of the service or its medical necessity.

Complicated disputes can take months to resolve, but persistence often pays off. Follow all appeals procedures carefully. Ask your employer's health benefits manager for help in dealing with an insurance company. Most public agencies have an appeals board that holds hearings to resolve disputes. Here are some strategies for resolving disputed claims:

Keep accurate records. The "Health Insurance Information" form in the directory of your personal health record provides spaces to record your policy numbers, public program identification numbers, and the names, addresses, phone numbers, and contact persons for each of your health care funding sources. Keep the form up to date, and have it handy when you call an insurance company or public agency.

In addition, save copies of all of your medical bills and receipts, and of all correspondence between you and your insurance company. Remember to save receipts for prescription medications, eyeglasses, and other medical costs in addition to bills from health care providers and hospitals. Staple receipts and documentation of insurance company payments to bills to make it easy to see what has been paid. Save all referral and preapproval forms. It is a good idea to keep a separate file for each family member.

Keep a log of telephone conversations, and keep the log in your personal health record for easy reference. Write down the name and title of the person you spoke with and the date of your conversation. Take notes on what was said. A sample "Telephone Log for Health Insurance Inquiries" is provided at the end of this chapter. (You may wish to make extra copies of this log for future use.)

Keep a log of outstanding medical bills in your personal health record. Record the date and type of service, the name of the provider, and the amount of the bill, as well as any payments made by you or your insurance company. A sample "Outstanding Medical Bills Log" is provided at the end of this chapter.

Do not delay. Contact your insurance company as soon as you find out that a claim has been denied. There may be a time limit on the period for filing appeals. Furthermore, you and your provider will have a better memory of details, such as the exact nature of the service received and the reason the service was medically necessary, which will help you deal more effectively with the insurer's objections.

Review medical bills for accuracy. Request itemized bills and examine them carefully. Errors are not unusual, particularly on hospital bills. Each type of medical service has an associated ICD-9 (International Classification of Diseases—9th Revision) code that must be listed on the bill sent to the insurance company. Contact the billing office if you have any questions about the nature of a coded service, or to report billing errors. If your insurance company has already paid a bill that contains an error, notify both the insurance company and the billing office. Erroneous charges paid by your insurance company can affect your benefit limits and lifetime maximum benefits.

Get it in writing. Any time an insurance company or billing department representative makes an oral agreement with you regarding payment for medical services, ask him or her to confirm the agreement in writing. This request is not an act of hostility or a show of distrust and will not be seen as such if you calmly explain that you would like a copy of the agreement for your files in the event that any questions arise in the future. In a similar vein, it's a good practice to follow up phone calls with a short note to the person you spoke with, summarizing the content of your conversation, any agreements reached, and any further action that is to be taken. Keep a copy of such letters for your records.

Ask for and record the name of the person handling your claim. If possible, speak with the same representative each time you call your insurance company about a claim, and address written correspondence to the same person. The claims representative will become familiar with your health insurance needs, and may be able to help you resolve similar disputes more easily in the future.

Get all necessary referrals and preapprovals before obtaining care. Except for emergency treatment, most insurance companies will not issue referrals retroactively. Even treatment that would normally be covered by your insurance can be denied if you fail to follow the required preapproval procedures. If you do forget to get a referral, file the claim anyway. You have nothing to lose, and a sympathetic insurance company representative may grant you an exception.

Ask for help from your health care providers. When you are denied coverage for a medical service, ask your pediatric rheumatologist, pediatrician, or other health care provider to write a letter explaining the nature of the service and why it is necessary. Speak with the clinic's social worker if you are having difficulty paying for health care that is not covered by your insurance or public health agency. Provider billing departments can also help you deal with insurance companies and public health agencies.

Ask for help from your employer. Your employer's health benefits manager can answer questions about your policy and help you present your case to the insurance company. Let your employer know if the company's plan does not meet your health insurance needs. Employers generally sign a new contract for health insurance each year. If employees are dissatisfied with a current plan, the employer may be willing to change plans, or may be able to negotiate better coverage under the existing plan.

Make a case for exceptions that can reduce the insurance company's costs. Occasionally, insurers will agree to pay for services that are not normally covered if you can show that by doing so you will avoid more expensive treatments that *are* covered by your plan. For example, your doctor may recommend intensive outpatient physical therapy to straighten a knee contracture, but your insurance does not cover physical therapy. An alternative treatment may be admission to the hospital for traction, which *would* be covered by your plan. If the outpatient physical therapy is less expensive than hospitalization and is equally (or more) effective, your insurance company may grant an exception and cover the costs of the physical therapy.

Understand and follow all procedures for filing an appeal. Insurance companies and public health agencies have established specific procedures for filing an appeal. To protect your rights, follow all procedures exactly. Be careful to meet time deadlines and promptly submit any additional information the insurer requests. Become familiar with appeals procedures before you actually need to use them. Your insurer can provide information about the appeals process.

File a complaint against your insurance company with your state's insurance commissioner.   The insurance commissioner is responsible for enforcing laws governing insurance practices. If your insurer does not honor the terms of your policy, you can file a complaint. The insurance commissioner's office will send you a description of the procedures for filing a complaint as well as documents that you will complete and return.

Form 14. Telephone Log for Health Insurance Inquiries

Date	Insurance Company or Agency Contacted	Name, Title, and Phone Number/Extension of Person Spoken With	What Was Discussed (For Specific Claims, Include Provider's Name, and Date and Type of Service	Action to Be Taken and Who Is Responsible

Form 15. Outstanding Medical Bills Log

Date of Service	Type of Service	Name of Provider	Amount of Bill	Amount You Have Paid	Amount Paid by Insurance	Check if Paid in Full

Chapter 9

•

The Child with Rheumatic Disease

All across the United States, bookstore shelves are stocked with materials offering childrearing advice to parents. These books and magazines describe and explain normal development and child behavior as well as specific childhood diseases and how to care for a child when he has one of these illnesses. For the most part, parents of a child with rheumatic disease will find that the advice offered in these materials applies perfectly to their child. In fact, the most important thing parents can do for their child with rheumatic disease is to raise him exactly as if he *did not* have a chronic disease.

The key to raising a child with chronic disease is to keep family life as normal as possible. If you have more than one child, treat your child with the rheumatic disease exactly the same as you do your other children. He should have the same responsibilities, be subjected to the same discipline, and complete his own set of household chores. If your expectations for your child are that he will grow into a happy, well-adjusted, and productive adult who will be independent and will be a contributing member of society—and this is what they should be—then the way you raise your child will convey to him your optimism and your confidence in him.

It's important to separate the illness from other aspects of childhood as much as possible. For example, you can expect and demand good behavior at all times, and you can assign appropriate household chores and expect your child to follow through on them. Be patient but firm in your expectations for your child. Don't allow your child to "get away" with unacceptable behavior just because he is feeling sick, or he may "use" his illness to justify misbehavior.

Because rheumatic diseases can lead to social isolation, it's important for school-aged children to participate in after-school activities and sports, with modifications when necessary. By the same token, younger children need to become part of a group of youngsters their own age. Most young children readily take part in normal childhood play groups, but some children are shy or reluctant and may need encouragement from you and the children in the group.

Finally, don't be preoccupied with your child's illness. If you are, your child will be, too. Let him go out into the world and try new things, even if you're afraid of the consequences.

As noted above, books and magazines describing normal childhood development and behavior and illnesses are useful resources for a parent of a child with rheumatic disease. This chapter, on the other hand, addresses some of the issues that are *different* for a child who is growing up with a rheumatic disease. It tries to explain what your child is feeling, and it provides guidance in how to help him with the obstacles he faces in his daily life. If you become concerned about your child's behavior, you may find it helpful to schedule a consultation with a mental health professional; the individualized advice you'll receive from him or her can make a huge difference. A social worker, a psychologist, or a psychiatrist located in the clinic or in your local community can help your child resolve his feelings and move on to healthy emotional development.

What Your Child May Be Feeling

Children learn from experience with acute illnesses (like ear infections and stomachaches) to expect their symptoms to go away if they follow their parents' and doctor's orders. It is very difficult for children to understand the notion of chronic illness. They may become discouraged when medication and therapy do not completely relieve their symptoms. They will also have trouble understanding that treatment must continue even when they are feeling well. Children who have chronic illness may feel sad, angry, frightened, or confused; they may experience a combination of these feelings, and their feelings are likely to change over time. It's not easy to adapt to daily routines of therapy and medication, frequent doctor visits, and uncertainty about the outcome of illness. Time, patience, and understanding will help.

Children who have rheumatic illnesses understandably have concerns about their health. They may be afraid of doctor visits, hospital stays, and blood tests and other medical procedures. They may also be worried that they will get sicker, become disabled, or even die. They may have fears that their parents or other family members will "catch" their illness. Teenagers, especially, are concerned about the impact of their illness on their future plans for careers, marriage, and children. Children are often reluctant to express their concerns, almost as if talking about it will make it come true.

Usually children imagine things to be much worse than they really are. To help them keep things in perspective, children need to receive honest information about their rheumatic illness. They should be told about likely outcomes, what to expect at the doctor's office, and when a procedure will be painful. To help children develop an optimistic outlook, they need to be told that their symptoms will likely get better even if they do not go away completely, that hospital stays and unpleasant procedures will come to an end, and that therapy will help them be able to do most of the things they enjoy doing.

Rheumatic illness can interfere with a child's developing sense of independence and competence. Even toddlers want to do things by themselves and make their own decisions, but the pain and stiffness caused by rheumatic illnesses can make it difficult for a child to dress, walk, and do other things by himself. It's tempting for parents to help too much. In the long run, however, it's much better to give the child extra time and provide whatever assistance is necessary, and *let him do things on his own.*

By encouraging a child to develop age-appropriate skills, adults can help the child develop self-confidence. Children should be given responsibility for doing home therapy, taking medications, and making decisions about their treatment plans in a manner appropriate to their age. Young children, for example, can decide whether they prefer to take medications in liquid or tablet form (when both forms are available), and they can be allowed to make decisions about what order to do their exercises in. Adolescents should be given the opportunity to participate in making decisions about their own health care whenever treatment options exist. They should also be responsible (with supervision) for taking their medications and doing their daily exercises.

Rheumatic illnesses can also make children feel isolated from their peers and classmates. Children want to "fit in": they want to look like other children their own age, and they want to do everything that other children their age enjoy doing. But rheumatic illness and the medications used in treating it can bring about unwanted changes in appearance (such as rash or weight gain) that threaten a child's body image and self-esteem. A child with a rheumatic illness may also be left out if he cannot run as fast or play as hard as other children. He also has less time for social activity because of frequent health care visits and daily home therapy programs.

Children may need help in dealing with teasing and in explaining their illness to friends and classmates. They also need encouragement in identifying their strengths and capabilities and in developing a strong sense of self-worth and accomplishment.

It is not uncommon for a child to feel guilty about having a chronic illness. Young children may believe that their illness is punishment for "bad" behavior, or that they caused the illness by something they did or failed to do. The child may blame himself when a new medication or treatment is ineffective. Older children sometimes feel guilty about the way their illness affects their families. They may worry about the high cost of their medical care and feel responsible when their illness interferes with family activities. Parents need to reassure their child that the illness is not his fault, and that he is important to the family and makes valuable contributions to the family despite his illness.

The following suggestions can help you help your child cope with his illness. It's essential to establish good communication at an early age, because it is often difficult to establish good communication for the first time as your child approaches adolescence and the teen years.

- Listen to your child. Talk to him about how he feels about the illness. Listen to his fears and concerns; allow him to express his feelings.
- Do not offer judgments or advice about his feelings. Don't try to talk him out of his feelings ("You don't need to be afraid, the disease will go away").
- Validate his feelings by conveying your understanding. Use phrases such as "I understand that you're angry about this disease." Avoid using phrases like "I know how bad you feel." You can't really *know* unless you have had the disease yourself, at the same age as your child. Instead, use phrases like "It must be awfully hard to have this disease at your age."
- Always think in terms of your child's *abilities* rather than his *limitations.* Emphasize what he *can* do rather than what he *can't* do; this will help him to develop a positive self-image. For example, if your child is concerned that he is the slowest runner in his gym class, gently remind him of what a strong swimmer he is. Encourage your child to develop interests that are appropriate for his illness.
- Help your child to understand his illness. Ask your child's doctor to help, too, by explaining what's going on and answering your child's questions.
- Don't hesitate to seek professional guidance to help your child deal with his emotions. The clinic's social worker or a community-based counselor can help your child resolve his feelings about the disease and move on to healthy emotional development. Ask your child's pediatrician or pediatric rheumatologist for advice about where you might go for professional counseling.

QUESTIONS AND ANSWERS ABOUT CHILD REARING

My older son has arthritis. Before arthritis he was active in sports. Now his younger brother is doing things that my son with arthritis can no longer do. Should I hold the younger brother back so that my older son won't feel bad about being unable to keep up?

In every family, different children develop in different ways, often with different interests and skills. It is important to encourage both children in areas that foster their self-esteem. The younger brother should be allowed to develop at his own pace; he should not be held back. You may need to explain to him why his older brother is unable to accomplish the same tasks or activities.

The older brother must learn to cope with the physical restrictions imposed by his JRA. Family members can help by acknowledging his frustration and possible anger while focusing on his abilities and accomplishments. He may need to receive some direction in identifying his own achievements or in choosing activities within his capacity to enable him to gain a sense of self-worth and confidence. If your son with arthritis is unable to participate actively in sports, encourage him to develop other interests and skills. The new activities may be equally rewarding to him. Perhaps your son with arthritis can play a musical instrument, become skillful in playing board games and video games, or keep statistics on professional ballplayers.

If he wants to, your son with arthritis can attend his brother's games; he may take pride in his brother's activities. If he resents his own inabilities, you can allow him to express his anger while gently steering him in other directions. Finally, if his distress impairs his relationships within the family or with peers, seek professional help for him in the clinic or in local agencies.

My daughter's pediatric rheumatologist has recommended that she attend "arthritis camp," which is a special one-week camp just for children who have arthritis. My daughter's arthritis really isn't that bad. Why should she go to arthritis camp instead of a regular camp with other children?

Arthritis camp can be a special experience for your child with arthritis, even if her arthritis is not severe. Arthritis camps usually last one week and are staffed by adults who have had JRA, medical professionals, and others with special interests in providing outdoor experiences for challenged individuals.

Arthritis camps provide a normal, fun camp experience for children with arthritis and encourage self-exploration and independence for children who may be dependent and overprotected in their daily lives. Staffers gently teach and remind campers how to ask for help, but they also give strong encouragement to allow them to achieve things they might not have thought they were capable of doing. Small victories, like swimming across the lake or conquering the zip-wire, can translate into confidence to reach goals in school and at home.

Perhaps the most important outcome of the camp experience is the enduring friendships established between campers. For many children, their week at arthritis camp is the first time they are in an environment in which they are not different, where no one cares if they move slowly (because everyone does), and where everyone understands what it's like to be stiff in the morning. Even for children who have mild arthritis, going to camp can be one of the most important experiences of their lives.

Being with a group of friends who are alike, and who understand without needing explanations, can be a powerful and positive experience, as this letter from Erika L. Lessard demonstrates. Erika wrote the letter in 1989 asking the nationally known radio disc jockey Casey Kasem to help her tell her friends from Camp Dartmouth-Hitchcock how much they meant to her. Not only did he play her request on his radio show, but he read her letter on the air.

Dear Casey Kasem:

I am a 14-year-old girl who has severe and chronic juvenile rheumatoid arthritis. I have had this disease since the age of 3. As I get older, the reality of the disease becomes more and more real.

In all of the pain and hard times, camp is a very special place to look forward to. This is a camp for kids with arthritis. I have been attending this camp for the past four summers. Kids from all over New England, New York, and Quebec, Canada, also attend. We don't like to think of it as a camp for kids who have arthritis. We like to think of it as a place for friends, who just happen to have the disease.

My best friends are from this camp, they are different from my friends I have at school, the ones from camp are very special to me. It's a good feeling to know that you have a friend who understands what you are feeling and going through. So Casey, could you please play "That's What Friends Are For" for everyone at camp, especially for Liz, Melissa, Frank, and Heather? They are the best friends a person could ask for.

Growing Up with a Rheumatic Disease

For the most part, developmental milestones such as learning to use the toilet, entering school, and expressing teenage rebellion will not be any different for a child with rheumatic disease than for healthy children. Occasionally, though, a child with rheumatic disease will have difficulty with one of the normal developmental tasks. It is not unusual for problems to arise, even if parents have made every effort to keep life as normal as possible. The following sections describe the range of issues encountered at different stages in childhood and offer tips on how to deal with them.

Infants and Toddlers

When a very young child develops arthritis or a rheumatic disease, it may be difficult to know how and when his medical problem impacts his behavior and development. Young children are unable to articulate their needs and problems. For example, your toddler may not be able to report where he feels pain, how severe it is, or whether it has improved or worsened after a treatment. Often, parents will report that their child with arthritis seems generally irritable or cranky and difficult to manage. It may not be until the arthritis is better controlled that the child's normal behavior returns, and it becomes clear that the cranky behavior was a result of discomfort from the arthritis.

Children who develop arthritis at the time of normal motor milestones may have delay in reaching their normal milestones. For example, a child who develops knee arthritis just after mastering walking may have diminished skill in walking and delay in beginning to run and climb. Children who develop arthritis in their hands or wrists may have delay in learning to dress or feed themselves. It is important to recognize that these delays are related to a physical difficulty, and to work specifically to encourage development of normal skills.

Frequent doctor visits, lab tests, taking medications, and doing therapy are understandably upsetting to a young child, who may show some emotional regression as one way of dealing with the disease. He may resume old habits you thought were gone, such as thumb-sucking, as a way of soothing himself. He may develop new behaviors, such as throwing temper tantrums when in the doctor's office, refusing to take medications, and so on. He may try to persuade you to help with activities such as feeding or dressing, even though he is able to do these things on his own. You cannot expect to be able to rationally explain your child's disease and need for treatment to your young child and thereby elicit his complete cooperation. Rather, you will need to work with him over time, comfort him when he needs it, and encourage him to do as much as he can on his own.

The Preschool Child

Developmental regression. Preschoolers often display regression in previously mastered developmental tasks when they develop a rheumatic disease or around the time of disease flares. For example, a previously toilet-trained toddler may begin to have accidents shortly after becoming ill.

If your child has this problem, the first thing to do is make sure that his difficulty with toilet training is not a result of physical problems caused by arthritis. His clothing should be easy for him to remove (elastic waists on pants are easier to handle than buttons or zippers). He should have a stepstool to support his feet while he sits on the toilet, and a stepstool or grab bar for standing in front of the toilet.

If you find that he is physically able to undress himself and get on the toilet, you may simply have to have patience, and resume the method of toilet training that was previously successful. Don't make a fuss about accidents, and be sure to praise or reward him for successful efforts.

Emotional regression. Preschoolers who become ill may start talking baby talk, sucking their thumb, or asking for a special blanket that they had previously given up. These activities can be comforting to a child. Although they are understandable at first, you should not encourage them to continue for a long time. The thing to do is ignore the regressive behaviors and praise mature behaviors and hope that your child abandons the regressive behaviors within a reasonable amount of time. If the regressive behaviors continue, gently but firmly encourage your child to give them up.

Separation difficulties. A preschool child may become clingy and fearful after developing the disease. For example, your child may refuse to play on the playground with other children, preferring to stay by your side. Your normal reaction may be to become overprotective in order to reassure your child and keep him from falling down. Instead, accompany your child onto the playground, help him to start playing with other children, and then gently step back to allow him to be independent.

The School-Aged Child

Emotional concerns. The school-aged child with rheumatic disease may develop excessive fear, anxiety, and timidity. Family difficulties, such as parental separation or divorce or financial problems, may have a greater effect on the child with a chronic illness, who may be more dependent on his parents than other children his age. Encourage your child to talk about his feelings, and try to reassure him while still being realistic. Establishing good communication between parent and child is important now and for the future.

Social activities. The child with rheumatic illness may not be able to participate fully in age-appropriate social activities such as hopscotch, jump rope, or baseball. Time taken up by frequent doctor visits and physical therapy may further limit his ability to play with friends. You need to encourage him to play with friends as much as possible, however, and make a special effort to invite friends over or make "play dates." Participating in community-oriented activities, such as Cub Scouts, Brownies, or 4-H Club, can be a real boost.

Self-image. Preteens may have significant concerns about the way they look and the effects of arthritis and their medications. Talk to your child about how he feels, and let him express his concerns. Help him in his efforts to look his best, perhaps by purchasing a special piece of clothing or getting a premium haircut.

School attendance. Attending school is vitally important both to help your child keep up with schoolwork and to allow him to have age-appropriate social interactions. Your child should be attending regular classes at school as much as possible. Home tutoring can increase social isolation and should be used only for rare occasions, such as following surgery, when a child cannot get to school.

Teenagers and Young Adults

Independence and responsibility. Every teenager matures and assumes responsibilities at his own pace, but at this age you can generally be successful in your efforts to encourage your child to become independently responsible for his own disease. Expect him to take his medications on time (and report any side effects to you) and perform his own exercise program. You will still need to monitor his activities to be sure medications are not missed and exercises are done.

This is also a good time to encourage your child to begin seeing the doctor independently, without having you in the examination room. This allows your child privacy during the examination and reinforces the message that he is the one who is ultimately responsible for taking care of himself. The doctor will still discuss his or her findings and recommendations with you, and will continue to seek input from you and answer your questions. Children should begin seeing an adult rheumatologist by age 21, or upon graduating from college.

Testing behavior. Teens often exhibit "testing" behavior as they begin to experience independence from their parents. Many chronically ill teens go through a period of experimentation with discontinuing their medications or refusing to perform necessary treatments such as physical therapy. If a medication is vitally important (prednisone, for example), you need to let your child's doctor know immediately if you suspect that your child is not taking it. If your teenager is experimenting with less risky behavior, like stopping his physical therapy or a nonvital medication, you should encourage him to discuss the issue with his doctor, but it may be up to you, again, to tell the pediatric rheumatologist about this behavior. It is usually better to allow the doctor to contract with your child to take his medicine, do his therapy, and so on, rather than allowing the issue to become a battleground at home. As worrisome as this behavior is to parents, it is very common, and most teens eventually develop a sense of personal responsibility about their disease.

Depression. Depression is common in adolescents with chronic illness. Parents need to be aware of the signs of depression, and to monitor their child's mood so they can detect depression and obtain timely professional help if it is needed. Parents who have established good communication with their child before the teenage years will find it easier to maintain an ongoing, open dialogue with their teenager; this both helps the parent monitor the child's moods and provides an outlet for the child. *The signs of depression are constant sadness, unexpected crying spells, withdrawal from previously important activities and friends, poor appetite, and trouble sleeping.*

Discipline. Continue to use appropriate discipline and establish firm rules at home. Don't be reluctant to establish and enforce rules for your child, even though he has a chronic illness. *Encourage age-appropriate social activities.* Being part of social groups is one of the most critical developmental tasks of adolescents, but chronic illness may keep a child from fully participating in such age-appropriate social activities as school dances or sports. Time needed for doctor visits or hospital stays may further limit his ability to socialize. Some teens may look like younger children because of short stature from arthritis or prednisone therapy. Parents can encourage age-appropriate social development by making it easy for their teenager to get together with friends and attend parties and other social events.

Employment. Encourage your child to get a part-time job when he turns 16. Work experience will give your child valuable skills and an expanded social circle. By working in high school, your child will learn responsibility and independence. He will also learn that he can be a valuable and contributing member of society. Studies have shown that chronically ill children who work part-time in high school are much more likely to go to college and become successful in jobs after graduation. Even younger children can have limited work experience through baby-sitting, news-paper routes, or helping with yard work.

Career planning. Talk with your teen about college and vocational training and employment plans following graduation. Your child's career choices may be limited by his disease. Be optimistic but realistic when considering career choices. Make use of appropriate vocational rehabilitation resources.

Self-image. Teens may have significant concerns about the way they look (body image) and the effect of arthritis and their medications. Talk to your child about how he feels, and let him express his concerns. If possible, help your child improve his appearance by purchasing clothing or getting a new haircut. Involve your child's doctor in discussions about appearance, as well, since he or she may be able to provide more information about the effects of illness and medications.

Sexuality and birth control. Teens with chronic illness frequently do not receive sex education comparable to that offered to their healthy peers, so it's especially important that you talk to your teenager about dating. Teenagers with rheumatic disease may be concerned about the effect of the disease and medications on future fertility, or they may have questions about birth control. Choices in methods of birth control may be restricted for sexually active teens with rheumatic diseases, and the disease or its medications may present specific concerns about pregnancy. Be sure that your child's pediatrician or pediatric rheumatologist discusses these medical issues with your teen.

Substance abuse. Talk with your teenager about alcohol and other drug use and abuse. *Children taking methotrexate should not drink alcohol.*

College. College presents a unique set of educational challenges for young adults with rheumatic diseases. In the college years, many children move away from home for the first time. They must deal with new living arrangements and a new school, and they must assume complete responsibility for their medical care. Planning ahead can help to ease the transition, and the Office for Handicapped Student Affairs at the college can usually help, as well. Here are some tips for college-bound students:

- If your child is taking an automobile to campus, he should plan to get a handicapped parking sticker.
- Your child needs to review his schedule with his advisor in advance to be certain that he will have enough time to get from one class to the next, keeping in mind that different classes meet in different buildings. Wearing high-quality athletic footwear will improve mobility on campus.
- If your child will be living in a dormitory without a reliable elevator, he should request a room on the first floor. A note from the doctor can help make sure that your child is given appropriate accommodations.
- A small tape recorder can help with note-taking, and a backpack is a must for carrying books. Access to a word processor will help with lengthy reports. For college students who have hand involvement, a laptop computer can be an essential tool.
- If the college is far from where he is currently living, he'll need to find a physician nearby as a contact. Your child's pediatric rheumatologist can help you and your child arrange the best plan for medical follow-up while away. He

should pack a good supply of the medications he is taking and a copy of his prescriptions that can be refilled at a pharmacy near the college.

The student health service at the college should be made aware of the diagnosis and any medical needs your child may have while at school, such as routine lab tests. Your child's pediatric rheumatologist should send medical records and any directions for necessary testing to the student health service.

Helping Your Child with Daily Life

Your child's rheumatic disease may cause him to have physical limitations that interfere with his ability to perform daily tasks. It may be hard for your child to dress, bathe, cut up food, or write and color. Performing household chores may be difficult. Although it is painful to watch your child struggle, it is important to let him do things for himself.

It is easy to fall into the trap of doing things for your child, because it is much easier and faster to do things yourself. Your child won't be late for school if you dress him in the morning, and you won't be late for your appointment if you carry him instead of waiting for him to walk. Most of all, it's hard to watch our children struggle.

Making your child do things for himself may be one of the hardest things you have to do, but it is very important. Your child needs to learn how to do things appropriate for his age, even if he does them in a way that is different from everyone else. It may be painful to watch him struggle to get into his clothes, but he will feel a tremendous sense of accomplishment when he achieves his goal. That sense of accomplishment is important to his developing self-esteem. Also, practice makes perfect; as he does these activities repeatedly, his speed and ease will improve.

You can still help your child; the important thing is *how* you help. Try to help in passive, unobtrusive ways rather than in an active, hands-on manner. For example, *do* buy clothes that are easy to put on and take off, but don't actually help him dress. Don't carry him to that appointment, but *do* be sure to allow extra time to get there and park close to the door to decrease the walking distance. The following sections address specific areas of daily life in which you may be able to assist your child toward independence.

Dressing

If your child has difficulty dressing or takes a long time to dress, try to analyze exactly what is causing the problem. Morning is often the worst time for stiffness, pain, and limited movement. A warm shower or a bath before dressing may relax muscles and joints enough to make dressing possible.

It's not unreasonable to expect your child to be fully dressed within 15 to 20 minutes of starting, unless your child is too tired afterward (this also assumes that your child doesn't get sidetracked with other things that take his attention away from the task at hand). If dressing takes longer than 20 minutes, or if your child is worn out after dressing, try organizing clothes in advance (the night before), and provide a chair at the right height for him to sit on to make the job easier. Use low drawers and shelves for storing clothes and shoes; use a low bar for hanging clothes in the closet.

Purchase loose-fitting clothes, elastic-waist pants, and shirts that pull on over the head rather than fasten. Look for clothes that fasten in the front rather than in the back. Velcro fasteners or snaps are easier to handle than buttons. Look for larger-sized buttons and zippers with large tabs; you might try adding a ring or loop to a zipper tab to make it easier to pull. Buy shoes with Velcro closures rather than ties, or try elastic shoelaces, so your child can slip his feet into his shoes without untying them; a long-handled shoehorn may also help. Attach cloth loops to socks so they can be pulled on more easily.

Your child may not be able to move his arms or legs easily enough to put on clothes as you do. In that case, you and your child should try to figure out an alternative way to dress. Enlist your child's curiosity when you ask him to solve his dressing challenges. You can also ask your child's occupational therapist about adaptive equipment that may make the job easier, such as a dressing stick, a sock aid, or a button aid. Praise and encouragement, as well as some tangible reinforcement (stickers, special time, or toy), help provide motivation for success.

Using the Bathroom

Mastering bathroom activities is critical to a child's self-esteem. It is important for your child to be able to use the toilet, wash his hands, and bathe independently, as appropriate for his age. Having the appropriate equipment available in your bathroom can help your child achieve the needed level of independence. Here are some tips to help your child be independent in the bathroom:

- Purchase a raised toilet seat for older children to make it easier to get on and off the toilet. A standard toilet is high enough for young children. Install grab bars next to the toilet, if needed.
- Place a nonslip bath mat in the tub. Try putting another bath mat, with a large piece of foam rubber attached to the back of it, over the edge of the tub to assist

in climbing in and out. A walk-in shower is often easier to use than a tub shower, so if it's desirable and possible, you might have a walk-in shower installed in your house.

- Your child may be able to shower independently if he can sit down to do it. Try using a shower bench or tub seat to make the job easier.
- A long-handled sponge can help him wash his feet and other parts of the body that may be difficult to reach. A bath pillow can make soaking in the bathtub more comfortable. A towel mitt can aid in washing and drying.
- Your child might find the push-button toothpaste dispensers to be easier to use than a tube with a screw-on top. An electric toothbrush with a built-up handle can help make thorough teeth cleaning easier.
- Provide your child with long-handled brushes and combs; build the handles up with pieces of foam rubber or sponge curlers to make them easier to grip.
- Be sure your child is able to use the toilet facilities independently at school, and be sure he actually uses them. Some children find it hard to use the school toilet. Consequently, they restrict their fluid intake and avoid using the toilet during the school day. If your child rushes into the bathroom immediately upon arriving home from school, this urgency may be a sign that he isn't able to use the bathroom facilities at school or doesn't feel comfortable using them.

Eating

Children with JRA who don't have enough dexterity in their hands to use utensils easily take more time to eat and may give up trying before they are full, just because eating is too much trouble. Many children with JRA have short stature and are underweight for their age. As noted earlier in this book, eating an adequate amount of nutritious calories each day is especially important for these children.

If your child has trouble using utensils, try the following suggestions, but don't abandon utensils altogether. Children need to learn proper table manners to avoid being embarrassed in public. Offer favorite foods like ice cream or pudding to encourage your child to practice using utensils, so that he will eventually feel confident about his skill in using them.

- Cook finger foods like pizza or chicken that are easy to manipulate and fun for your child to eat.
- Serve raw carrots and celery sticks instead of cooked vegetables.
- Allow your child to pick up his food with his fingers, rather than forcing him to use a knife and fork. Chicken can easily be eaten with the fingers, but even salad, cooked vegetables, and meats should not be off limits at home.

- Pack school lunches with foods that your child can easily eat, including sandwiches, raw vegetable sticks, and fresh fruit. Your child may feel uncomfortable eating with his fingers at school, and may have difficulty using utensils to eat a hot school lunch.
- Serve foods in a sandwich so your child won't have to cut them. Serve hamburgers and hot dogs on a bun, or steak in a sandwich.
- Choose foods that are easy to eat with utensils. For example, macaroni is easier to eat than spaghetti, and stew is easier to eat than soup.
- Ask your occupational therapist about special built-up utensils that are easy to use. You can also build up utensils yourself—by wrapping a sponge curler around the handle, for example.
- Cut firm foods like meat and potatoes into small pieces before serving them. Butter bread before serving it.
- Put a mug or glass with a handle at your child's place setting, because it will be easier to grasp. Provide him with a flexible straw if holding the cup is difficult.
- Place a disk of rubber or a damp cloth under dishes to keep them in place.

Getting Around

Children with arthritis need to walk in order to keep their muscles and bones strong and to keep their joints moving. You should encourage your child to walk independently whenever possible, whether or not he is uncomfortable. It is not healthy for a child's social or emotional development to be carried for extended periods of time. Carry your child only as much as is appropriate for his age; school-aged children should not be carried, and preschoolers should be carried only occasionally. Many of the things you do will now take longer, so plan to allow extra time whenever possible.

Footwear. One way of helping your child to walk more easily is to purchase appropriate footwear. Appropriate footwear can help a child with arthritis walk for longer distances with less pain. Shoes with rigid soles or high heels should be avoided. Desirable features include flat heels, flexible soles, a wide toe box, and plenty of cushion. Well-built athletic shoes are usually the best choice, as they have all of these features plus certain biomechanical advantages. Price is often (but not always) an indication of quality. Ask your physical therapist if there are specific features you should look for in shoes.

Handicapped license plates. Handicapped parking spaces are provided, by law, at most places of business, schools, and shopping areas. Handicapped spaces are wider than traditional parking spaces and are located near curb cuts and building entrances. In a parking garage, the handicapped parking spaces may be located on the ground floor or near elevators. Only cars bearing an official handicapped plate or placard are permitted to park in these spaces. Others risk being ticketed or towed away.

If your child has significant problems with mobility, or if he uses crutches or a wheelchair, you may be able to obtain a handicapped plate or placard. Contact your state's Registry of Motor Vehicles or Department of Motor Vehicles to request an application form. The form contains different parts that must be completed by both you and your child's physician. Generally, successful applicants are required to have a permanent disability that causes substantial difficulty with usual activities, such as work for adults or school in the case of children. Many parents of children who have rheumatic illnesses have been successful in obtaining handicapped plates or placards.

The handicapped plate attaches permanently to your car, in place of your old license plate. The handicapped placard has the advantage of portability: it can be placed on the dashboard of any vehicle your child is riding in. If your child frequently rides in two or more vehicles, the placard may be a better choice for you. Occasionally, when a vehicle with a standard license plate parks in a handicapped space, it is ticketed by a police officer who forgets to check the dashboard for the handicapped placard. The New England Chapter of the Paralyzed Veterans of America offers bright yellow and black bumper stickers with the message "Handicapped Parking Permit on Dash" to help placard users avoid this problem. There is no charge for the first sticker. Up to three additional stickers may be purchased for a charge of fifty cents each. To obtain the bumper stickers, send a business-size, self-addressed stamped envelope to Paralyzed Veterans of America, New England Chapter, Suite 101R, 1600 Providence Highway, Walpole, MA 02081.

Mornings

Mornings are chaotic in every household. Parents need to get ready for work, children need to get ready for school or day care, and there never seems to be enough time. When your child has arthritis, mornings deserve special consideration. Because of morning stiffness, it can take much longer for your child to get ready for the day. Getting him into a warm bath and seeing him through a series of range-of-motion exercises to relieve morning stiffness may seem impossible given the time constraints you are under. Letting your child wash and dress independently may seem hopeless. Here are some ideas to help mornings go more smoothly:

- Prepare in advance. Have your children pick out their clothes the night before. Be sure your child has any equipment he needs. Pack lunches and book bags before going to bed at night. Have the coats by the door and the breakfast materials laid out on the table.

- Have your child get up early enough so there is time to get everything done without feeling rushed. If you are concerned about the amount of sleep he gets, have him go to bed earlier at night rather than wake him up later.
- Give the morning dose of medication to your child a half hour before he needs to wake up. This will give the medicine time to work while he sleeps a bit more, and will help to minimize the morning stiffness.

Assistive Devices

Assistive devices are used to increase independence in daily living skills. They include a wide variety of equipment, some of which may be permanently installed in your home. Dressing aids, bathroom equipment, and crutches are examples of assistive devices. The use of assistive devices has both benefits and drawbacks. The obvious benefit is increased independence for the child, which improves self-esteem. Some assistive devices, however, may discourage the child from using his joints normally. This can lead to increased disability and dependence on the equipment. For this reason, most assistive devices are recommended only when they are absolutely necessary. Ask your physical or occupational therapist for advice regarding assistive devices that may be useful for your child.

Looking Good with SLE and Scleroderma

Many teenagers who have SLE or scleroderma are concerned about the effect of the disease on their appearance. Here are some ideas to help your teen look his best:

- Cover skin rashes. Use foundation to cover rashes or uneven skin tone. Lightly tinted foundation will also add healthy color to pale skin. To hide dark- or light-colored spots, apply foundation followed by a light dusting of face powder. Then brush a colored blusher on and around the spots and blend in with the other areas.
- Acne. Use over-the-counter astringents and soaps to cleanse the skin. If these do not work, ask your pediatric rheumatologist or dermatologist for assistance.
- Thinning hair. Your child should use a mild shampoo to slow hair loss from SLE. Ask your hairdresser about safe, gentle products available. Rubber bands and hair clips that might pull on hair should be avoided. Rubber brushes and combs with rounded rubber tips are more gentle than hard plastic. Hair should not be brushed while wet; comb tangles out gently, starting at the ends of the hair and gradually working toward the scalp. Soft sponge rollers should be used

in place of brush rollers. Avoid using strong chemicals (hair dyes, permanents, or sprays), curling irons, and hot rollers. Fun hats and scarves can be used to camouflage thinning hair. A natural-looking wig that will successfully cover severe hair loss can be purchased ready-made or can be custom made.

QUESTIONS AND ANSWERS ABOUT DAILY LIVING

Should my child wear a Medic Alert bracelet?

Any child whose medical condition requires special treatment in an emergency should wear a Medic Alert bracelet or necklace. This includes children who are taking prednisone, because they must receive special care and may need additional steroids in the event of an accident or other medical emergency. If you are uncertain of your child's need for a Medic Alert identification tag, speak with the nurse in your child's pediatric rheumatology clinic, the pediatric rheumatologist, or your child's pediatrician.

A Medic Alert identification can help your child receive appropriate emergency care, especially if you are not available to provide important medical information yourself. The identification necklace or bracelet is engraved with your child's own identification number, critical medical information, and Medic Alert's 24-hour emergency hot line. Medic Alert maintains additional, confidential medical information in its data base, including the name and phone number of your physician and pharmacy, and family phone numbers. Each year, Medic Alert sends you a wallet card copy of your medical information and a reminder to keep the information up to date. Emergency medical personnel are familiar with the Medic Alert system and will know how to obtain emergency medical information about your child.

Medic Alert application forms are available at most pharmacies. You can enroll in the system by phone or mail. There is a one-time charge that covers the cost of the identification bracelet or necklace and lifetime access to the emergency hot line. You can update your emergency medical information at any time by phone or mail for a service fee. The standard identification tag is made of stainless steel. For a higher fee, you can purchase tags made of sterling silver or 22-karat gold plate. For more information, contact the Medic Alert Foundation International, 2323 Colorado Avenue, Turlock, CA 95380, or call 800-ID-ALERT.

My employer recently offered a new life insurance plan with an option to purchase a low-cost rider for my children. I was shocked when coverage was denied for my daughter, who has JRA. It turns out that she was denied coverage because of the insurance company's policy about rheumatoid arthritis, not JRA. I am worried that my daughter may have to face a lifetime of being denied life insurance because of her illness. What can I do?

You would be smart to take action now, rather than waiting until your daughter is older. Obtaining life insurance for her now will give you peace of mind and will serve as a precedent for your daughter to use in the future as she faces this issue again in employment situations.

- Begin by writing a letter to the insurance company requesting an appeal of their decision.
- Call the human resources department of the company that's giving you the problem, and obtain the name and title of the person in charge of this area. Then write a letter to that person and ask for assistance. Include a reference to any case or policy numbers that were included in the company's correspondence with you.
- Be firm but polite with your requests. Avoid making hostile or emotionally charged statements. Type the letter in a business format. A well-written, professional-looking letter will be given much more attention than a scribbled note.
- Request that the medical review board fully differentiate between JRA and rheumatoid arthritis. Include quotes from the literature that support your claim that JRA in children is not as severe as rheumatoid arthritis in adults.
- Enclose a letter from your child's doctor stating that there is a negligible probability that JRA will reduce your child's life span.
- Include the names and addresses of all of your child's physicians (pediatric rheumatologist, pediatrician, and ophthalmologist). Include a signed statement that gives your insurance company permission to contact these physicians as needed regarding your child's case. This both lets them know that you are not alone in making your appeal and makes it easier for them to make a decision.
- Send the letter by registered, return-receipt mail. This provides confirmation of delivery of the letter and indicates that your claim is not to be taken lightly.
- Include your name, address, and a daytime phone number. Say that you will call 3 weeks after receiving confirmation of delivery of the letter to check on the status of the appeal.
- Keep a copy of the letter (and enclosures, if applicable). Send copies of the letter to your employer's benefits department or to any other party who can act as an advocate for your case.

- Follow up in 3 weeks' time, as indicated in your letter. With any luck, before the 3 weeks have elapsed, you will hear from your insurance company that their original decision has been reversed. If the insurance company will not change its decision, you will have to decide whether it's worth it to you to appeal the decision one more time, or whether you would prefer to seek life insurance for your daughter elsewhere.

Sports and Other Recreational Activities

Children with rheumatic disease must have the opportunity to participate in sports and other recreational activities that are so very important in a child's life. It is through these activities that children develop new physical skills as well as develop balance and coordination and gain confidence in their physical abilities. They also give children a chance to learn how to interact in group situations.

Performed in conjunction with a prescribed exercise program, certain sports and recreational activities can help a child achieve the goals of therapy: they help to maintain normal joint movement, preserve muscle strength, and bolster overall fitness. In short, sports and recreational activities help your child to exercise his muscles, develop important social skills, and have fun, as the following narrative illustrates. It was written by Kendra Staudinger when she was 12 years old.

I am 12 years old and I have had arthritis since I was 6. Even though I have this disease, I still try to do all the things I want to do. My favorite sport is horseback riding. I have been riding for 3 years. At first it was scary. My mom and dad thought that I could get hurt, but my doctor said that if I wanted to ride, I should do it. I am glad that she helped convince my parents that I could start riding. I have been able to compete in many horse-riding shows over the past 3 years, and have won several blue ribbons and champion trophies. My suggestion is to try to do whatever you enjoy doing, and to do your best!

As Kendra's story illustrates, it's best to let your child choose his own activities, since he is most likely to enjoy activities that interest him and that he has chosen himself. You can encourage him to choose activities that exercise the joints and muscles without putting too much stress on them, however. Swimming and bike riding are excellent choices. In the long run, refusing to let your child participate in an activity he likes may be worse for him than the arthritis itself. Achieving success at the new activity can be extremely rewarding, and a series of small successes will help your child to develop confidence in himself and his abilities. Be sure to check with your doctor or therapist before your child begins a new physical activity.

Your child's discomfort will usually be the only factor limiting physical activities. Children can usually tell if they have done too much by the way they feel the next day, but they may not always tell you how they feel. Some children push themselves too hard, trying to keep up with their peers. Others learn to "use" fatigue and soreness to avoid activities they don't want to do. As a rule, you can tell whether an activity has been too much for your child by whether or not he complains of increased pain for more than 2 hours after the activity; another indication would be a significant decrease in his functional abilities. If this occurs, it doesn't mean the activity is off limits. It does mean that it would be a good idea for him to participate for a shorter period of time or in a less aggressive manner the next time.

Finally, sports and other recreational activities are *not* a substitute for your child's therapy program. Only therapeutic exercises can provide the specific stretching and strengthening that is necessary to improve joints and muscles. Sports are a good adjunct to therapy, and the therapy will help your child perform better in sports, but they are not interchangeable. Here are some more guidelines:

- Avoid activities that put full body weight on a normally non-weight-bearing joint that has arthritis. For example, children who have neck arthritis should not perform somersaults and headstands. Children with hand and wrist arthritis should not perform handstands and cartwheels.
- Contact sports such as football should be avoided.
- Toe ballet (pointe) should be avoided by children with foot and ankle arthritis, although regular ballet or other dance is a helpful activity.
- Evaluate whether new activities are appropriate by asking yourself the following questions: Which joints are stressed by this particular activity? Do these joints have arthritis? What is the general state of your child's arthritis (acute or controlled)? What is his overall physical condition?

Recreational Activities

It is important for your child to be able to participate in recreational activities along with children his own age. Swimming, bike riding, and dancing are excellent activities for children of all ages; they help a child increase strength and endurance without causing too much stress to any joints. Swimming or splashing and kicking in a wading pool allows a child to freely move his arms and legs. Water provides buoyancy, which makes it easier for the child to move. If your child doesn't know how to swim, he can wear flotation devices to help him move in the water. Children with arthritis usually relax more easily and feel less stiff in a heated pool.

Bike riding helps maintain joint motion and muscle strength in the legs. It also builds endurance. For preschoolers, a standard tricycle is an excellent way of building both motion and strength; it can also come in handy if your child is having difficulty walking during a flare. Other beneficial recreational activities include kick-ball, dodge-ball, tag, hide-and-seek, kick-the-can, softball, badminton, and golf.

Some of the popular recreational activities can be difficult for children with arthritis because they place stress on certain joints that may have arthritis. Jumping rope and playing hopscotch are tough on ankles that have arthritis. Volleyball can be hard on children with wrist and hand arthritis, as can ice skating or roller skating (because you fall on your hands). You may want to ask your doctor or therapist for guidelines in these situations. Protective equipment may be used to reduce the chance of injury.

Skill-Based Exercise Classes

Organized exercise classes such as ballet, karate, and gymnastics are splendid choices for children with arthritis, who may not be able to maintain the same activity level as their healthy peers and therefore may have difficulty developing balance, coordination, and physical skills at the rate of other children their age. Organized exercise classes promote healthy development by providing a controlled and safe environment where children with arthritis can try new physical activities. Success at the new activities can be extremely rewarding and may help the child to develop new confidence in himself and his abilities. Always check with your child's doctor or therapist before your child undertakes a new physical activity.

Sports

Having strong muscles to provide joint protection is the key to participating safely in sports. Although contact sports are not recommended, even very aggressive sports like soccer and basketball may not be off limits. Before your child takes up any new sport, however, you should consult with your child's doctor and therapist. They will determine whether or not the sport is appropriate for your child by assessing his level of pain and physical ability. Some types of arthritis are severe, and engaging in sports may not be wise if this is the case. On the other hand, your child may be able to do special exercises to *train* for the sport he likes. Protective equipment can further reduce the risk of injury.

Training. Proper training is the key to both safety and performance in sports. Training is very important for *all* athletes and is doubly so for children with rheumatic diseases. Proper training will improve athletic performance, prevent injuries, speed the healing of injuries that do occur, and prevent arthritis flares.

Training should consist of flexibility exercises, muscle strengthening, and aerobic training. Training should begin 6 to 8 weeks in advance of starting the sport. For example, if a child wants to ski in January, he must begin strengthening in mid-November.

Warm-up and cool-down. Your child should learn warm-up and cool-down stretches to do before and after participating in a sport during the athletic season. Heat and cold can also be useful adjuncts to warm-ups and cool-downs. Heat is used before doing warm-up stretches. Warming a joint up before engaging in a sport helps to make the joint more flexible and "ready" for the sport. Applying a heating pad or immersing in a whirlpool or warm bath lasting 20 minutes is usually sufficient.

Ice can be applied immediately after cool-down (right on the field, if possible). A joint becomes inflamed and experiences microtrauma during vigorous sporting activities. Applying ice directly to the joint for 10 minutes immediately after cool-down can help to reduce the swelling, pain, and stiffness that might occur. The benefits of the icing will be reduced if the child waits until he gets home to apply it.

Game time. When your child is ready to start playing, gauge his activity by the way he feels later. Rather than playing a full game at the start, have him play for 20 to 30 minutes and see how he feels that evening and the next day. If your child finds that his joints are extremely sore, he may need to play for a shorter period next time. If he feels fine, he can play longer. Keep in mind that a new sport usually results in some discomfort later, even for people who do not have arthritis.

When a child has arthritis he is more likely to injure his joints during sport activities. The injuries that occur are similar to those in a child without arthritis, but they may be more severe and they may take longer to heal. These injuries rarely result in long-term disability, however. Some children find that their arthritis flares when they play a new sport that is more vigorous than they are accustomed to. Once they become adept in the new sport, however, they are able to perform it without a flare of their disease. Take Maria Bruno, for example, an honor roll student and one of only 10 girls chosen to play on the Massachusetts Patriots Regional Volleyball team, who describes her own career in group sports this way:

I was first diagnosed as having JRA at the age of three and a half. My knuckles, both hips, and both knees were affected. Throughout the years, I have led a pretty normal life. I took ballet and tap-dancing lessons and was a happy kid. I had a few flare-ups in the second and fourth grades, yet they only involved my left knee. Things went along pretty smoothly during the sixth and seventh grades. I was playing basketball for my junior high school team and my arthritis wasn't stopping me from participating. Everything seemed too good to be true.

Well, everything was too good to be true! At the beginning of the eighth grade I experienced a major flare-up. The arthritis spread from my left knee to several other joints, such as my neck, jaw, two fingers, and my right wrist. It was horrible as well as terribly frightening. I thought I would be confined to a wheelchair. My dreams of being a basketball star were shattered. My therapy was not helping. Something else had to be done. Why was this happening after my arthritis was doing so well for so long?

The only thing that I could try now was gold injections. I was scared. Would it hurt terribly? Would I experience some of the side effects of the medication? And most of all, would it work? God, I prayed it would. After 6 months of weekly injections and endless blood and urine tests, the medication started to show its effects. My joints were less stiff and painful, and things were looking a lot brighter! The following summer my arthritis was being controlled by this wonderful drug.

In the fall, I entered my freshman year at Bishop Feehan High School, in Attleboro, Massachusetts. I tried out for the volleyball and basketball teams. I made both teams. I chose to play these sports despite my arthritis. I didn't want to baby the disease because that would do more harm than good. Now, today, as my volleyball team goes into the state championship finals, I look back and wonder how I did it. I am the starting setter-hitter on the Bishop Feehan volleyball team and I play the entire game. I believe, from my experience, that nothing is impossible, even if you have JRA. But still to this day, my doctor wonders why I couldn't have chosen something "safe" like joining the high school debating team or the math team!

Coaching, Refereeing, and Timekeeping

Children who aren't able to participate in sports because of arthritis but who are very interested in them and want to be involved should be encouraged to get a position as scorekeeper, timekeeper, assistant coach, trainer, referee, or umpire. These positions are often available in school intramural and competitive athletics as well as in recreational leagues or councils. The following story was written by Christopher Sadler, a student at the Massachusetts Maritime Academy, who was not able to participate in team sports due to active arthritis while in high school but nevertheless found plenty of things to do:

When diagnosed with JRS, I was 15 years old and enrolled as a freshman in high school. Since I was unable to participate in sports and socialize with girls, I combined the two by offering my services to the coaches of female sports teams. I had the best of both worlds by being involved with a sports team and being surrounded by girls; almost the whole time, I was the only male around. I was also the envy of many other guys because of that fact. I felt it gave me an advantage in my life, especially when I needed all I could get.

My parents and doctor backed me on important decisions that might not have turned out to have a positive outcome. Before my flare, I was involved in a scuba class. When it was time to get my certification, I was not in condition to be on my own at 30 feet under water. I beat the odds, earned my certification, and look back on that as a major achievement in my life, even to this day. At the time it meant more because there was not that much that I could do, and every little thing was magnified somehow in importance. If I was not allowed to do it, I would probably regret it for a very long time. When my condition grew worse, I did have to quit my part-time job because it was too physically demanding. I missed having extra money and having something to do on the weekends or at night.

I was also lucky enough to have friends at an athletic club, which allowed me to get a membership allowing me to use a pool, hot tub, and weights. I found that swimming relieved much of the pressure on my joints. I could do my exercises and stretches with better results.

QUESTIONS AND ANSWERS ABOUT SPORTS AND OTHER RECREATIONAL ACTIVITIES

My 15-year-old-son has arthritis in one knee but still wants to play baseball with his school team in the spring. Could he make his disease worse by doing this?

Many children who have arthritis participate in competitive sports, and your son may be able to, as well. This will depend on how active he is now, and whether he is willing to train in advance to prepare for the baseball season. In the long run, baseball may not make his arthritis worse if he takes proper precautions to protect himself. With advance planning, your son may be able to play competitive baseball with little difficulty. Here are the things you need to do:

- Consult with your child's doctor to be sure baseball is appropriate for your son.
- Be certain that your son participates in an adequate training program *before* the start of the baseball season. Training should consist of a comprehensive program of stretching, strengthening, and aerobic exercises. The training exercises should begin 6 to 8 weeks prior to starting practice and should be done daily for at least 30 to 45 minutes. Ask your son's therapist for advice regarding specific exercises that would help.
- At the start of the season, have your son start by playing only one or two innings and see how he feels that evening and the next day. If he experiences significant

pain, he may need to play for a shorter period of time; if he has no difficulty, he can extend his play time to five or six innings in the next game.

In Their Own Words

We have seen many, many children with rheumatic diseases throughout our years of practice. One message we want to convey, and we hope that we have done so in this book, is that these children do well. They accomplish, they achieve, they go to college, they outperform their peers, and more. Perhaps the best way to demonstrate what these children are capable of is to share their testimonies about how their lives have gone. That's what we've done in the remainder of this chapter.

I am your average American kid. You know, blond hair, blue eyes, glasses, and well, freckles (just a few, though). I've got a pretty good life except for one little setback: I have JRA. I was diagnosed with JRA when I was 18 months old, so I've had a lot of practice learning to live with it. Sure, I wake up stiff and take medications, but like the song says, "I haven't got time for the pain." JRA is a bit inconvenient, but I sure don't let it get the best of me. I still have a lot of living to do.

I enjoy swimming. In fact, I was a member of the YMCA 1991 swim team. I also bike ride, play piano, roller skate, and I once tried to ice skate and ski. I even have a paper route. My JRA can get in the way of my papers, but I have a "back-up." Sometimes I have flare-ups and I hurt so much that my mom and brother help me out. My dad's really great too, he does them for me when I have doctors' appointments. So all you kids with JRA, get off your couches and enjoy life. After all, you only live once!!

Written by Andrea Dubois when she was 13 years old.

When I was little, I dreamed of being an Olympic track runner. I was the fastest in my class. I could beat practically anyone. At age 10, my dream was shattered. I came down with dermatomyositis. My muscles were stiff and sore. I could hardly walk. I got horrible stomachaches and could hardly eat. My skin got all scaly, red, and sore. For 3 years I was up and down on prednisone, and I felt awful. In September 1987 I went to the hospital and stayed for one month. Now, in April, I am almost totally off prednisone and I feel great. I know I'm not always happy, and I am shorter than I should be, but it is like they say in a song from Les Miserables, "The world is big but little people turn it around." P.S. Watch out 1992 Olympics. I'm running again!

Written in 1988 by Lyndsley Wilkerson when she was in the eighth grade at the Peck School in Morristown, New Jersey, where she published a biweekly newspaper. Lyndsley had recently received the Johns Hopkins University Gifted and Talented Youth Program State Award.

When I was 10 years old, I had a terrible reaction to erythromycin. I vomited for hours. Approximately 6 months went by before the doctors could figure out why I wasn't getting well. I was diagnosed as having systemic lupus erythematosus after having all kinds of tests. I had never heard of lupus before I got sick. Now it seems like everyone I know knows someone who has it. I have many friends who were diagnosed with lupus at an early age.

I had joint and muscle pain, and the doctor removed fluid from my right knee. There was heart and liver damage and lesions (sores) in my mouth. After that, they started me on prednisone and I had frequent blood tests, EKGs, echocardiograms, and chest X rays. From there I bounced up and down on prednisone doses with all the usual side effects. In May 1987, the doctors found my kidneys were also affected. I started chemotherapy (Cytoxan) every month for 7 months, then every 2 months. I started losing my hair. I found that when I was unhappy and nervous about Cytoxan treatments I got sick. The calmer I am, the better the treatment goes.

I'll be 14 years old in May. School's going great and I feel great. Our goal is to get me completely off prednisone. I live a very normal life except for a few minor setbacks, such as staying out of the sun, not being too active, and watching my salt intake. I don't know what the future holds for me. They may find a cure for lupus, or at least find better ways of treating it. My goal is to stay as healthy and happy as I possibly can.

Written by Elizabeth Ramsey, an honor-roll student and a recipient of the President's Award for Fitness. This is excerpted from a report she wrote that won first place in her school's project fair.

For the past year and a half now I've been very ill with a rare disease called dermatomyositis. I spent a total of 7 months in the hospital. Those were the hardest months of my life. I was confined to a wheelchair and was extremely weak. While in the hospital, I learned many ways to adapt myself to my new life-style.

I had planned to go away to college and live on campus. I intended to study journalism. But due to my illness I wasn't able to fulfill my plans. I felt so much frustration at that point because I was really looking forward to going away for college and now everything was put on hold because of my disease.

The importance behind this event in my life is that my self-esteem was completely uplifted to a higher degree. Before all of this I was very shy and insecure. I never thought anything I did was right or even beautiful. The only thing that I did properly all of the time was my schoolwork. I also thought that I wasn't an important person to either my family or friends. I always felt left out.

But over time I've learned that I'm smart, interesting to others, and beautiful. So I no longer see myself as a dark shadow. I see myself as a rainbow that shines after every storm.

> *Written by Eva Aquino when she was 16 years old. Eva now studies journalism at the University of Massachusetts.*

You have probably never heard of it, yet scleroderma is five times more common than muscular dystrophy or multiple sclerosis. It's nothing new. Evidence of it has been discovered even on ancient Egyptian mummies. Scleroderma, from the Greek meaning "hard skin," is a connective tissue disease involving the collagen-forming tissues. It is a chronic disease which affects as many as 250,000 people in the United States. My reason for writing this report is because I have generalized scleroderma and I want to let people know that there are other diseases out there that are just as bad as cystic fibrosis and multiple sclerosis. I was diagnosed as having this disease when I was 13 years old. The doctors can't give me a prognosis; my mother says, one day at a time.

> *Excerpted from a science report written by Michael Strothman when he was 15 years old and in the tenth grade at Malden High School, Malden, Massachusetts.*

Every Wednesday after school I go to the hospital near my house and volunteer as a candy striper. I have been doing it for one and a half years and I really enjoy it. When I first started, I did courier work, which consisted of running errands for different departments in the hospital and delivering flowers. After one year of that, I switched to working in the pediatric department, in the playroom that is there, because I wanted to work with kids.

The types of things I do with the children are varied. We can play Nintendo, make arts and crafts projects, play games, or just have fun talking and laughing. When I don't feel well there are a lot of people who help me, and it makes it easier to feel better. They are helping me and making life a little easier. I know that when I volunteer, I am helping others, and that I am making a difference in their lives. So even when you don't feel your best, there are a lot of things you can do, so get up and go make a difference.

> *Written by Lyndsley Wilkerson when she was a sophomore at Kent Place High School in Summit, New Jersey. Lyndsley has dermatomyositis.*

When I was 2 years of age I was diagnosed as having juvenile rheumatoid arthritis. Until I was about 8 I was pretty much a "normal" child. By "normal" I mean I had no deformities and no noticeable handicap. Since then, the deformities have become noticeable, and I have had several joint replacement surgeries.

Throughout my life, I have dealt with many people staring and younger children saying to their parents, "What's the matter with him?" I always heard older people remarking, "That poor child" or "I feel so bad for him." If I accepted help from everybody who has ever offered, then I would always be relying on somebody. And eventually, I would become dependent on the help of others, and that is far from what I want.

It may appear that I deal with my handicap very easily, but it isn't always so easy. At times I have been saddened at being unable to do like the others, and sometimes I ask myself "Why me?" or "What did I ever do to deserve this?" There are no answers to these questions. I was once told by a close friend, "God only gives us what He believes we can handle, and He must believe you can handle a lot." I always say this to myself when I'm disappointed with my condition. I also remind myself of how lucky I am compared to others.

Excerpted from an essay written by Paul Scanlon when Paul was a senior in high school preparing for college in the fall.

I want to pursue a career in Special Education in order to help children who are physically challenged and have a learning disability. I am physically challenged, and since the ninth grade, I have been involved with the special education program. I have an Individual Educational Plan (IEP) so I can get assistance if I need it. I am enrolled in college-level courses and doing well.

I once had a problem with a special education teacher who told me that I should not push myself in school. She said that if I took a full load of courses, it would be too stressful. She said that I could take a couple of courses a year and graduate in 6 years or so, and that it won't matter if I graduated with my class. When she told me that I got angry. I thought she was supposed to encourage, not discourage, me. I said, "I am graduating with my class in 1992. It might be hard, but I can do it. I have faith in myself." She still thought that I could not do it. The next year, I won a Mathematics Achievement Award and an English Achievement Award. In my junior year, I won the United States National Mathematics Award. I was chosen for Who's Who Among American High School Students.

I have proven my detractors wrong. When I told my special education teacher about the United States National Mathematics Award, she was pleasantly shocked. I know now that I can do whatever I want to do if I put my mind to it, despite what other people think. I really want to encourage children to try as hard as they can, to speak up for themselves. I know how they feel, I have been through adversity already.

Written by Melissa Schaffer.

Chapter 10

•

Rheumatic Disease and the Family

A child's chronic illness affects every member of the family. It consumes the family's time and financial resources, and it changes how family members interact with one another. Frequent visits with health care providers and the daily demands of home therapy programs can use up much of a busy family's spare time. Active disease can further restrict leisure opportunities if the child's illness makes it difficult for the child and other family members to take part in activities that they had previously enjoyed. Finally, it's only natural that every member of the family will have concerns and worries about the chronically ill child.

The good news is that families do eventually learn to adapt to a child's rheumatic illness, and they have full and rewarding family lives. Shortly after the initial diagnosis, when illness is the focus of everyone's attention, this may not seem possible. It will almost certainly take some time to develop new ways of thinking about illness and dealing with the necessary changes in the family's routines. You should not be discouraged by temporary setbacks. Learn as much as you can about your child's illness, and encourage frequent and honest communication among all family members. The remainder of this chapter discusses some of the specific ways that families are affected by chronic illness, and offers some suggestions for dealing with difficult situations.

What You May Be Feeling

As parents, we often expect too much of ourselves. We feel guilty if we become angry or frustrated with a child who complains about doing his exercises or takes too long to dress and misses the school bus. We may overindulge the ill child to make up for our inability to prevent or cure his illness. Even though our children place us high on pedestals and believe that we can do no wrong, we should forgive ourselves if we occasionally fail to achieve perfection. We did not cause our child's illness; we cannot make it go away; we do not know everything; and we cannot always be in control of our emotions.

Parents experience a wide range of emotions when a child is chronically ill. Disbelief, fear, guilt, anger, sadness, and frustration are all common and normal. You may be surprised at the range of feelings that you have:

- Anger at yourself, your spouse, God, doctors, or even at your child for what has happened to you and your family.
- Anger at your friends for their good fortune in having healthy children.
- Guilt that you may be in some way responsible for your child's illness.
- Anxiety over upcoming events, or general anxiety.
- Grief over the loss of your child's good health.
- Helplessness that you could not prevent what happened.
- Resentment because "It happened to me."
- Confusion over the information your child's doctors give you.
- A constant feeling of sadness that may worsen at important milestones in your child's life.
- The desire to "run away" and escape your situation.
- Lack of confidence in your ability to protect and care for your child.
- Concerns about health care costs, changes in the family's daily routine, and employment.

All of these emotions are normal and, while they will continue to come and go, and to increase and decrease in intensity, it is true that things will get easier over time. As your child and family adjust to the illness, you may feel the satisfaction, comfort, and even exhilaration that can come from managing a difficult situation, growing together, and seeing your child make progress. You may feel that because of your growing understanding of your child, you and your family have a greater understanding for other people who are in some way different, or who have special needs.

Coping with Your Emotions

It takes time to develop new routines that accommodate the needs of a chronically ill child without making illness the focus of everyone's life. Other parents of children with rheumatic illnesses can offer helpful suggestions from their own experience. All families are different, however, and each family will discover new strengths and develop their own mechanisms for dealing with chronic illness. Through trial and error, parents learn what will work best for their own families. Here are some tips to help you cope with your emotions and deal with the stresses in your life:

- Take good care of your own physical needs. You can be the most help to your child when you are feeling your best. Be sure to eat properly every day and get good physical exercise at least three times a week. Exercise is an excellent way of decreasing stress. You can ride a bike, swim, jog, play golf or tennis, or take brisk walks.

- Arrange for some time to be by yourself every day, and encourage your spouse to do the same. Don't feel selfish about your time alone. Time alone can help you to rejuvenate. You will feel happier and more at peace, and you will be better able to cope with your child's special problems. Also spend time together as a couple, without the children, once a week.

- Participate in fun recreational activities or hobbies that you enjoy. You may feel so determined to manage well that you ignore your own needs for relief, fun, and relaxation. You will be a better parent to your child if you continue to participate in the activities that you enjoy.

- Keep close relationships with supportive family and friends, and work at having a social life for yourself. The many demands of chronic illness can leave parents with little time or energy to address their own needs for adult company. Caring family members, friends, and neighbors can provide support that makes a great difference.

- Talk things over regularly with all members of your family. Keeping the lines of communication open helps prevent the buildup of tensions and fears that can add stress to family life.

- Make contact with parents who have had similar experiences. Many parents find it helpful to talk to another parent who has gone through the same thing with their child. Support groups and telephone networks provide opportunities for parents to exchange information and offer mutual support. Ask the team at your pediatric rheumatology center if they have a parent-to-parent telephone network or support group, or if they can give you the phone number of another parent who attends the clinic. Your local Arthritis Foundation chapter office is another good resource; many of these chapters organize parent support groups, hold informational meetings, or oversee parent telephone networks.

- Seek information about your child's medical condition and ways to care for your child. This may help you deal with your feelings and give you a positive sense of accomplishment.

- Participate in advocacy organizations related to your child's health problem, such as the Arthritis Foundation and the American Juvenile Arthritis Organization (AJAO). The AJAO is a membership organization within the Arthritis Foundation that is composed of families of children with rheumatic diseases.

- Don't hesitate to seek professional help, especially if your feelings of grief and sadness begin to become overwhelming. The social worker on your child's health care team can help you to work through your feelings, or can suggest a professional counselor in your community who can help on a more regular basis.

Giant Little Steps

A mother of a child with JRA wrote the following narrative describing her feelings about her child's illness.

Our son Skippy was 11 months old when he was diagnosed with pauciarticular JRA, and I remember it with very mixed emotions. For weeks he had had a slightly swollen knee following a fall. We consulted an orthopedic surgeon who felt it was an isolated problem. One Thursday morning he awoke with an unexplained swollen ankle, and at our doctor's suggestion we brought him to the hospital. The surgeon told us that she had been concerned about the continued swelling in the right knee and now that there was an additional joint involved she wanted to admit him and do some tests in the hospital. My husband and I were shocked. She told us that she suspected JRA, but because Skippy was not in one of the usual groups of children who get the disease, she felt that she should rule out some more serious possibilities, like a malignancy or a bone infection. No matter how hard we tried to concentrate on what she said she was pretty sure it was, we just stopped dead when she mentioned cancer. We spent the night with Skippy praying for arthritis. "God," we prayed, "just give him arthritis and we'll deal with it." We made deals with God all night long, and all the while Skippy was having the tests.

When the tests came back negative we were thrilled. "Oh, he's only got arthritis," we said. "No problem." Well, that lasted about 2 weeks before the reality of that diagnosis began to take hold. Unfortunately, because his knee flared before he began to walk, Skippy stopped even trying to bear weight on it. In fact, he was 2 years old before he could walk five consecutive steps. I found that I became obsessed with getting him to walk. I think I tried every push or pull toy, every incentive I could imagine to get him up on his feet. It was especially hard to see other children much younger, running and jumping around while Skippy could barely move without pain.

All of these feelings were doubly hard to take because I had grown up with a brother with muscular dystrophy and was well aware of the difficulties that could be ahead for any child with a physical disability. It just didn't seem fair. Hadn't my family had its share of illness? Why did it have to be *my* son? Of course, we eventually saw the other side of this: Why *not* us? Who better than we who are sensitive, educated, and aware of the needs of the disabled? Who better than we to raise this extra-special child? We've come to terms with the loss of the fantasy of our "perfect" child, but the real one we've come to understand and appreciate for his very own special self is far better than any "fantasy" child we could have created.

The bottom line is this: in his 4 years Skippy has already taught us many lessons. We have learned to accept him unconditionally. Our hopes and dreams for him remain; we have learned to be tough but realistic in our expectations for his progress and we've accepted that we may be in this for a long haul. Above all things, though, we've learned to be flexible. Yesterday, Skippy could walk through the supermarket by himself; today he might need a helping hand. Skippy has taught us to appreciate every little step. Many small milestones in his motor development have actually been tremendous achievements. We have plenty of opportunity with Skippy to celebrate the small things.

As I watch him roller skate away from me, face beaming with pride, I have to wonder. If we were given a chance to do all of this again, I know for sure that I would always want to take his pain away forever, but I'm not sure I'd want to lose the lessons I've learned from him, the joy we've felt from some very small but hard-won victories.

Brothers and Sisters

Siblings of all ages suffer when their brother or sister becomes ill. Worry, fear, guilt, anger, resentment, and loneliness are just some of the feelings that a brother or sister of a child with a rheumatic disease may experience at various times during the course of the illness. All of the following emotions are common among children who have a brother or sister with a rheumatic illness:

- Worry about their sibling's health, or that their sibling might die
- Worry about their own health, fearing that they, too, may develop a serious illness
- Worry that they somehow caused the illness
- Concern that the illness is punishment for "bad" behavior
- Resentment because the ill child receives extra attention or because her illness interferes with family outings or recreational activities
- Embarrassment that their brother or sister needs help with activities of daily living or looks different
- Guilt and shame that they have negative feelings about their chronically ill brother or sister

Siblings who are not ill may face disruptions in normal daily routines, and may experience repeated separations from one or both parents as well as from their ill sibling. Confused, concerned siblings can develop physical and emotional problems when they do not have the opportunity to discuss their feelings with someone. Conflicts with parents, school phobia, learning problems, stomachaches, sleeping difficulties, and other behavior changes may occur.

What can be done to help a child cope with his brother's or sister's rheumatic disease? Here are some suggestions:

- Provide honest information about the sibling's condition and reassurance that other children in the family will not "catch it," and that they did not cause the illness.
- Schedule "special" time alone with your well child on a regular, planned basis, and have your spouse do the same. By spending individual time with each child, parents can limit a sibling's feelings of resentment over special treatment of the ill child.
- Be available to listen to the concerned sibling.
- Keep open communication within the family about the progress of the child with the rheumatic disease.
- From time to time allow the siblings to accompany the child with the rheumatic disease on visits to the clinic or hospital, even if this means an absence from school. Health care providers should welcome their questions and discuss any concerns they have about their own or their sibling's health.
- Encourage siblings to continue their usual activities, especially with peers.
- Talk directly to the sibling about his feelings. "How are *you* doing, (child's name)?"
- Drawing pictures of the illness may give younger children an outlet if they do not yet have the words to describe what they are feeling.
- Acknowledge that siblings are also affected by their brother's or sister's illness. Tell them that their negative feelings are legitimate.
- Help your children to recognize and appreciate the individual talents of each member of the family. Healthy siblings may feel guilt about their own good health and physical abilities. They may give up sports or other recreational activities for fear of hurting the feelings of the chronically ill child. Instead, healthy children should be encouraged to excel in all areas of talent, including physical skills.

Finally, it is reported that many brothers and sisters claim their experience with chronic illness has helped them to develop more compassion and sensitivity to the needs of others. They become wise and strong as a result. Families can learn the importance of interdependence and connectedness while living with a chronic illness.

When my 10-year-old daughter became ill, my younger son began acting out in school. I've tried disciplining him, but nothing seems to work. Why is he misbehaving, and what can I do about it?

This type of change when an older sibling gets sick is quite common. There are changes in the way a family functions when an older sibling gets sick that might give some insights into why a younger sibling's behavior might change. In many families, the child who becomes ill requires extra attention from parents. This can include trips to the doctor, administration of medicine, special exercises, special comforting moments between parent and child, or extra help by parents with homework. This change in family functioning is difficult on everyone. For a younger sibling, whose emotional functioning is less mature and who is more dependent on parents' support and supervision, such a change could be very troubling.

Since younger siblings do not have the ability to adapt to changes within the family as easily as older siblings and adults, changes in their behavior might occur. The younger child's behavior might change by becoming more problematic or by becoming too good (he or she might turn into the "perfect" child). Although the impact of these two options is quite different, they both appear to represent the younger child's struggle to regain his "lost" position in the family and regain attention from parents and siblings. Discipline at this point should not be very different from what it was before the other sibling's illness, but additional steps are often needed to solve the problem.

Once you recognize why your younger child is acting out, it will be easier for you to help him deal more appropriately with his feelings. Try to return to old patterns of interaction and to the activities you used to enjoy together. Spend time alone with the younger sibling doing things that are mutually enjoyable and that reflect the unique characteristics of the younger sibling. If the younger child's behavior does not improve within 4 to 8 weeks, you may want to consult with his pediatrician, school counselor, or other mental health professional.

Your Spouse and Your Marriage

Having a child with a rheumatic disease can have dramatic effects on a marriage. On the one hand, it can be a test of the strength of your relationship. As much as you may have relied on each other for support as parents in the past, you will need to support each other more than ever now. A husband and wife may have different needs when it comes to coping with the stress of having a child with illness, and they may not always be able to support each other. Some people need to pull back from a close relationship from time to time while they attempt to manage difficult feelings.

On the other hand, having a child with a rheumatic illness can strengthen a marital relationship. Couples who manage to work through such stressful times can develop bonds of great depth and lasting strength. It will take some experimenting to find out what works best for you, but here are a few tips to help you and your spouse get started in supporting each other during these trying times:

- Talk with your spouse. Listen to his or her ideas and feelings. Try to understand what he or she is thinking or feeling about your child's illness. Talking can help, even if you have different feelings and responses. Make decisions about treatment and other matters together.
- Accept each other's feelings and different ways of dealing with the illness. Some parents choose to minimize their child's illness as a way of coping with the strong emotions they feel, while others may want to talk and read a great deal about the illness. Try to be honest with each other about these differences, and work on a compromise that allows each partner to support the other.
- Each spouse needs someone with whom he or she can relate or talk, a person who will listen and give support. Sometimes, a husband and wife need support persons beyond each other. Using the support offered by other relatives or friends may take the pressure off the marital relationship.
- Find some time to be alone with your spouse. This may mean sharing in hobbies or recreational activities, going for walks, going out to dinner, or taking weekend trips without the kids. Your marriage needs tending and time together is important.
- Divide your child's special care between the two of you. This gives both parents the opportunity to have a break once in a while and helps both parents feel they are taking an active and important role in managing the child's illness.
- If needed, seek professional counseling with a therapist, minister, counselor, or mental health professional.

Special Concerns of Working Families

Finding appropriate and safe day care for your child while you work can be a daunting process when your child has special health needs. Job restrictions may make it difficult to take needed time off work for doctor's visits, hospitalizations, or to care for a sick child. Parents may wonder if perhaps one of them should leave their job to stay home and take care of their child. This section will help you sort through work-related issues that may come up when you have a child with special health needs.

Should I Work?

The decision to work or not is an intensely personal one that may be influenced by a variety of personal, family, and economic factors. There is no right or wrong answer. Traditional families, in which one parent (usually the mother) stays home, are becoming rare in our society. After having children, some women return to work because they want to. Many women return to work for more pragmatic reasons: the family simply cannot maintain their current standard of living unless both parents have an income. Whatever your reason for working, you should not feel guilty about doing so. The key to success is to find a reliable, compassionate, and responsible day care provider, and train him or her in providing the care your child needs. If you achieve this, your child will do just fine.

Your Rights in Day Care

The Americans with Disabilities Act (ADA) prohibits discrimination in places of business on the basis of disabilities. This law explicitly extends to both day care centers and family day care programs. This means that a day care program cannot refuse to enroll your child just because she has special health needs, nor can they expel your child should special needs develop during the course of an existing relationship. The ADA mandates that the day care provider must make reasonable modifications to accommodate your child's special needs, and prohibits the day care provider from charging any additional fees just because your child is disabled. Programs operated by religious organizations (for example, parochial schools) are exempt from this ruling unless they receive federal funding.

Locating a Day Care Provider

Good day care is hard to find for healthy children; the prospect of finding day care for a child with a rheumatic illness may seem impossible. With adequate preparation and lots of homework, however, you should be able to find a day care provider who is right for your child.

In general, day care for a child with a rheumatic disease does not need to be very different than it would be for a healthy child. It is not necessary to find a center that has a registered nurse on staff unless you feel uncomfortable having a nonmedical person administer your child's medications. Because your child has special needs, you may want to consider looking for a program that has a lower child-to-staff ratio;

you might also consider having care provided in your own home. These situations are often more expensive, but it may be worth a few extra dollars to ensure that your child's needs are adequately addressed.

When interviewing prospective child care providers, be clear, concise, and realistic about all of your child's special needs. Although a provider cannot refuse to accept your child just because she has a disability, your child may be most happy with a provider who really wants to care for her. Describe your child's illness and the effects it has on her day-to-day life. Be certain to itemize all of the illness-related tasks the day care provider will be expected to perform, and be certain that the care provider feels comfortable in handling the extra responsibility your child requires. The day care provider may need to administer medication, put on splints, do exercises, or modify your child's activity in some way. If the prospective day care provider seems hesitant to accept your child, look elsewhere for someone who will take on her care willingly.

Training the Day Care Provider

Once you locate a day care provider, you will need to train him or her in caring for all of your child's needs. Here are some steps you can take to help accomplish this task:

- Educate your provider about your child's illness. Describe her condition and how it affects her on a daily basis. Describe how her activity level may vary over the course of a day (stiffness in the morning, fatigue after a period of activity). Describe physical limitations and activity restrictions. Ask your doctor or therapist for help with this if you are unsure.
- Describe any special help your child needs that most children her age usually do not require, such as assistance with toileting, dressing, eating, using scissors, or making arts and crafts.
- Describe any limitations your child has that might prevent her from doing activities that the other children routinely participate in, such as picking up toys at the end of the day, carrying a cot for nap time, or sitting on the floor.
- Specify whether your child needs to restrict her activity in any way on the playground, or if she needs special supervision.
- Provide explicit instructions about your child's need for rest, and schedule additional nap times or rest times if needed. Specify whether your child needs to wear splints during her nap.
- Be certain that the day care provider understands your child's dietary restrictions if he or she will be supplying your child's food.

- Demonstrate any special procedures the care provider will be expected to perform, such as doing therapy exercises, administering medications, or putting on splints. Have the provider try the procedures while you observe so that you can offer a gentle correction if needed.
- Give the provider written instructions and a schedule for your child that includes all of her illness-related needs. Provide a list of emergency phone numbers and the physician's name and telephone number. Indicate when medications need to be given, the dosage, and specific instructions (for example, "take with food"). Also write down when nap or rest times should occur, when splints need to be put on, and when exercises need to be performed. ("The Baby-sitter Information Form" at the end of this chapter can be modified for day care providers.)
- Give your provider a written log book that can be filled in daily. Have him or her record all the treatment provided, such as the time and dose of medications administered and whether the exercises were done. She or he should also briefly outline your child's activities for the day.

Dealing with Your Employer

Having a child with a rheumatic disease can cause additional work-related stresses. Parents may require frequent time off from work to take their child to doctors' visits or therapy, during periods of hospitalization, or to care for a sick child. The Family and Medical Leave Act of 1993 (FMLA) protects a parent's job during such absences. The FMLA entitles each parent to 12 weeks of unpaid, job-protected leave each year to care for a child who has a *serious health condition*. A serious health condition is defined as a chronic health condition that requires treatment by a health care provider (such as any of the childhood rheumatic diseases) or a condition that requires hospitalization.

To be eligible for FMLA benefits, you must work for a covered employer. The FMLA explicitly extends to all public agencies and to private-sector employers with fifty or more employees. You must have worked for the employer for at least 12 months, and you must have worked at least 1,250 hours over the previous 12 months.

For part-time employees or those who work variable hours, the FMLA entitlement is calculated on a proportional basis. FMLA leave may be taken all at one time (for 12 consecutive weeks) or periodically as needed (such as for intermittent visits to the pediatric rheumatologist, physical therapist, or other health providers, or during hospitalizations).

Your employer will probably require a letter from your child's doctor that names your child's diagnosis and states that this is a chronic health condition. The letter may be more helpful if the doctor specifies in it how much time the parent will need to miss from work. For example, the letter could state that you need 1 week off to be with your child during a planned hospitalization, or that you need an afternoon off from work once every 6 weeks to take your child to outpatient clinic visits.

Using a Baby-sitter

All parents need to have time away from their children to participate in social activities and enjoy each other's company. Parents who take time for themselves can keep their child's illness in better prospective, and are more relaxed and better able to address their children's needs.

Finding the time can be difficult for any busy couple, but chronic illness can make getting away even more complicated. Parents may feel guilty about leaving a child who has an illness, or worry about finding a reliable baby-sitter. These barriers can be overcome with a little planning. With thorough instruction, older teenagers, adult neighbors, or relatives can provide appropriate short-term care for children with chronic rheumatic conditions. Here are a few tips for locating a baby-sitter in your neighborhood:

- Ask other parents about reliable sitters in the area. Invite prospective sitters over to meet your child. Describe your child's needs and find out if the sitters would be interested in caring for her.
- Nursing students or child development majors may be especially interested in caring for your child. Contact nursing students at local hospitals or schools of nursing or child development majors at nearby colleges.
- Look for a mature adult or other parent with children close to your own child in age.
- Form a babysitting co-op with friends and neighbors and teach them about your child's special needs.
- Investigate respite or temporary care facilities in your community.

Once you have identified a sitter, be sure to inform him or her about your child's condition and treatment regimen. The form on the next page can be used to provide important information for baby-sitters, neighbors, or relatives when they take care of your children. You may wish to make additional copies of the "Baby-sitter Information Form" for your own use. Because much of the information in the emergency section of the form will not change very often, it may be more convenient to fill in this information before copying the form.

Form 16. Baby-sitter Information Form

We are at (address)_____

Phone number _____   We will be home by _____

General Instructions	
Meals	Snacks
Medications	Bedtime (hour, splints, usual routine)
Other instructions	

Emergency Information		
Police	Fire	Ambulance
Doctor	Phone	
Neighbor or relative	Phone	
Our home address is	Phone	
Child's name and age	Medical condition	Current medications
Health insurance (company name, phone, and ID number)		

Appendix 1

●

Sample Clinic Guide

THE PEDIATRIC RHEUMATOLOGY CLINIC AT THE FLOATING HOSPITAL FOR CHILDREN

Welcome to the Pediatric Rheumatology Clinic at the Floating Hospital for Children. This clinic guide will answer many questions you may have about how the clinic works, such as how to contact the doctor, what to do in an emergency, or what to expect during a clinic visit.

The Pediatric Rheumatology Clinic and the Floating Hospital for Children offer a variety of services, including comprehensive care, care coordination, translator services, and family support programs. Many additional services are listed in this section, along with conveniences such as banking machines and cafeterias. Clinic and medical center billing procedures are explained. Directions to the medical center and a map showing buildings and parking areas are included at the end of the section.

The Clinic Team

All of the members of the pediatric rheumatology team are listed below. Please note that phone numbers are included only if the direct line is different from the main number. All team members, however, can be reached through the main telephone number (555) 555-1234.

Pediatric Rheumatologists
Jane G. Schaller, M.D.
Laurie C. Miller, M.D.
Lori B. Tucker, M.D.

Pediatric Rheumatology Fellows
Bradley Bloom, M.D.
Mikhail Harjacek, M.D.

Nurse
Judi DiNardo, M.S., R.N.
(555) 555-4567

Physical Therapist
Bethany A. DeNardo, M.P.H., P.T.
(555) 555-5678

Occupational Therapist
Madelon Visser, O.T.R./L.
(555) 555-6789

Social Worker
Susan Hollis, LICSW
(555) 555-9101

Parent Consultant
Sheila Rubino

Nurse's Aide
Beulah Davis

Secretaries
Patricia Davis
Marcia Healy

Clinic Operations

Where and When

The Pediatric Rheumatology Clinic is located on the second floor of the Floating Hospital for Children at 755 Washington Street, Boston, Massachusetts. Visits are by appointment; regular clinic hours are as follows:

Monday:	9:00 a.m. to 12:00 a.m.
Tuesday:	1:00 p.m. to 5:00 p.m.
Wednesday:	1:00 p.m. to 5:00 p.m.

Note:

✓ The Monday morning clinic is an "abbreviated" clinic, only attended by the physicians. The other members of the health care team are not available during Monday clinic hours.

✓ The last clinic appointments on Tuesday and Wednesday are scheduled at 4:00 p.m. If your child is scheduled to see the occupational or physical therapist, it is best to ask for an appointment no later than 3:00 p.m.

What to Expect during a Clinic Visit

Your child will usually be seen by a number of health care providers during the visit to the pediatric rheumatology clinic. The nurse's aide will weigh and measure your child and then assign you to an individual examining room. The other members of your team (nurse, therapists, social worker, dietitian, etc.) will come to the room to speak with you and examine your child. Usually, your child will be examined by one of the pediatric rheumatology fellows. Often, the pediatric rheumatologist is the last health care provider you will see. The pediatric rheumatologist will examine your child, review the findings and recommendations of the other team members, and answer any questions you have. You may be sent to other areas of the hospital for tests and procedures such as labs and X rays.

The clinic visit often takes an hour or more because of the many specialists involved in caring for your child. Coordinating the schedules of so many team members is difficult, but we try very hard to keep your waiting time to a minimum. Even so, it is likely that you will have to wait to be assigned to an examining room and that there will be some waiting between visits from team members. You may find it helpful to bring along a favorite toy or book to help your child pass the time.

Laboratory Tests

- Blood tests are performed in the Clinical Laboratory on the third floor of the Floating Hospital daily from 8:30 a.m. to 5:00 p.m. A laboratory technician who has special experience working with children generally staffs the facility.
- It is the policy of the hospital that no more than two attempts to draw blood will be made by the same person during a visit to the clinical lab. In this event, your child will be returned to the clinic where one of the pediatricians will draw the blood.
- Children who are fearful of blood tests may be more relaxed during their visit with the doctor if they have their blood drawn before the clinic visit. If this is the case with your child, ask the physician if the lab slips can be drawn up in advance. Not all children can have their blood drawn in advance. Sometimes the exact set of tests needed cannot be determined until the doctor has examined your child.

X Rays and Ultrasound

- X rays and ultrasound tests are performed in the Department of Pediatric Radiology, on the fourth floor of the Floating Hospital.

Eye Exams

- Eye exams are performed by the pediatric ophthalmologist, on the first floor of the Boston Dispensary Building. This is a brief walk from the Floating Hospital.
- Eye appointments can be coordinated with your child's clinic visit. Ask one of our secretaries to schedule the eye exam for you.
- If you prefer, eye exams can be performed by an ophthalmologist in your local community, if he or she is comfortable examining young children. Please have your ophthalmologist send us the results of each visit for our records.

Other Tests and Services

The Floating Hospital is a full-service hospital with a full range of pediatric subspecialty services. All testing and physician consultation can be performed within the Floating Hospital or at varying locations within the medical center.

The Care Coordination Service

The Pediatric Rheumatology Division offers a complete care coordination service to help prevent numerous visits to the hospital for tests and procedures. In most cases, all of your child's appointments can be scheduled on one day.

- Call (555) 555-1213 and give a list of all the appointments you wish to schedule to our division secretary. Also tell the secretary which days you are *not* available.
- The secretary will call you back after scheduling the appointments.
- Once an appointment is made for your child, you are responsible for keeping the appointment or canceling the appointment yourself, if necessary.

Other Clinic Services

The Pediatric Rheumatology Division offers a range of additional services for patients and their families. These include:

- *The Joint Report* is a quarterly newsletter for children with rheumatic disease and their families. Your name should be placed on our mailing list automatically, shortly after your child's first visit. If you are not receiving the newsletter, call the office at (555) 555-1415 to add your name to the mailing list.
- A *Lupus Parent Support Group* meets the first Tuesday of every month. Contact the pediatric rheumatology nurse at (555) 555-1617 for information.
- A *Lupus Teen Support Group* meets the first Tuesday of every month. Contact the pediatric rheumatology social worker at (555) 555-1718 for information.
- *Arthritis Parent and Teen Support Groups* are offered as interest warrants. If you would like to participate in a support group, please contact the pediatric rheumatology social worker at (555) 555-1819.
- The *Parent Telephone Network* puts parents in touch with other parents whose children have had similar experiences. Parents may ask to speak with another parent about medications, other therapies, school issues, health insurance, or other topics of particular concern. Ask any member of your health care team to connect you with the Parent Telephone Network.
- Our *Lending Library* has a selection of reading materials available for parents and children, including educational materials and fictional works about the lives of children with arthritis. Speak with the Parent Consultant or nurse to check out library materials or to see what is available.

Other Hospital Services

The Floating Hospital offers a variety of additional services to assist families.

- *Transportation assistance* is available to families with financial need. Subway tokens and parking and taxi vouchers are available from the clinic social worker.
- *Parking* for clinic visits is available in the Tremont Street garage, which connects directly to the Floating Hospital from the second and third floor. *Handicapped*

parking is located on the third floor of the garage. Additional patient parking is available at other Medical Center locations. When you arrive at the clinic, please ask the secretary to validate your parking ticket for a reduced parking rate. The patient parking rate is $2.00 per hour, with a $7.00 maximum per day.

- *Interpreter services* are available through the hospital at no charge to families. If you need an interpreter, please notify the secretary at the time the appointment is made.
- *Lodging* is available at the Tremont House across the street from the hospital at discounted rates for patients and their families. In addition, the clinic social worker can help locate low-cost accommodations in the Boston area through programs that provide these services to patients and their families. When a child is hospitalized, one parent may stay with him in his hospital room.
- *Financial assistance* for medically related expenses is available to families with financial need. The clinic social worker is available to discuss a family's financial resources and need for assistance.
- The hospital *pharmacy* is located on the street level next to the elevators. The pharmacy is open from 9:00 a.m. to 5:00 p.m. To save time, call in your prescription refills before leaving home. The phone number is (555) 555-1920. The pharmacy accepts payment in cash, check, Master Card, Visa, and American Express, as well as Medicaid, Mass Health, and PCS coverage for prescriptions. The PCS card is issued by a number of different health insurance companies. Check with your insurance carrier if you have questions regarding your prescription coverage.
- A *Shawmut ATM* is available in the Floating Hospital, on the Plaza level. A *BayBank ATM* is located in the Farnsworth Building at the Harrison Street entrance.
- A full-service *cafeteria* is located on the Plaza level. Hot and cold meals are served daily from 6:00 a.m. to 10:00 p.m. weekdays, and 6:00 a.m. to 8:00 p.m. weekends and holidays. Ample seating is available. A *Dunkin' Donuts,* located near the elevators on the first floor of the Proger Building, is open weekdays from 6:00 a.m. to 8:00 p.m.
- The *gift shop,* on the Plaza level just to the right of the front doors, is open Monday through Friday, from 8:00 a.m. to 8:00 p.m. Saturday and Sunday the gift shop is open from 8:00 a.m. to 6:00 p.m.

Contacting the Office

To Make a Clinic Appointment Call (555) 555-1234

The Pediatric Rheumatology office is open between 8:30 a.m. and 5:00 p.m., Monday through Friday. Please call during regular business hours to schedule an appointment.

To Speak with a Doctor

- For routine calls during regular work hours call (555) 555- 1234:

  ✓ Tell the secretary who answers the phone which physician you wish to speak with, and briefly summarize the nature of the call. The secretary will pass the message along to the doctor.

  ✓ Usually, your call will be returned within an hour or two. Your call will *always* be returned by a physician prior to the end of the work day, which may be as late as 8:00 or 9:00 at night. Please keep this in mind, and leave both daytime and evening phone numbers where you can be reached.

  ✓ Most routine phone calls are returned by the clinical pediatric rheumatology fellow, who may not be your child's personal physician. Please tell the secretary if you need to speak with a specific physician. You should be aware, however, that the physicians in our division practice a team approach to care. All patients seen during the week are presented at a Friday afternoon conference attended by all of the physicians. Thus, every physician in our division is aware of your child's case and is adequately prepared to answer most of your questions.

- For routine calls during non-work hours call (555) 555-1234:

  ✓ An answering machine is always connected to the line in our office. While we prefer to receive routine calls during work hours, you may leave a message on our answering machine at any time.

  ✓ Your call will be transmitted to the physician at 9:00 a.m. on the next regular work day.

- For *urgent calls* during regular work hours call (555) 555-1234:

  ✓ Please tell the secretary who answers the phone that your call is urgent in nature. The secretary will page a physician to answer your call without delay, while you wait on the line.

  ✓ Urgent calls are answered by whichever physician is immediately available, not necessarily your child's personal physician.

- For *urgent calls* during non-work hours call (555) 555-2021:

  ✓ A physician from the Pediatric Rheumatology staff is *always* available to answer your call.

  ✓ Tell the page operator who answers the phone that you are a patient's parent, and that you would like to speak with "the pediatric rheumatology fellow-on-call."

✓ You will be put on hold for several minutes while the operator pages the fellow. Please do not hang up. If you get disconnected, call back immediately.

✓ Occasionally, the operator will take your number and have the fellow return your call. Your call will be returned within 20 minutes. If it is not, call again, and tell the operator that you have been waiting for the fellow to return your call.

✓ It is helpful to have a list of your child's current medications and dosages on hand when you call.

To Obtain Test Results Call (555) 555-1234

- Physicians from the Pediatric Rheumatology staff are available to speak with you regarding test results on Friday afternoons after 4:00 p.m. Please tell the secretary who answers the phone that you are calling for test results.
- If the physician is not immediately available, please leave both day and evening phone numbers. Also tell the secretary when you will be in transit and not available.

For Prescription Refills Call (555) 555-1234

Please have the following information available when you call:

- The name of the physician who prescribed the medication
- The name of the medication to be refilled
- The dose and frequency of the medication
- The name and phone number of the pharmacy
- Your child's approximate weight

Emergency Visits

In case of an emergency or significant medical event, you may bring your child to the Emergency Room at any time, day or night. It is best to call first if possible. If an acute emergency arises or you have difficulty calling the fellow, you should just come immediately to the Floating Hospital Emergency Room. A pediatrician is present in the Emergency Room at all times.

Call First: (555) 555-2021 (when possible)

- Tell the operator who answers that you would like to speak with the pediatric rheumatology fellow-on-call.

- The fellow will help you decide if your child needs to be seen immediately in a local hospital, if she is able to come to the Emergency Room at the Floating Hospital, or if you should contact your local pediatrician.
- The fellow-on-call will be prepared for your arrival in the Emergency Room if it is necessary to bring your child to the hospital immediately.

Emergency Room Location

- Monday through Friday, 8:00 a.m. to 11:00 p.m., go to the Pediatric Walk-In Clinic on the street level of the Floating Hospital.
- Saturday, Sunday, or weeknights after 11:00 p.m., go to the New England Medical Center general Emergency Room at 185 Harrison Avenue.

What to Expect in the Emergency Room

Upon your arrival, your child will *always* be examined by a pediatrician, who will discuss your child's situation with the pediatric rheumatology fellow-on-call. If your child has a rheumatic complaint, he will be examined by the pediatric rheumatology fellow-on-call, and possibly by one of the attending pediatric rheumatologists. The pediatric rheumatology fellow does not always come to the Emergency Room if the child's complaint is not a rheumatologic problem (stomach pain, for example), but will always discuss the problem with the pediatrician who has examined your child.

Our Philosophy of Care

Traditional medicine often diagrams the health care team by using a pyramid. The doctor is on the top of the pyramid and the other health professionals (nurses, therapists, etc.) are arranged below. The family is often not even included. Our pediatric rheumatology service employs a different philosophy; we put the family in the top spot on our pyramid. We have a strong commitment to family-centered care and we strive to develop strong partnerships with the families we serve. It is our goal to provide the following type of care for your child:

- High Quality: We keep abreast of all new developments in the field of pediatric rheumatology so that we can offer your child the most current and scientifically tested treatments. Often, clinical and laboratory research conducted by our own faculty and staff is directly responsible for advances in the field.
- Comprehensive: The core team in our clinic is made up of health professionals from a variety of specialties. The members of the "interdisciplinary" team work

together to develop a comprehensive plan to provide the care your child needs. Specialty, laboratory, and diagnostic testing services that may be needed are also available at the Floating Hospital.

- Coordinated: We make every effort to make your child's medical care as convenient as possible for your family. Special tests or services can usually be scheduled on the same day as your clinic appointment. Our division secretary will coordinate your clinic visit and other services for you.
- Family-Centered: Our staff are experts in the treatment of rheumatic illnesses in children, but you are the expert when it comes to understanding the impact of rheumatic illness on your child and family. Together we can develop a plan for treating your child's illness that works best for your family. We value your observations and opinions, and encourage you to be involved in all treatment decisions.
- Community-Based: Much of your child's care will be provided in your own community by your child's pediatrician and other local health professionals. We are in contact with these care providers regularly to ensure that your child is receiving appropriate and effective treatment. We are also available to meet or talk with teachers or other school personnel to explain the effect the disease may have on your child in the classroom.
- Compassionate: We know it is hard for children to be sick, that many children are frightened of doctors and clinics, and that clinic visits upset family schedules. We all try our very best to make your visit with us as pleasant and as helpful as possible.

Growing Up in the Pediatric Rheumatology Clinic

We care for many teenagers and young adults in the Pediatric Rheumatology Clinic. We feel that it is very important for teenagers who have a chronic disease such as JRA to learn how to take responsibility for their health care as part of becoming independent and responsible adults. In addition, it is important for teenagers to have personal time with their doctors to bring up any concerns they might not feel comfortable discussing with their parents present, and to have privacy during their physical examination if desired.

When children reach adolescence, we frequently ask their parents to step out of the examination room during the physical examination. Generally, parents will be present during the initial part of the visit to offer any interval history since the last clinic visit, or to express their questions and concerns. After the physical examination is completed, the doctor will ask the parents to rejoin their teen so the care plan can be discussed with the entire family and everyone's questions answered. The age at which children are ready for more independence in their clinic visits is variable, but generally, by the age of 14–15, most children should have some private time with their doctor.

We frequently care for young adults who have been followed in our clinic through their college years. The right time to transition to the care of an adult rheumatologist is a very individual decision. Some teenagers are ready to move on to an adult rheumatologist after high school graduation, and others at college graduation. When your young adult is ready for this transition, we will provide our best advice concerning a referral, and we will communicate with the adult rheumatologist to help make this transition as smooth as possible.

Billing Procedures

Availability of Free Care

All patients receive care in the pediatric rheumatology clinic regardless of their ability to pay. If you do not have health insurance, or cannot pay for a service that is not covered by your health insurance, please notify one of the team members.

Clinic Fees

Fees for all services obtained at New England Medical Center are billed through the central billing office. The medical center bills most insurers directly, and sends the patient a copy of the bill.

- There is a range of usual fees for a visit to the pediatric rheumatology clinic depending on the type of visit (initial or follow-up), the length of the visit, and the nature of the visit (complicated or routine). Additional time spent by the pediatric rheumatologist in care coordination and follow-up is included in the determination of the fee. The basic clinic fee includes all charges for the pediatric rheumatologist, nurse, social worker, and nutritionist. There may be additional charges for special tests (such as a tuberculosis test) or procedures (such as joint injection) performed in the clinic.
- Physical therapy is billed as part of the clinic visit, but is a separate charge. There is a range of charges for physical therapy, based on the service that was performed (range of motion assessment, muscle strength testing, therapeutic exercises, or other). Parents should speak with the physical therapist if they are having any difficulty obtaining insurance coverage of PT charges in clinic. Many steps can be

taken to assure insurance coverage for this service and prevent the family from incurring out-of-pocket costs.

- Occupational therapy is billed separately from the clinic charge, through the hospital rehabilitation department. The cost of an OT visit depends on the length of time the OT works with your child; there is a cumulative charge for each 15 minutes of care.
- All laboratory work, X rays, and tests performed outside of the clinic area are billed independent of the clinic charge.

Your Health Insurance

It is important for you to alert the pediatric rheumatology team if your HMO requires permission to do lab tests or X rays. If you are considering changing your health insurance, you may want to ask your child's pediatric rheumatologist's advice about the new plan. Once a change in health insurance is made, please notify the clinic secretary and your child's pediatric rheumatologist.

Assistance with Billing Problems

Sometimes there is a delay in the insurance company's payment of your bill. If you get an overdue notice or a collection notice on your bill, *don't panic!* Call the proper billing office to clarify the status of your account.

- If you have a problem with your bill for IN-patient services, contact: Claire Curran, Coordinator, IN-Patient Financial Coordination (555) 555-2122
- If you have a problem with your bill for OUT-patient services, contact: Emily Barron, Coordinator, OUT-Patient Financial Coordination (555) 555-2223
- If you are experiencing difficulty in paying for hospital services, please contact the Pediatric Rheumatology office at (555) 555-1234 and ask to speak with the social worker. The social worker will help you determine your eligibility for assistance with your medical bills through programs such as SSI or free care.

Appendix 2

•

Other Sources of Help

Agencies and Organizations

Childhood Rheumatic Disease Membership Organizations

The Arthritis Foundation and *The American Juvenile Rheumatoid Arthritis Organization*, 1314 Spring Street, NW, Atlanta, GA 30309; (404) 872-7100. The Arthritis Foundation is a national volunteer organization that supports research into the causes and treatments of all rheumatic illnesses and provides information and support services for individuals who have arthritis or other rheumatic illnesses. A chapter of the Arthritis Foundation is located in each state. The local chapters provide a variety of services, including information and referral, support groups, and seminars for the public and for professionals. They will provide medical referrals by sending a list of doctors in your area who care for children with rheumatic diseases, but they will not make recommendations among the health care providers. The physician list will not necessarily indicate whether an individual physician is board certified in pediatric rheumatology. The Arthritis Foundation also provides numerous books and brochures for parents; call your local chapter office for a list of these resources.

The American Juvenile Arthritis Organization (AJAO) is a council of the national Arthritis Foundation that is concerned with childhood rheumatic illnesses. This organization holds an excellent annual conference for parents and distributes a quarterly newsletter. It maintains a partial directory of pediatric rheumatology centers in the United States but will not make specific recommendations; the directory does not include information on whether physicians are board certified in pediatric rheumatology.

The Association for the Care of Children's Health, 7910 Woodmont Avenue, Suite 300, Bethesda, MD 20814; (301) 654-6549. This is a multidisciplinary association of professionals and parents that promotes a family-centered approach to health care for children with special health needs and their families. Services include education, research, advocacy, and networking. Numerous books and brochures will be provided to parents who call or write to ACCH at the above address.

The Federation for Children with Special Needs, 95 Berkeley Street, Boston, MA 02116; (800) 331-0688. A national, nonprofit organization for parents of children with special health needs, the federation has established parent information and training centers in each state. These centers offer workshops in special education law. Many also provide Individualized Education Plan (IEP) clinics and telephone information and referral services. They may be able to help you locate the services of a volunteer advocate who can assist you in working with the school district to obtain educational services for your child.

The Lupus Foundation of America, Inc., 4 Research Place, Suite 180, Rockville, MD 20850-3226; (800) 558-0121. This is a national volunteer organization that supports research into the causes and treatments of SLE and provides information and support services for individuals who have SLE. The Lupus Foundation has ninety local chapters throughout the United States. Services at local chapters include information and referral, support groups, and educational seminars.

The Scleroderma Federation, Peabody Office Building, 1 Newbury Street, Peabody, MA 01960; (800) 422-1113. This is a national volunteer organization that provides information, physician referral and support services for individuals who have scleroderma. They publish a quarterly newsletter and have a collection of educational materials for individuals with scleroderma and their families, which can be obtained by calling or writing the above address.

The Spondylitis Association of America, P.O. Box 5872, Sherman Oaks, CA 91413; (800) 777-8189. This national volunteer organization provides information and support services for persons who have ankylosing spondylitis. They distribute a quarterly newsletter and educational materials; call the organization or write to them at the above address.

Resource Agencies and Professional Organizations

The Affiliated Children's Arthritis Centers of New England, 750 Washington Street, Box 286, Boston, MA 02111; (617) 636-5071. This is a nonprofit organization for families of children with rheumatic diseases in New England, and for health professionals with a special interest in the childhood rheumatic diseases. Family services include referrals for medical care and distribution of information on camp programs for children and other subjects of interest. The organization sponsors seminars for professionals in the area of childhood rheumatic diseases. Publications available for parents and professionals can be obtained by calling or writing to the above address. Recommended publications include the following:

- *Learn about JRA*, A module for classroom use to instruct the peers of a child with JRA about the disease (1993)
- *Just One of the Kids*, a videotape to educate teachers and school personnel about JRA (1994)
- *Physical Therapy Practice Guidelines for Children with Chronic Arthritis*, second edition (1993)
- *Occupational Therapy Practice Guidelines for Children with Chronic Arthritis*, second edition (1993)
- *Care Coordination Practice Guidelines for Children with Chronic Arthritis*, second edition (1993)
- *School Nurse Standards of Care for Children with JRA* (1993)
- *Social Work Standards of Practice for Pediatric Rheumatology* (1994)
- *Medical Care for Children with Chronic Arthritis: Guidelines for Coordination of Primary and Specialty Care* (1994)

The American Academy of Pediatrics, 141 Northwest Point Boulevard, P.O. Box 927, Elk Grove Village, IL 60009-0927; (708) 228-5005. The national membership organization for pediatricians and pediatric subspecialists, the American Academy of Pediatrics is the agency responsible for board-certifying of pediatric rheumatologists. The academy provides information about board-certified pediatric rheumatologists in your area and can tell you whether or not a specific physician is board certified in pediatric rheumatology.

The American College of Rheumatology and *The Association of Rheumatology Health Professionals*, 60 Executive Park South, Suite 150, Atlanta, GA 30329; (404)-633-3777. The national membership organizations for physicians and health professionals, respectively, with a specialty or interest in rheumatology, these organizations publish the scientific journals *Arthritis and Rheumatism* and *Arthritis Care and Research*, sponsor conferences and seminars for professionals in the area of rheumatology, and fund research. Both organizations have pediatric rheumatology sections that can provide information about health care professionals.

Glossary

Acetylsalicylic acid.   The chemical name for aspirin.

Activities of daily living.   Everyday tasks such as eating, dressing, bathing, and walking.

Acute illness.   Illness of limited duration, usually days or weeks, such as ear infections and chicken pox.

Acute joint.   An arthritic joint which is very painful, warm, swollen, and stiff in the morning. Also called *highly inflamed.*

Adaptive physical education (APE).   Physical education classes that are modified to meet the individual physical education needs of children with chronic health conditions or disabilities.

Aerobic exercise.   Exercise done to increase general fitness; aerobic exercise requires sustained vigorous activity to increase the heart rate.

Aid to Families with Dependent Children (AFDC).   A program of the federal government that provides supplemental income and Medicaid benefits for qualified families.

Americans with Disabilities Act (ADA, P.L. 101-336).   Federal legislation that protects the civil rights of individuals with disabilities.

Analgesic.   Pain-relieving medication.

Anemia.   A condition in which the number of red cells in the blood is decreased, or the oxygen-carrying capacity of red blood cells is diminished.

Anesthetic.   Medication that causes loss of sensation; used to prevent pain from medical procedures. A general anesthetic causes loss of consciousness; a local anesthetic causes loss of sensation in a limited area of the body without loss of consciousness.

Ankylosing spondylitis.   A rheumatic disease that causes stiffness and fusion in the spine.

Annual maximum. The maximum amount an insurance company will pay for covered services in a single year, the annual maximum may apply to specific types of services or to the total of all covered health care costs.

Antibiotic. Medication used to treat bacterial infections.

Antibody. A protein produced by the immune system to recognize and destroy foreign substances like viruses and bacteria.

Antinuclear antibody (ANA). An antibody that attacks the nucleus of certain cells of the body.

Antipyretic. A medication that reduces fever.

Arthralgia. Pain or discomfort in a joint without arthritis.

Arthritis. Inflammation of the joints, characterized by redness, swelling, heat, and pain.

Arthrocentesis. Removal of fluid from a joint.

Arthrodesis. A surgical procedure to fuse the bones of a joint in a functional position.

Arthroplasty. A surgical procedure to replace or repair a damaged joint.

Arthroscopic surgery. Joint surgery performed by inserting viewing and surgical instruments through a small incision.

Aspirate. To remove fluid from a joint or other body cavity using a needle.

Aspirin. Nonsteroidal anti-inflammatory medication that also has pain-relieving and fever-reducing effects; chemically known as acetylsalicylic acid.

Asymmetric arthritis. Arthritis that affects one joint on one side of the body but not the same joint on the opposite side of the body.

Atrophy. A wasting away or shrinking of a part of the body, such as a decrease in muscle mass caused by loss of use.

Autoantibody. An antibody that reacts with an individual's own body tissues or cells. See *antinuclear antibody* and *rheumatoid factor.*

Autoimmune disease. A disease in which the body produces autoantibodies that attack the individual's own tissues or cells.

Avascular necrosis. A condition in which the blood supply to the bone is cut off, causing part of the bone to die.

Blood urea nitrogen (BUN). A blood test done to detect abnormalities in kidney function.

Body mechanics. The performance of daily activities such as sitting, standing, and lifting in a way that places the least amount of stress on joints and muscles.

Calcinosis. A condition that occurs in some people with dermatomyositis in which calcium deposits develop under the skin.

Care coordination. The process of organizing health care resources to ensure access to and efficient delivery of services.

Cartilage. Smooth, shock-absorbing connective tissue that lines the ends of the bones within a joint and also makes up part of the nose and outer ear.

Case management. Another term for care coordination.

Cataract. A condition in which part or all of the lens of the eye becomes cloudy; a cataract can impair vision.

Cervical spine. The seven vertebrae of the neck.

Children with Special Health Care Needs (CSHCN) Programs (Title V). Programs funded by the Maternal and Child Health Bureau under Title V of the Social Security Act and matching funds from the state. Services provided vary from state to state.

Chronic illness. Illness that persists for a long period of time, perhaps months or years.

COBRA (P.L. 99-272). Federal legislation that permits continuation of insurance coverage for individuals and their dependents who lose employee health benefits due to loss of job or death; the individual pays the full insurance premium.

Collagen. The main structural protein of connective tissues.

Community-based care. Services obtained in the local community or as close to home as possible.

Complete blood count (CBC). A series of tests done on a small sample of blood; includes red and white blood cell counts, differential white cell count, platelet count, and a smear to detect abnormalities in the appearance of red cells.

Conjunctivitis. Inflammation of the eyes.

Connective tissue. The tough, fibrous tissue that connects body parts and provides support; includes tendons, ligaments, cartilage, skin, and bones.

Contracture.   A joint that becomes fixed in a bent position, making it impossible for the person to move the joint through its normal range of motion due to stiffness or shortening of the soft tissues surrounding the joint.

Controlled joint.   An arthritic joint that was previously inflamed but is now only barely uncomfortable, mildly swollen, and has little morning stiffness.

Copayment.   The amount you must pay for covered health care services; usually a small fixed amount for HMOs and a percentage of the fee for traditional health insurance plans.

Coping strategies.   The problem-solving efforts that individuals make when faced with situations that cause stress, anxiety, fear, or grief.

Cornea.   The transparent covering of the front of the eye.

Corticosteroid.   A powerful anti-inflammatory hormone produced naturally by the body; also available in synthetic form as a medication to treat severe inflammation.

Creatinine.   A blood test done to detect abnormalities in kidney function.

Deductible.   The amount of out-of-pocket costs you must incur for covered health services before your insurance benefits begin.

Deformity.   A malalignment of a joint.

Dermatomyositis.   A rheumatic disease characterized by inflammation in the skin and muscles that results in muscle weakness.

Diagnosis.   The identification of the specific disease or condition responsible for causing symptoms; a diagnosis is based on the patient's complaints, clinical findings upon physical examination, and the results of laboratory and other tests.

Diarthrodial joints.   Joints that normally allow free movement in almost any direction.

Differential diagnosis.   A diagnosis made by ruling out all other causes of illness.

Discoid lupus.   A condition that causes scaly, red, disk-shaped sores on the face, neck, and chest. Discoid lupus is not systemic lupus erythematosus; it affects only the skin, not the other organ systems.

Distal interphalangeal joints (DIP).   The joints near the tip of the fingers.

Drug interaction.   A change in the effectiveness or action of a drug caused by another drug; a drug interaction may occur when certain drugs are used together.

Drug overdose. An accidental or intentional ingestion of an excessive amount of a medication.

Durable medical equipment. Medical equipment that an individual will use for an extended period of time, such as a wheelchair. Health insurance plans usually limit the amount they will pay for durable medical equipment.

Early intervention. Medical or educational services for children from birth to 3 years of age that are designed to prevent or limit developmental disabilities.

Edema. The accumulation of fluid in body tissues or cavities, including the joints; swelling.

Education for All Handicapped Children Act (P.L. 94-142). A federal law passed in 1975 that guarantees a free, appropriate public education for children who need special education and related services.

Education of the Handicapped Act Amendments of 1986 (P.L. 99-457, Part H). Federal legislation that addresses the early intervention needs of children from birth to 3 years of age.

Endurance. The ability to perform an activity repetitively over a period of time, such as walking for 20 minutes.

Enthesopathy. Inflammation at the site of attachment of a ligament or tendon to a bone (called the *entheses*), resulting in pain in these areas.

Erosion. Damage to the surface of a joint or destruction of parts of the bones caused by long-term inflammation.

Erythrocyte. Another name for a red blood cell.

Erythrocyte sedimentation rate (ESR). A blood test that provides a nonspecific measure of inflammatory activity; also called *sed rate* or *sedimentation rate.* Elevated ESR can occur in a number of conditions other than rheumatic illness.

Extension. A movement that causes straightening of a joint, or a measure of the degree to which a joint can be straightened.

Extra-articular. Literally, "outside of the joint"; refers to symptoms, such as eye inflammation, that do not involve the joints.

Family-centered care. Care that takes into account the effect of illness and its treatment on the entire family, actively seeks input from the family, and promotes normal living patterns.

Family physician.   A physician who provides primary care for the entire family, both adults and children.

Fellow.   A physician who has completed residency training for general practice and is in a training program to become a specialist.

Flare.   A period of increased disease activity, or return of symptoms after a remission.

Flexion.   A movement that causes bending of a joint away from the straight position, or a measure of the extent to which a joint can be bent.

Flexion contracture.   An inability to straighten a joint fully, or fixing of the joint in a bent position. See *contracture*.

Functional splint.   A splint worn during the day, usually on the wrist, to provide support for a joint and permit use of the affected part of the body.

Gait.   The manner or speed of walking.

Gastritis.   Inflammation of the lining of the stomach.

Gelling (or gel phenomena).   Stiffness that results from periods of inactivity, such as in the morning upon awakening.

Generic drugs.   Medications called by their common names.

Glaucoma.   Increased pressure in the eyes.

Goniometer.   An instrument used to measure joint range of motion.

Health care team.   An interdisciplinary group of health care providers and family members who plan and provide health services; the health care team includes the child and parents, the pediatrician and other providers in the community, and the pediatric rheumatology team.

HLA-B27.   A substance found on the surface of cells that is present in a number of children with ankylosing spondylitis and that also occurs not uncommonly in the general population.

Immunosuppressant drug.   A drug used to control severe rheumatic disease that works by suppressing various elements of the immune system.

Individualized education plan (IEP).   A written plan that details the special education and related services provided to address the child's individual needs.

Individuals with Disabilities Education Act (IDEA, P.L. 101-476).   A federal law passed in 1990 which is an amended version of P.L. 94-142 (see above) and which guarantees a free, appropriate public education for children with special educational needs.

Inflammation.   A response of the body to injury or infection that is usually protective; it is characterized by redness, swelling, heat, and pain. Uncontrolled inflammation is the major cause of symptoms in rheumatic diseases.

Inflammatory bowel disease.   A disease associated with chronic inflammation of the intestines, causing diarrhea and abdominal pain (also called *Crohn's disease*).

Internist.   A physician who provides primary medical care for adults.

Iridocyclitis.   Inflammation of the iris and ciliary body of the eye.

Iris.   The colored part of the eye surrounding the pupil that regulates the amount of light entering the eye.

Iritis.   Inflammation of the iris.

Isometric exercise.   Exercise done to strengthen muscles; the muscles are contracted without moving the joints.

Isotonic exercise.   Muscle-strengthening exercise done by moving the joint against resistance, such as gravity, weights, or pressure applied by another person.

Joint.   An area of the body where two bones meet, usually to permit movement, although immovable joints are located in some parts of the body, such as in the skull.

Joint contracture.   See *contracture* and *flexion contracture*.

Joint replacement surgery.   A surgical procedure to replace a joint with an artificial joint made of plastic and metal.

Joint space.   A space between the bones in a joint that is visible on X rays.

Juvenile rheumatoid arthritis (JRA).   A rheumatic disease characterized by chronic arthritis that begins before the age of 16. There are three major onset-subtypes of JRA: polyarticular, pauciarticular, and systemic disease.

Leg length discrepancy.   A finding common in JRA, in which one leg is longer than the other.

Lifetime maximum.   The total amount an insurance company will pay for health care services during an individual's lifetime.

Ligament.   A band of tough fibrous tissue that connects bones or other tissues.

Linear scleroderma.   Scleroderma that occurs in a linelike pattern over an extremity.

Lyme arthritis.   Arthritis associated with Lyme disease, which is caused by the bite of an infected deer tick and is treated with antibiotics.

Lymphocyte.   A type of white blood cell involved in the production of antibodies to protect the body from infection.

Magnetic resonance imaging (MRI).   An imaging technique that permits visualization of internal organs and does not use radiation.

Malar rash.   A butterfly-shaped rash over the cheeks and across the bridge of the nose, common in systemic lupus erythematosus.

Managed care.   A system of health care delivery that contains costs by restricting an individual's access to services; in a managed-care environment, services must be ordered by the primary physician.

Manual muscle examination.   A test performed by a physical or occupational therapist to quantitatively measure muscle strength.

Medicaid (Title XIX).   A public health program jointly funded by the federal and state governments that pays covered health care costs for individuals who meet eligibility requirements.

Medicare.   A federal public health program for individuals over the age of 65, individuals under 65 who have been eligible for Social Security Disability Income for 2 years, and children with chronic kidney disease who require dialysis or kidney transplant.

Metacarpophalangeal joint.   The joint where the fingers meet the palm of the hand.

Monoarticular.   Literally, one joint. JRA involving a single joint is sometimes referred to as monoarticular JRA.

Monocyte.   A type of white blood cell that protects the body from infection by engulfing and removing foreign substances.

Morning stiffness.   A period of stiffness experienced after waking in the morning because of prolonged inactivity while sleeping.

Morphea.   Scleroderma that occurs in round spots.

Myalgia.   Muscle pain.

Night splint.   A splint worn at night to maintain or correct joint position. Also called a *resting splint.*

Nonsteroidal anti-inflammatory drugs (NSAIDs).   A class of anti-inflammatory drugs, including aspirin, ibuprofen, naproxen, and tolmetin sodium, that do not contain steroids.

Occupational therapist.   A health care provider who assesses strength and function of the upper limbs and ability to perform activities of daily living, and prescribes appropriate exercises.

Occupational therapy.   Therapeutic strengthening and stretching exercises done to improve range of motion and function in the hands, arms, and shoulders.

Onset subtypes.   The three different types of JRA, which are determined during the first 6 months of a child's disease.

Ophthalmologist.   A medical doctor (M.D.) who specializes in the diagnosis and treatment of eye diseases. Nonphysician specialists who assess vision and prescribe corrective eyeglasses and contact lenses are called *optometrists.*

Optometrist.   A nonphysician specialist who assesses vision and prescribes corrective eyeglasses and contact lenses.

Orthopedic surgeon.   A physician who performs surgery to repair bone or joint damage, including joint replacement surgery.

Orthotics.   Custom-made shoe inserts used to relieve foot pain.

Osteoporosis.   A thinning and weakening of the bones.

Paraffin bath.   Melted wax into which affected parts of the body (usually hands or feet) are dipped to provide deep heat for the relief of pain or stiffness.

Pauciarticular JRA.   A subtype of juvenile rheumatoid arthritis that begins in four or fewer joints, and is the JRA subtype likely to result in eye inflammation (iritis).

Pediatric rheumatologist.   A pediatrician who has completed a fellowship training program in pediatric rheumatology and has passed (board certified) or is eligible to take (board eligible) the pediatric rheumatology board certification exam of the American Academy of Pediatrics.

Pediatrician.   A physician who has completed pediatric residency training and specializes in the treatment of children and adolescents.

Pericarditis.   Inflammation of the sac surrounding the heart (pericardium) that can lead to an accumulation of fluid around the heart.

Physical therapist.   A health care provider who assesses posture, gait, and strength and range of motion of the lower limbs, and prescribes appropriate exercises.

Physical therapy.   Therapeutic strengthening and stretching exercises done to improve range of motion and function in the feet and legs, and improve posture and gait.

Placebo.   A substance that is given as medicine but contains no active medical ingredients (also called a *sugar pill*), a placebo is often used as a control in studies to test the effectiveness of new drugs.

Platelets.   Elements occurring in large numbers in the blood that are crucial to the clotting process; also called *thrombocytes.*

Pleuritis.   Inflammation of the lungs.

Podiatrist.   A nonphysician health care provider who cares for problems of the feet and fabricates custom-made shoe inserts (orthotics).

Polyarticular JRA.   A subtype of juvenile rheumatoid arthritis that begins in five or more joints.

Pre-existing condition.   An illness or health condition that exists at the time of application for insurance, or one that was treated or known about before the application.

Preferred Provider Organization (PPO).   A system of health care delivery in which the insurer contracts with health care providers to provide services at the negotiated rate. PPO subscribers have higher copayments and deductibles when they obtain services from providers outside of the plan.

Primary care.   Health care that includes routine checkups, treatment for acute illness, and preventive medicine. Primary care is provided by pediatricians, family physicians, and internists.

Prognosis.   A forecast of the likely course, duration, and result of an illness or injury.

Prolonged illness clause.   A clause that extends insurance benefits (usually to 100% coverage) for covered services needed to treat a chronic illness or condition.

Psoriasis.   A chronic skin condition that results in a scaly, red rash, and occurs commonly in the scalp or near joints.

Pulse therapy.   A treatment strategy using several smaller doses of medication, rather than one larger dose.

Pupil.   The opening in the center of the iris through which light enters the eye.

Range of motion.   All of the normal movements that a joint can make in different directions, from fully flexed to fully extended; range of motion is frequently limited in arthritis.

Range-of-motion exercises.   Exercises done to maintain and increase flexibility by moving each involved joint through all of its motions, with gentle pressure applied where movement is restricted.

Raynaud's phenomenon.   A condition in which the blood vessels in the fingers and toes constrict when exposed to cold or stress, causing the fingers and toes to turn blue, white, and then red.

Red blood cell.   Oxygen-carrying cell of the blood; also called an *erythrocyte.*

Related services.   Services such as transportation and physical, occupational, and speech therapy that are necessary to meet a child's special educational needs.

Remission.   A period during which there are no active signs of disease.

Resident.   A physician (M.D.) who is in training to become a pediatrician, internist, or other specialist.

Resting splint.   A splint worn at night to maintain or correct joint position.

Retina.   Light-sensitive tissue in the back of the eye.

Reye's syndrome.   A serious, rare childhood illness affecting the liver and nervous system, Reye's syndrome usually develops following a viral illness, especially flu or chicken pox. Aspirin should not be given to children with the flu or chicken pox because it increases the likelihood that Reye's syndrome will develop.

Rheumatic fever.   An acute childhood illness that develops after a strep infection and usually subsides within a few weeks but that may cause permanent damage to the heart valves. Symptoms include rash, fever, arthritis that moves from one joint to another, and inflammation of the valves of the heart.

Rheumatoid factor (RF).   An autoantibody that reacts with a person's own normal antibodies, Rf is found in a small percentage of children with JRA, but also in a small number of people without arthritis.

Rheumatoid nodules.   Lumps beneath the skin caused by chronic inflammation, nodules are more common in adult rheumatoid arthritis but are occasionally found in children with JRA.

Rheumatologist.   A physician who specializes in caring for adults with rheumatic diseases.

Salicylate level.   A blood test that measures the amount of salicylates in the blood; helpful in determining correct dosage and monitoring for toxicity.

Second-line drugs.   Powerful drugs, also known as disease-modifying antirheumatic drugs, that may slow down or modify the course of arthritis.

Section 504 of the Rehabilitation Act of 1973 (P.L. 93-112).   Federal legislation that prohibits discriminating against a student on the basis of disability.

Seronegative.   A term used to describe children with polyarticular JRA who have a negative rheumatoid factor blood test.

Seropositive.   A term used to describe children with polyarticular JRA who have a positive rheumatoid factor blood test.

Serositis.   Inflammation of the lining around the heart or lungs, which may cause fluid to develop in these areas.

Serum glutamic oxaloacetic transaminase/serum glutamic pyruvic transaminase.   Blood tests done to detect damage to the liver.

Shoe lift.   A device worn on the shoe of the shorter leg when there is a medically significant difference in leg lengths.

Side effect.   An undesirable effect of a drug.

Slit lamp.   An instrument with a magnifying lens and bright light used to examine the interior of the eye.

Slow-acting antirheumatic drugs (SAARDs).   A class of antirheumatic drugs that accumulate slowly in the body, requiring 4 to 6 months before their effects are apparent: includes methotrexate, sulfasalazine, gold, hydroxychloroquine, and d-penicillamine.

Social Security Disability Income (SSDI).   A federal program that provides supplemental income for disabled individuals who have paid into the Social Security system for the required number of quarters. SSDI recipients become eligible for Medicare after 2 years.

Social worker. A health care provider who assists families with practical matters, such as transportation and financing, and provides counseling for the emotional adjustment to chronic illness.

Sphygmomanometer. An instrument used to measure blood pressure.

Spleen. An abdominal organ that stores blood and functions as part of the immune system.

Splint. A device used to keep joints in a good position and to relieve pain. See *functional splint* and *night splint.*

Steroid. See *corticosteroid.*

Still's disease. Another name for systemic JRA.

Stretching exercises. Exercises that move a joint or muscle through its available motion and then apply pressure to help it move farther.

Subluxation. Malalignment of the bones in a joint; a partial or incomplete dislocation.

Supplemental Security Income (SSI). A federal government program that provides supplemental income for individuals over 65, and disabled or blind individuals under 65 who satisfy financial eligibility criteria. In most states, SSI recipients are automatically eligible for Medicaid benefits.

Support group. A group of parents or children who meet to exchange information about an illness and provide mutual support.

Symmetric arthritis. Arthritis that affects the same joints on both sides of the body.

Synovial fluid. The clear, thick fluid inside the joints that provides lubrication.

Synovial joint. A joint enclosed in a synovial membrane.

Synovial membrane. A thin layer of connective tissue that surrounds the joint, also called *synovium.*

Synovitis. Inflammation of the synovial membrane, synovitis results in an increase in synovial fluid within the joint.

Systemic illness. An illness that affects the body as a whole.

Systemic lupus erythematosus (SLE). An autoimmune disease affecting nearly every system of the body; skin rashes, fever, arthritis, kidney abnormalities, and abnormalities of the blood-forming elements can occur.

Systemic JRA.   A subtype of juvenile rheumatoid arthritis that is characterized by a high, spiking daily fever and rash. Arthritis may not be present until some time after the other symptoms appear.

Temporomandibular joint (TMJ).   The joint connecting the lower jaw to the skull, the TMJ may be inflamed in some children with JRA.

Tendinitis.   Inflammation of a tendon.

Tendon.   A thick band of fibrous tissue that connects a muscle to a bone.

Tenosynovitis.   Inflammation of the synovial membrane surrounding a tendon.

Traction.   A method of treatment that involves pulling on the joints by attaching a series of weights and pulleys to them, traction is used to stretch soft tissues to relieve a contracture or to correct misalignment of the bones.

Training.   A special set of exercises performed to prepare the body for participation in sports.

Ultrasound.   The use of sound waves to produce an image of the internal organs. Also a form of deep heat used by physical therapists to reduce pain and inflammation.

Unproven remedy.   A substance or procedure used to treat illness whose safety and efficacy have not been scientifically proven.

Urethritis.   Inflammation of the urethra.

Urinalysis.   Evaluation of the urine for the presence of blood, sugar, and other substances that can indicate infection or a kidney abnormality.

Uveitis.   Inflammation of the parts of the eye. Anterior uveitis (occurring in the front of the eye) causes iritis. Posterior uveitis (occurring in the back of the eye) may occur in children with ankylosing spondylitis.

Vasculitis.   Inflammation of the blood vessels.

Weight-bearing joint.   Joints that support the weight of the body when standing, such as the hips, knees, and ankles.

White blood cell.   Any of a number of different cells of the immune system circulating in the blood, including neutrophils, lymphocytes, and monocytes. Leukocyte is a general term for any type of white blood cell.

X ray.   An image of a bone (usually) or other organ of the body made using ionizing radiation.

Bibliography

Annas, G. J., L. H. Glantz, and B. F. Katz. *The rights of doctors, nurses and allied health professionals: A health law primer.* Cambridge: Ballinger Publishing, 1981.

Arnett, F., G. E. Solomon, and D. Yu. *Reiter's syndrome.* Atlanta: Arthritis Foundation, 1988.

Barnes, E., C. Berrigan, and D. Biklen. *What's the difference? Teaching positive attitudes toward people with disabilities.* Syracuse, N.Y.: Human Policy Press, 1978.

Beckett, J. *Health care financing: A guide for families.* Iowa City: National Maternal and Child Health Resource Center, 1989.

Bowyer, S., N. Ilowite, A. Kovalesky, D. Magilavy, L. Pachman, and P. Rettig. *Meeting the challenge: A young person's guide to living with lupus.* Atlanta: Arthritis Foundation, 1990.

Bowyer, S. L., and C. H. Spencer. *Juvenile dermatomyositis.* Atlanta: Arthritis Foundation, 1988.

Bradshaw, J. *Bradshaw on: The family.* Deerfield Beach, Fla.: Health Communications, 1988.

Brewer, E. J., and K. C. Angel. *Parenting a child with arthritis.* Los Angeles: Lowell House, RGA Publishing Group, 1992.

Brown, S., and M. Moersch (eds.). *Parents on the team.* Ann Arbor: University of Michigan Press, 1978.

Buckley, D., E. Fudge, E. Hazlett, and B. Morreo. *School nurse standards of care for children with JRA.* Boston: Affiliated Children's Arthritis Centers of New England, 1993.

Colby, L. A., M. Rapoff, E. S. Shear, A. Johnson, F. Donivan, A. Kovalesky, S. K. Amondsum, and S. Hoch. *We Can: A guide for parents of children with arthritis.* Atlanta: Arthritis Foundation, 1990.

Conn, D. L., and J. S. Sergent. *The vasculitides.* Atlanta: Arthritis Foundation, 1987.

DeNardo, B. A., S. H. Allaire, D. Buckley, et al. *Care coordination practice guidelines for children with chronic arthritis,* 2d ed. Boston: Affiliated Children's Arthritis Centers of New England, 1993.

DeNardo, B. A., V. Rhodes, and B. Gibbons. *Physical therapy practice guidelines for children with chronic arthritis,* 2d ed. Boston: Affiliated Children's Arthritis Centers of New England, 1993.

DeNardo, B. A., J. A. Stebulis, L. B. Tucker, and J. G. Schaller. Parents of children with rheumatic disease as peer counselors. *Arthritis Care and Research 1995* 8(2):120–25.

DeNardo, B. A., and I. S. Szer. Managing childhood arthritis: A framework for health service delivery. *Journal of Musculoskeletal Medicine* 6(7):58–70, 1989.

Epstein, S. G., A. B. Taylor, A. S. Halberg, et al. *Enhancing quality: Standards and indicators of quality care for children with special health care needs.* Boston: New England SERVE, 1989.

Featherstone, H. A. *Difference in the family: Life with a disabled child.* Bethesda, Md.: ACCH Clearinghouse, 1980.

Federation for Children with Special Needs. *The parent manual: A guide to parents' and children's rights under federal and state special education laws.* Boston: Federation for Children with Special Needs, 1990.

Fisher, R., and W. Ury. *Getting to yes: Negotiating agreement without giving in.* New York: Penguin Books, 1981.

Ginzler, E. M. *Systemic lupus erythematosus.* Atlanta: Arthritis Foundation, 1990.

Goldfarb, L. A., M. J. Brotherson, J. A. Summers, et al. *Meeting the challenge of disability or chronic illness: A family guide.* Baltimore: Paul H. Brookes Publishing, 1986.

Hafeli, D., D. Hafeli, P. Slutsky, N. Liburd, and T. H. Caldwell. *When your student has arthritis.* Atlanta: Arthritis Foundation, 1992.

Hobbs, N., J. M. Perrin, and H. T. Ireys. *Chronically ill children and their families.* San Francisco: Jossey-Bass, 1985.

Holland, M. *Guide to low sodium, low calorie foods for children.* Boston: New England Medical Center, The Francis Stern Nutrition Center, 1987.

Hollis, S. S., K. Ayers, A. Baird, et al. *Social work standards of practice for pediatric rheumatology.* Boston: Affiliated Children's Arthritis Centers of New England, 1994.

Jacobs, J. C. *Pediatric rheumatology for the practitioner,* 2d ed. New York: Springer-Verlag, 1992.

Joint Movement. A newsletter on RA research for people with rheumatic diseases. Arthritis Foundation 2(3), 1990.

The Joint Report: The official newsletter of the Affiliated Children's Arthritis Centers of New England. Distributed quarterly, 18 issues; October 1987 through October 1993.

Katz, J. *The silent world of doctor and patient,* New York: Free Press, Macmillan, 1984.

Kovalesky, A., M. Boutaugh, D. Erlandson, et al. *Understanding juvenile rheumatoid arthritis: A health professional's guide to teaching children and parents.* Atlanta: Arthritis Foundation, 1987.

Kriegsman, K. H., E. L. Zaslow, and J. D'Zmura-Rechsteiner. *Taking charge: Teenagers talk about life and physical disabilities.* Rockville, Md.: Woodbine House, 1992.

Larson, G. (ed.). *Managing the school age child with a chronic health condition.* St. Paul: Pathfinder Resources, 1988.

Larson, G., and J. A. Kahn. *Special needs, special solutions: How to get quality care for a child with special health needs.* St. Paul: Lifeline Press, 1991.

Leroy, E. C. *Scleroderma.* Atlanta: Arthritis Foundation, 1983.

Manes, J., and L. S. Carry. *SI new opportunities for children with disabilities.* Washington, DC: Mental Health Law Project, 1991.

May, J. *Fathers of children with special needs: New horizons.* Bethesda, Md.: ACCH Clearinghouse, 1990.

McCaffrey, F. D., and T. Fish. *Profiles of the other child: A sibling guide for parents.* Columbus, Ohio: The Nisonger Center Publication Department, 1989.

McCollum, A. *The chronically ill child: A guide for parents and professionals.* Bethesda, Md.: ACCH, 1981.

McManus, M. *Understanding your health insurance options: A guide for families who have children with special health care needs.* Bethesda, Md.: ACCH, 1988.

Meyer, D. J., P. F. Wadasy, and R. R. Fewell. *Living with a brother or sister with special needs: A book for sibs.* Seattle: University of Washington Press, 1985.

Miller, M. L., A. P. Tanchyk, A. Kovalesky, et al. *Arthritis in children,* 2d ed. Atlanta: Arthritis Foundation, 1994.

Moore, M. E., C. H. McGrory, and R. S. Rosenthal (eds.). *Learning about lupus. A user friendly guide.* Ardmore, Pa.: Lupus Foundation of Delaware Valley, 1991.

Neill, A. J. *Meeting the challenge: A young person's guide to living with lupus.* Atlanta: Arthritis Foundation, 1990.

Neville, K. M. *Strategic insurance negotiation: An introduction to basic skills for families and community mental health workers.* Boston: Federation for Children with Special Needs, 1991.

Peterson, R., and D. Tenenbaum. *Fighting back health insurance denials.* Madison, Wis.: Center for Public Representation, 1992.

Phillips, R. H. *Coping with lupus.* Rockville, Md.: Lupus Foundation of America, 1984.

Porter, S., J. Burkley, T. Bierle, et al. *Working toward a balance in our lives.* Boston: The Children's Hospital, Project School Care, 1992.

Powell, T. H., and P. A. Gallagher. *Brothers and sisters: A special part of exceptional families.* Baltimore: Paul H. Brookes Publishing, 1993.

Senécal, J. L. *Lupus: The disease with 1000 faces.* Calgary, Alberta: Lupus Canada, 1990.

Sharples, A. C., J. A. Stebulis, and M. Weafer-Hodgins. *Just one of the kids: A video for teachers and school personnel.* Boston: Affiliated Children's Arthritis Centers of New England, 1994.

Shelton, T. L., E. S. Jeppson, and B. H. Johnson. *Family centered care for children with special health needs.* Bethesda: Association for the Care of Children's Health, 1992.

Southwood, T. R., and P. N. Malleson (eds.). *Arthritis in children and adolescents.* London: Baillière Tindall, 1993.

Stark, S. L. *Health insurance made easy: How to understand your health insurance so you start saving your money and stop wasting your time.* Shawnee Mission, Kan.: Stark Publishing, 1989.

Stebulis, J. A. (ed.). *The handbook for families.* Boston: Affiliated Children's Arthritis Centers of New England, 1993.

Stebulis, J. A., R. Cummings, L. Denner, et al. *Learn about JRA: A module for classroom use to instruct the peers of a child with JRA about the disease.* Boston: Affiliated Children's Arthritis Centers of New England, 1993.

Stebulis, J. A., B. A. DeNardo, D. Price, I. S. Szer, and L. B. Tucker. *The parent telephone network: Network coordinators manual.* Boston: Affiliated Children's Arthritis Centers of New England, 1990.

Thiele, C. *Jodie's journey.* Scranton, Pa.: Harper Collins Publishers, 1988.

Tiger, S. *Understanding disease: Arthritis.* New York: Simon & Schuster Juvenile Division, 1986.

Troy, M. B., B. Borr, M. A. Burns, et al. *Occupational therapy practice guidelines for children with chronic arthritis,* 2d ed. Boston: The Affiliated Children's Arthritis Centers of New England, 1993.

Tucker, L. B., R. J. McKay, E. Kaplan, M. Luloff, and J. A. Stebulis. *Medical care for children with chronic arthritis: Guidelines for coordination of primary and specialty care.* Boston: The Affiliated Children's Arthritis Centers of New England, 1994.

Turnbull, H. R. III, et al. *Disability and the family: A guide to decisions for adulthood.* Baltimore: Paul H. Brookes Publishing, 1989.

Virgen, L. *Same and different.* Columbia, Mo.: UMC Arthritis Center, 1989.

Warren, R., and R. Petty. *Juvenile ankylosing spondylitis.* Los Angeles: Ankylosing Spondylitis Association, 1989.

Wells, E., M. Mitchell, M. Cole, et al. *Paying the bills: Tips for families on financing health care for children with special needs.* Boston: New England SERVE, 1992.

Wetherbee, M. S., and A. J. Neil (eds.). *Educational rights for children with arthritis: A manual for parents.* Atlanta: Arthritis Foundation, 1989.

Williams, G. F. *Children with chronic arthritis: A primer for patients and parents.* Littleton, Mass.: PSG Publishing, 1981.

Ziebell, B. *As normal as possible: A parent's guide to healthy emotional development for children.* Tucson: Arthritis Foundation, Southern Arizona Chapter, 1976.

Index

Pages on which a record-keeping form appears are in **boldface**. *Definitions of terms may be found in the Glossary.*

About the Authors

Lori B. Tucker, M.D., is a pediatric rheumatologist and assistant professor in pediatrics at the Floating Hospital for Children, New England Medical Center, and Tufts University School of Medicine in Boston, Massachusetts. Dr. Tucker was the Project Director for the Affiliated Children's Arthritis Centers of New England, a regional pediatric rheumatology program funded between 1984 and 1994 by the Bureau of Maternal and Child Health to promote family-centered care for children with rheumatic diseases.

Bethany A. DeNardo, M.P.H., P.T., is a licensed physical therapist and research associate for the Division of Pediatric Rheumatology at the Floating Hospital for Children, New England Medical Center. Ms. DeNardo has over 12 years of experience in working with children with rheumatic diseases and their families. She has been providing clinical physical therapy to children with rheumatic diseases since 1982 and served for 10 years as the Associate Director of the Affiliated Children's Arthritis Centers of New England.

Judith A. Stebulis, M.A., is the parent of a child with arthritis. In 1983, her son Matthew was diagnosed with juvenile rheumatoid arthritis, at the age of three. Ms. Stebulis spent six years as the Outreach Coordinator for the Affiliated Children's Arthritis Centers of New England. A past member of the Executive Committee of the American Juvenile Arthritis Organization (AJAO), Ms. Stebulis is currently attending the University of Massachusetts Medical School; it is her goal to become a general pediatrician.

Jane G. Schaller, M.D., is the Chief of Pediatric Rheumatology, David and Leona Karp Professor of Pediatrics, and Pediatrician-in-Chief of the Floating Hospital for Children, New England Medical Center, and Tufts University School of Medicine. Dr. Schaller is a recognized international expert in the field of pediatric rheumatology. She initiated the development of the Affiliated Children's Arthritis Centers of New England and served as the principal investigator for 10 years.

Library of Congress Cataloging-in-Publication Data

Your child with arthritis : a family guide for caregiving / Lori B. Tucker ... [et al.] :
foreword by Barbara M. Ansell.
p.   cm.
Includes bibliographical references and index.
ISBN 0-8018-5293-5 (alk. paper)
1. Rheumatism in children—Popular works.   2. Rheumatoid arthritis in children—
Popular works.   I. Tucker, Lori B.
RJ482.R48Y68   1996
618.92'723—dc20   95-49212
CIP